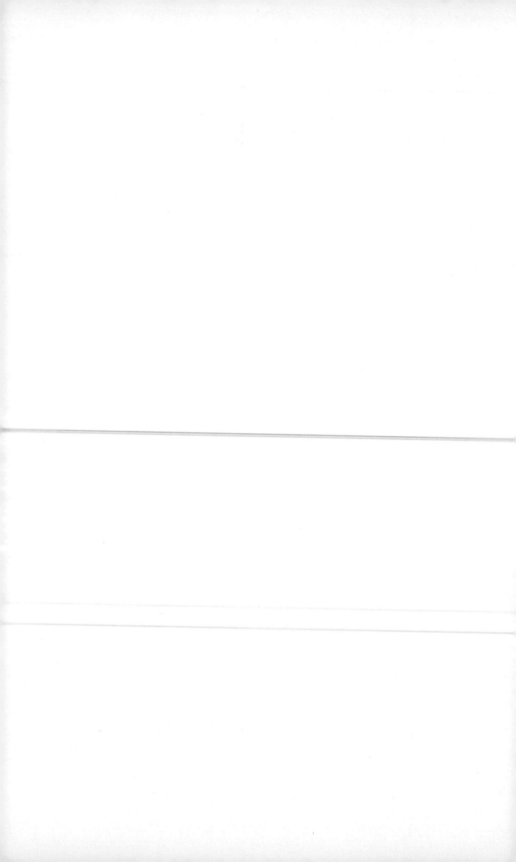

# Obsessive Compulsive and Related Disorders

*Editor*

WAYNE K. GOODMAN

# PSYCHIATRIC CLINICS
# OF NORTH AMERICA

www.psych.theclinics.com

September 2014 • Volume 37 • Number 3

**ELSEVIER**

1600 John F. Kennedy Boulevard ● Suite 1800 ● Philadelphia, Pennsylvania, 19103-2899

http://www.theclinics.com

**PSYCHIATRIC CLINICS OF NORTH AMERICA Volume 37, Number 3**
**September 2014 ISSN 0193-953X, ISBN-13: 978-0-323-32341-3**

Editor: Joanne Husovski
Developmental Editor: Stephanie Carter

*Psychiatric Clinics of North America* (ISSN 0193-953X) is published quarterly by Elsevier Inc., 360 Park Avenue South, New York, NY 10010-1710. Months of issue are March, June, September, and December. Business and Editorial Offices: 1600 John F. Kennedy Blvd., Suite 1800, Philadelphia, PA 19103-2899. Periodicals postage paid at New York, NY and additional mailing offices. Subscription prices are $300.00 per year (US individuals), $546.00 per year (US institutions), $150.00 per year (US students/residents), $365.00 per year (Canadian individuals), $687.00 per year (Canadian Institutions), $455.00 per year (foreign individuals), $687.00 per year (foreign institutions), and $220.00 per year (international & Canadian students/residents). Foreign air speed delivery is included in all *Clinics'* subscription prices. All prices are subject to change without notice. **POSTMASTER:** Send address changes to *Psychiatric Clinics of North America*, Elsevier Health Sciences Division, Subscription Customer Service, 3251 Riverport Lane, Maryland Heights, MO 63043. Customer Service: 1-800-654-2452 (US). From outside the United States, call 1-314-447-8871. Fax: 1-314-447-8029. E-mail: journalscustomerservice-usa@elsevier.com (for print support) and journalsonlinesupport-usa@elsevier.com (for online support).

*Reprints.* For copies of 100 or more, of articles in this publication, please contact the Commercial Reprints Department, Elsevier Inc., 360 Park Avenue South, New York, New York 10010-1710. Tel.: 212-633-3874, Fax: 212-633-3820, E-mail: reprints@elsevier.com.

*Psychiatric Clinics of North America* is covered in *MEDLINE/PubMed (Index Medicus)*, *Current Contents/Social and Behavioral Sciences, Social Science Citation Index, Embase/Excerpta Medica,* and PsycINFO.

# Contributors

## EDITOR

**WAYNE K. GOODMAN, MD**
Professor and Chair, Department of Psychiatry, Icahn School of Medicine at Mount Sinai, New York, New York

## AUTHORS

**MELISSE BAIS, MD**
Department of Psychiatry, Academic Medical Center, Amsterdam, The Netherlands

**MICHAEL H. BLOCH, MD, MS**
Assistant Professor in the Child Study Center and Instructor in Psychiatry; Associate Director of the Yale OCD Research Clinic and of the Yale Child Study Center TS/OCD Clinic, Yale University, New Haven, Connecticut

**HEIDI A. BROWNE, BSc**
OCD and Related Disorders Program, Division of Tics, OCD, and Related Disorders, Department of Psychiatry, Icahn School of Medicine at Mount Sinai; Friedman Brain Institute, Icahn School of Medicine at Mount Sinai, New York, New York

**BARBARA J. COFFEY, MD, MS**
Director, Tics and Tourette's Clinical and Research Program, Division of Tics, OCD and Related Problems, Icahn School of Medicine at Mount Sinai, New York, New York; Professor, Department of Psychiatry; Research Psychiatrist, Nathan Kline Institute for Psychiatric Research, Orangeburg, New York

**DAMIAAN DENYS, MD, PhD**
Department of Psychiatry, Academic Medical Center; Netherlands Institute for Neuroscience, Royal Netherlands Academy of Arts and Sciences, Amsterdam, The Netherlands

**ANGELA FANG, MA**
Clinical Fellow in Psychology/Psychiatry, OCD and Related Disorders Program, Department of Psychiatry, Massachusetts General Hospital, Harvard Medical School, Boston, Massachusetts

**MARTIJN FIGEE, MD, PhD**
Department of Psychiatry, Academic Medical Center, Amsterdam, The Netherlands

**SHANNON L. GAIR, BA**
OCD and Related Disorders Program, Division of Tics, OCD, and Related Disorders, Department of Psychiatry, Icahn School of Medicine at Mount Sinai, New York, New York

**DIANA M. GERARDI, MA**
Rothman Center for Pediatric Neuropsychiatry, USF Pediatrics, St Petersburg, Florida

**WAYNE K. GOODMAN, MD**
Professor and Chair, Department of Psychiatry, Icahn School of Medicine at Mount Sinai, New York, New York

**DOROTHY E. GRICE, MD**
Professor of Psychiatry, OCD and Related Disorders Program, Division of Tics, OCD, and Related Disorders, Department of Psychiatry, Icahn School of Medicine at Mount Sinai; Friedman Brain Institute, Icahn School of Medicine at Mount Sinai, New York, New York

**DAVID C. HOUGHTON, MS**
Department of Psychology, Texas A&M University, College Station, Texas

**KYLE A.B. LAPIDUS, MD, PhD**
Department of Psychiatry, Icahn School of Medicine at Mount Sinai, New York, New York

**JAMES F. LECKMAN, MD, PhD**
Child Study Center, Yale University School of Medicine, New Haven, Connecticut

**ADAM B. LEWIN, PhD, ABPP**
Associate Professor and Director, OCD Program, Department of Pediatrics, Rothman Center for Neuropsychiatry, University of South Florida, St Petersburg, Florida; Department of Psychiatry and Behavioral Neurosciences, University of South Florida; Department of Psychology, University of South Florida, Tampa, Florida

**NATALIE L. MATHENY, BA**
Clinical Research Coordinator, OCD and Related Disorders Program, Department of Psychiatry, Massachusetts General Hospital, Harvard Medical School, Boston, Massachusetts

**JOSEPH F. McGUIRE, MA**
Department of Pediatrics, Rothman Center for Neuropsychiatry, University of South Florida, St Petersburg, Florida; Department of Psychology, University of South Florida, Tampa, Florida

**TANYA K. MURPHY, MD, MS**
Rothman Center for Pediatric Neuropsychiatry, USF Pediatrics, St Petersburg, Florida

**CHRISTOPHER PITTENGER, MD, PhD**
Associate Professor of Psychiatry, Psychology, and in the Child Study Center; Director, Yale OCD Research Clinic, Yale University, New Haven, Connecticut

**JEREMIAH M. SCHARF, MD, PhD**
Assistant Professor of Neurology, Psychiatric and Neurodevelopmental Genetics Unit, Departments of Neurology and Psychiatry, Massachusetts General Hospital, Harvard Medical School, Boston, Massachusetts

**ZOEY A. SHAW, BA**
Clinical Research Coordinator, Tics and Tourette's Clinical and Research Program, Icahn School of Medicine at Mount Sinai, New York, New York

**EMILY R. STERN, PhD**
Assistant Professor, Department of Psychiatry, Icahn School of Medicine at Mount Sinai; Fishberg Department of Neuroscience, Friedman Brain Institute, Icahn School of Medicine at Mount Sinai, New York, New York

**ERIC A. STORCH, PhD**
Professor and All Children's Hospital Guild Chair, Department of Pediatrics, Rothman Center for Neuropsychiatry, University of South Florida, St Petersburg, Florida; Department of Psychiatry and Behavioral Neurosciences, University of South Florida; Department of Psychology, University of South Florida, Tampa, Florida

**STEPHAN F. TAYLOR, MD**
Professor, Department of Psychiatry, University of Michigan, Ann Arbor, Michigan

**SABINE WILHELM, PhD**
Director, OCD and Related Disorders Program, Department of Psychiatry, Massachusetts General Hospital; Professor, Harvard Medical School, Boston, Massachusetts

**DOUGLAS W. WOODS, PhD**
Professor of Psychology, Texas A&M University, College Station, Texas

**MONICA S. WU, BA**
Department of Pediatrics, Rothman Center for Neuropsychiatry, University of South Florida, St Petersburg, Florida; Department of Psychology, University of South Florida, Tampa, Florida

# Contents

This article reviews the clinical features and neurochemical hypotheses of obsessive-compulsive disorder (OCD) with a focus on the serotonin system. In DSM-5, OCD was moved from the anxiety disorders to a new category of Obsessive-Compulsive and Related Disorders. OCD is a common, typically persistent disorder marked by intrusive and disturbing thoughts (obsessions) and repetitive behaviors (compulsions) that the person feels driven to perform. The preferential efficacy of serotonin reuptake inhibitors (SRIs) in OCD led to the so-called serotonin hypothesis. However, direct support for a role of serotonin in the pathophysiology (e.g., biomarkers in pharmacological challenge studies) of OCD remains elusive. A role of the glutamatergic system in OCD has been gaining traction based on imaging data, genomic studies and animal models of aberrant grooming behavior. These findings have spurred interest in testing the efficacy of medications that modulate glutamate function. A role of glutamate is compatible with circuit-based theories of OCD.

Tourette syndrome is a childhood onset neurodevelopmental disorder characterized by multiple motor and vocal tics. Although many youth experience attenuation or even remission of tics in adolescence and young adulthood, some individuals experience persistent tics, which can be debilitating or disabling. Most patients also have 1 or more psychiatric comorbid disorders, such as attention-deficit/hyperactivity disorder or obsessive-compulsive disorder. Treatment is multimodal, including both pharmacotherapy and cognitive-behavioral treatment, and requires disentanglement of tics and the comorbid symptoms.

Body dysmorphic disorder (BDD) can be a severe and often debilitating psychiatric disorder that has been largely under-recognized and under-diagnosed. Pharmacologic and nonpharmacologic treatment options are available but limited. This review aims to provide an updated overview of the psychopathology and epidemiology of BDD, with an emphasis on current pharmacologic and nonpharmacologic treatment options for BDD.

Trichotillomania, or chronic hairpulling, is a common condition that affects primarily women. The disorder can cause significant psychosocial impairment and is associated with elevated rates of psychiatric comorbidity. In this article, the phenomenology, etiology, assessment, and treatment of the disorder are discussed.

Heidi A. Browne, Shannon L. Gair, Jeremiah M. Scharf, and Dorothy E. Grice

Twin and family studies support a significant genetic contribution to obsessive-compulsive disorder (OCD) and related disorders, such as chronic tic disorders, trichotillomania, skin-picking disorder, body dysmorphic disorder, and hoarding disorder. Recently, population-based studies and novel laboratory-based methods have confirmed substantial heritability in OCD. Genome-wide association studies and candidate gene association studies have provided information on specific gene variations that may be involved in the pathobiology of OCD, though a substantial portion of the genetic risk architecture remains unknown.

Emily R. Stern and Stephan F. Taylor

Cognitive neuroscience investigates neural responses to cognitive and emotional probes, an approach that has yielded critical insights into the neurobiological mechanisms of psychiatric disorders. This article reviews some of the major findings from neuroimaging studies using a cognitive neuroscience approach to investigate obsessive-compulsive disorder (OCD). It evaluates the consistency of results and interprets findings within the context of OCD symptoms, and proposes a model of OCD involving inflexibility of internally focused cognition. Although further research is needed, this body of work probing cognitive-emotional processes in OCD has already shed considerable light on the underlying mechanisms of the disorder.

Tanya K. Murphy, Diana M. Gerardi, and James F. Leckman

Whether some instances of obsessive-compulsive disorder are secondary to infectious and/or autoimmune processes is still under scientific debate. The nosology has undergone an iterative process of criteria and acronyms from PITANDS to PANDAS to PANS (or CANS for neurology). This review focuses on the clinical presentation, assessment, proposed pathophysiology, and treatment of pediatric autoimmune neuropsychiatric disorders associated with streptococcus (PANDAS), and the newest iteration, pediatric acute-onset neuropsychiatric syndrome (PANS). Children who have these symptoms, which have become known as PANS, have been described by their parents as "changed children."

Christopher Pittenger and Michael H. Bloch

Obsessive-compulsive disorder (OCD) affects up to 2.5% of the population over the course of a lifetime and produces substantial morbidity. Approximately 70% of patients can experience significant symptomatic relief with appropriate pharmacotherapy. Selective serotonin reuptake inhibitors are the mainstay of pharmacological treatment. These drugs are typically used at higher doses and for longer periods than in depression. Proven second-line treatments include the tricyclic clomipramine and the addition of low-dose neuroleptic medications. OCD refractory to available treatments remains a profound clinical challenge.

# PSYCHIATRIC CLINICS OF NORTH AMERICA

**FORTHCOMING ISSUES**

*December 2014*
**Stress in Health and Disease**
Daniel L. Kirsch and
Michel Woodbury, *Editors*

**Young-onset Dementia**
Chiadi Onyike, *Editor*

**Current Topics in Psychiatry**
David Baron, *Editor*

**RECENT ISSUES**

*June 2014*
**Sexual Deviation: Assessment and Treatment**
John M.W. Bradford and
A.G. Ahmed, *Editors*

*March 2014*
**Neuropsychiatry of Traumatic Brain Injury**
Ricardo E. Jorge and
David B. Arciniegas, *Editors*

*December 2013*
**Late Life Depression**
W. Vaughn McCall, *Editor*

DOWNLOAD Free App!

*Review Articles*
THE CLINICS

**NOW AVAILABLE FOR YOUR iPhone and iPad**

# Preface

# Obsessive Compulsive and Related Disorders

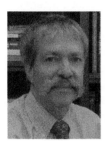

Wayne K. Goodman, MD
*Editor*

One of the most striking changes in DSM-5[1] is the introduction of a new section called Obsessive Compulsive and Related Disorders.[2] It contains obsessive compulsive disorder (OCD), body dysmorphic disorder (BDD), trichotillomania (hair-pulling disorder), hoarding disorder, and excoriation (skin-picking) disorder. OCD was previously classified among the anxiety disorders; BDD was a somatoform disorder, and trichotillomania was an impulse control disorder. Both hoarding disorder[3] and excoriation disorder are new diagnostic entities. The common feature of these disorders is the presence of persistent interfering obsessions, preoccupations, or repetitive behaviors. Although tic and Tourette disorders are listed elsewhere in DSM-5, these neurodevelopmental disorders are also characterized by repetitive motor or vocal behaviors and share considerable comorbidity with OCD. The well-established relationship between tics and some forms of OCD[4] has been codified in the DSM-5 criteria for OCD by asking the clinician to specify if the case is "tic-related" (current or past history of a tic disorder).

The purpose of this issue is to provide concise expert reviews on current understanding of the clinical features, etiology, and treatment of OCD, BDD, trichotillomania, and tic disorders. Several articles are devoted to OCD, so that topics related to pathophysiology (cognitive neuroscience theories and immune-mediated etiologies) and different treatment modalities (behavioral, pharmacologic, and device-based) could be covered in greater depth.

Although the impetus for this issue was the aforementioned changes in DSM-5, a radical change in the way we approach psychiatric diagnoses is also underway. The National Institute of Mental Health has launched the Research Domain Criteria initiative that takes a dimensional rather than a categorical approach to mental disorders.[5] Instead of a focus on clusters of symptoms that form the clinical syndromes delineated in DSM, domains of behavior are identified that cut across conventional diagnoses and can be characterized at different levels of analysis: from genes to molecules to cells to circuits to neurophysiology to behaviors. As further research is conducted using this

Psychiatr Clin N Am 37 (2014) xi–xii
http://dx.doi.org/10.1016/j.psc.2014.06.005
0193-953X/14/$ – see front matter © 2014 Elsevier Inc. All rights reserved.

framework and reliable biomarkers are developed, it is conceivable that the disorders listed in the Obsessive Compulsive and Related Disorders section of DSM will prove less related than they appear currently at the clinical surface.[6]

In the meantime, clinicians in the field need to grapple with our revamped DSM. Some of the changes embodied in DSM-5,[7] including the move of OCD out of the anxiety disorders,[8,9] have met with controversy. Because these nosologic issues are abundantly covered elsewhere in the literature,[8,9] this volume does not concern itself with that debate. Thankfully, many of the world's leading authorities on these disorders agreed to contribute to this review of obsessive compulsive and related disorders and share their clinical and scientific expertise with the reader.

Wayne K. Goodman, MD
Department of Psychiatry
Icahn School of Medicine at Mount Sinai
One Gustave L. Levy Place, Box 1230
New York, NY 10029, USA

E-mail address:
wayne.goodman@mssm.edu

## REFERENCES

1. American Psychiatric Association, DSM-5 Task Force. Diagnostic and statistical manual of mental disorders: DSM-5. 5th edition. Washington, DC: American Psychiatric Association; 2013.
2. Stein DJ, Craske MA, Friedman MJ, et al. Anxiety disorders, obsessive-compulsive and related disorders, trauma- and stressor-related disorders, and dissociative disorders in DSM-5. Am J Psychiatry 2014;171:611–3.
3. Frost RO, Steketee G, Tolin OF. Diagnosis and assessment of hoarding disorder. Annu Rev Clin Psychol 2012;8:219–42.
4. Cohen SC, Leckman JF, Bloch MH. Clinical assessment of Tourette syndrome and tic disorders. Neurosci Biobehav Rev 2013;37:997–1007.
5. Cuthbert BN, Insel TR. Toward the future of psychiatric diagnosis: the seven pillars of RDoC. BMC Med 2013;11:126.
6. Monzani B, Rijsdijk F, Harris J, et al. The structure of genetic and environmental risk factors for dimensional representations of DSM-5 obsessive-compulsive spectrum disorders. JAMA Psychiatry 2014;71:182–9.
7. First MB. Diagnostic and statistical manual of mental disorders, 5th edition, and clinical utility. J Nerv Ment Dis 2013;201:727–9.
8. Storch EA, Abramowitz J, Goodman WK. Where does obsessive-compulsive disorder belong in DSM-V? Depress Anxiety 2008;25:336–47.
9. Phillips KA, Stein DJ, Rauch SL, et al. Should an obsessive-compulsive spectrum grouping of disorders be included in DSM-V? Depress Anxiety 2010;27:528–55.

# Obsessive-Compulsive Disorder

Wayne K. Goodman, MD*, Dorothy E. Grice, MD, Kyle A.B. Lapidus, MD, PhD,
Barbara J. Coffey, MD, MS

## KEYWORDS

- Obsessive-compulsive disorder (OCD) • Obsessions • Compulsions • Serotonin
- Serotonin reuptake inhibitors (SRIs) • Glutamate
- Cortico-striato-thalamo-cortical (CSTC) circuit • History

## KEY POINTS

- Obsessive-compulsive disorder (OCD) is marked by recurrent and disturbing thoughts (obsessions) and repetitive behaviors (compulsions) that the person feels driven to perform.
- Patients with OCD generally recognize the senselessness of their obsessions and the excessiveness of their compulsive behaviors.
- OCD affects up to 2.3% of the population over the course of a lifetime and can be disabling.
- The 2 prevailing neurochemical based theories of OCD pathophysiology implicate the brain serotonin and glutamate systems, with the latter gaining traction.
- Based largely on brain imaging and neurosurgical experience, frontal–striatal pathways have been proposed as the dysfunctional neurocircuit underlying obsessive-compulsive behavior.

## INTRODUCTION

Obsessive-compulsive disorder (OCD) is a common, typically chronic disorder marked by intrusive and disturbing thoughts (obsessions) and repetitive behaviors (compulsions) that the person feels driven to perform. Typical themes include fears of illness and contamination, unwanted aggressive thoughts, other taboo thoughts involving sex or religion, and the need for symmetry or exactness. Compulsions, such as excessive cleaning, arranging, checking, counting, repeating, or reassurance

Disclosures: Roche, Research Support; Medtronic, donated devices (W.K. Goodman); Brain and Behavior Research Foundation and Simons Foundation, Research Support; Halo Neuro, Advisory Board; Medtronic, donated devices (K.A.B. Lapidus).
Department of Psychiatry, Icahn School of Medicine at Mount Sinai, One Gustave L. Levy Place, Box 1230, New York, NY 10029, USA
* Corresponding author.
E-mail address: wayne.goodman@mssm.edu

Psychiatr Clin N Am 37 (2014) 257–267
http://dx.doi.org/10.1016/j.psc.2014.06.004
0193-953X/14/$ – see front matter © 2014 Elsevier Inc. All rights reserved.
psych.theclinics.com

seeking, generally serve to neutralize the distress of obsessions. However, sometimes the compulsions themselves can become so time consuming or onerous that they engender anxiety. Avoidance of triggers to obsessions and compulsions is a common feature of OCD.

Starting with the fifth edition of the *Diagnostic and Statistical Manual for Mental Disorders* (DSM-5), OCD was removed from the anxiety disorders and added to a new section termed obsessive-compulsive and related disorders.[1] A common feature of disorders in this category is the presence of repetitive behaviors. This nosologic revision reflects growing neurobiological and treatment response data that distinguish OCD from anxiety disorders such as panic disorder, generalized anxiety disorder or social anxiety disorder.[2] This change does not imply that anxiety is absent in OCD; in fact, anxiety is often a prominent feature of the illness. On the other hand, marked physiologic arousal or specific fears that are often present in anxiety disorders are less evident in some forms of OCD. For example, patients with OCD involving exactness or symmetry obsessions may report that they perform their associated rituals until they feel "just right," instead of describing relief from anxiety. Similarly, patients concerned with bodily waste may not experience a "fear" of a dreaded consequence, such as disease; rather, they may report "disgust"[3] as the primary emotional driver. Such examples raise the question whether these phenotypic differences also point to distinct neurobiological circuits that distinguish some forms of OCD from anxiety disorders.[4–6] Future research on the validity of the DSM criteria and, more important, investigations that adopt dimensional approaches such as the Research Domain Criteria[7] will tell us whether DSM-5 got it right or not.[8,9] New to the DSM-5 criteria for OCD are specifiers for level of insight and for tic relatedness.

This article provides an overview of the clinical features and pathophysiologic theories of OCD at the neurotransmitter and circuit levels of analysis. Separate articles within this issue address etiologic theories based on infection-triggered immune dysfunction, genetic factors, and cognitive neuroscience (see articles by Murphy, Gerardi, Leckman, Scharf and Grice, as well as Stern and Taylor, respectively). Treatment interventions (pharmacologic, behavioral, and device based) for OCD are also covered elsewhere in this issue.

## EPIDEMIOLOGY AND COURSE

OCD is a leading cause of disability worldwide.[10–12] According to the National Comorbidity Survey Replication, the lifetime prevalence of OCD is 2.3%, and during the prior 12 months. In addition, 1.2% of respondents met criteria for a full DSM-IV diagnosis.[11] The prevalence of subthreshold OCD symptoms was much higher.[11] Other epidemiologic studies have estimated the lifetime prevalence of OCD as ranging between 1.9% and 3.0%.[13] The modal onset of OCD is usually in early adulthood with nearly 50% of cases presenting during childhood or adolescence[11,14]; onset after the age of 40 is unusual.[14] Males tend to have an earlier age of onset than females, but by adulthood females outnumber males by a small margin. If untreated, OCD is usually chronic and follows a waxing and waning course.[15,16] Only about 5% to 10% of OCD sufferers have a spontaneous remission.[14,16] Another 5% to 10% experience progressive worsening of their symptoms.[14] Some cases in childhood may follow an episodic course.[17,18]

## CLINICAL FEATURES

OCD is characterized by persistent disturbing thoughts, images, or impulses (obsessions), or repetitive, ritualized behaviors that the person feels driven to perform (compulsions), or both. The majority of patients have both obsessions and compulsions, but a diagnosis can be made without both present. Most patients are able to acknowledge their symptoms as senseless or excessive at some point during the illness. In practice, there is a range of insight from good to poor to absent at times; DSM-5 calls for specifying degree of insight accordingly. Symptoms produce subjective distress, are time consuming (>1 h/d), or interfere with function.

Obsessions are experienced as intrusive and attempts are made to ignore, suppress, or neutralize them with another thought or action. Compulsions are repetitive behaviors or mental acts the person feels driven to perform, either in response to an obsession (eg, to prevent a dreaded event from occurring), or according to rigid rules designed to prevent or reduce distress. The acts are clearly excessive or senseless. Compulsions usually reduce distress, but are not inherently pleasurable.

Common types of obsessions include concerns about contamination (eg, fear of dirt, germs or illness, disgust with bodily waste), safety or harm (eg, being responsible for a fire), unwanted acts of aggression (eg, unwanted impulse to harm a loved one), unacceptable sexual or religious thoughts (eg, sacrilegious images), and the need for symmetry or exactness. Common compulsions include excessive cleaning (eg, ritualized hand washing), checking, ordering and arranging rituals, counting, repeating routine activities (eg, going in/out of a doorway), and hoarding (eg, difficulty parting with possessions, regardless of their actual monetary or sentimental value). (See the article by Frost, Steketee, and Tolin for a further discussion of this topic.) Although most compulsions are observable behaviors (eg, hand washing), some are performed as unobservable mental rituals (eg, silent recitation of prayers to neutralize a horrific image). Detailed examples of obsessive-compulsive symptoms can be found in the Symptom Checklist of the Yale-Brown Obsessive Compulsive Scale.[19]

## SCREENING AND DIFFERENTIAL DIAGNOSIS

The presence of insight distinguishes OCD from a psychotic illness, such as schizophrenia, although comorbid obsessive-compulsive symptoms are not uncommon in schizophrenia.[20] Obsessions may involve unrealistic fears, but unlike delusions, they are not fixed, unshakeable, false beliefs. Patients with OCD recognize the thoughts as emanating from their own minds as opposed to the way auditory hallucinations are experienced. Occasionally, an obsession can be misdiagnosed as an auditory hallucination when the patient, especially a child, refers to it as "the voice in my head," even though it is recognized as his or her own thoughts. The symptoms of OCD may be bizarre, but the patient recognizes their absurdity. However, the DSM-5 allows for a range of insight as reflected in the following specifiers: Good or fair insight, poor insight, or absent insight/delusional OCD beliefs. Poor or absent insight is not uncommon in young children with OCD.[21]

Patients are often reluctant to disclose unwanted thoughts or odd behaviors because they are embarrassed. Therefore, clinicians should probe for OCD symptoms in patients or parents of children presenting with commonly comorbid mood or anxiety complaints. A simple screening question follows: "Sometimes people will be bothered by unwanted or repetitive thoughts or sudden, strong urges to check, wash, or count things. Does anything like that ever happen to you?" More comprehensive and validated self-report screening instruments are available for identifying cases of OCD.[22] Confirmation of the diagnosis requires a clinical assessment that should include a rating of symptom severity.[23] Patients may not seek treatment until social, work, or school impairment is significant or comorbid depressive symptoms have developed. Childhood OCD is often recognized by parents or teachers who become aware of ritualized behaviors or reassurance seeking that interferes with functioning.

Much of the confusion in the professional and lay literature regarding the differences between OCD and other conditions stems from the varied uses of the words obsession and compulsion. To be true symptoms of OCD, obsessions and compulsions are strictly defined as described in this article. A key point to remember is that the compulsions of OCD are not considered inherently pleasurable; at best, they relieve anxiety. As a contrasting clinical example, patients seeking treatment for "compulsive" eating, gambling, or sexual behavior may feel unable to control behaviors they acknowledge as deleterious, but at some time in the past these acts were experienced as gratifying.

Individuals with OCD have a 7% lifetime risk of Tourette syndrome (TS) and a 20% risk of tics.[24] Distinguishing between complex motor tics and certain compulsions (eg, repetitive touching) can be problematic. By convention, tics are distinguished from "ticlike" compulsions (eg, compulsive touching or blinking) based on whether the patient attaches a purpose or meaning to the behavior. For example, a patient feeling an urge to repeatedly touch an object would be classified as having a compulsion only if it was preceded by a need to neutralize an unwanted thought or image; complex motor tics can be often distinguished by sensorimotor urges that precede the motor behavior.[25] Tics are often identified by "the company that they keep"; if a complex motor act is accompanied by clearcut tics (eg, head jerks), it is most likely a tic itself. However, there are many exceptions to this rule in which the same patient with OCD and TS may have both simple and complex motor tics as well as compulsions. The types of obsessive-compulsive symptoms present in patients with comorbid tics often can be distinctive.[26] Patients with TS and OCD often describe a need or feeling to get things "just right," and repeat behaviors to achieve a feeling of symmetry or exactness in touch or appearance.[27] Conversely, in patients with OCD without TS, contamination or illness concerns are more common. (See the article by Shaw and Coffey in this issue for a detailed discussion of relationship between OCD and tic disorders.)

## ETIOLOGIC HYPOTHESES OF OCD

The intellectual climate and scientific tools of the period have influenced each stage in the history of OCD. Until the 1850s, obsessive-compulsive phenomena were undifferentiated from other forms of insanity.[28] The earliest descriptions of a malady resembling OCD correspond with what would be called "scrupulosity" today.[29] For example, Robert Burton reported a case in his compendium, the Anatomy of Melancholy (1621)[30]: "If he be in a silent auditory, as at a sermon, he is afraid he shall speak aloud and unaware, something indecent, unfit to be said." French 19th-century accounts of cases resembling OCD emphasized the central role of doubt ("folie du doute") and indecisiveness.[28] Later French writers, including Pierre Janet in 1902, stressed the loss of will and low mental energy ("psychasthenia") underlying the formation of obsessive-compulsive symptoms.[28]

Meanwhile in Germany, Westphal was the first to distinguish obsessions from delusions in 1877.[31] Freud adopted a similar viewpoint when he introduced the term "obsessional neurosis" in 1895.[31] The greater part of the 20th century was dominated by psychoanalytic theories of OCD. According to psychoanalytic theory, obsessions and compulsions reflect maladaptive responses to unresolved conflicts from early stages of psychosexual development. Psychoanalytic treatment focused on unraveling the symbolic meaning and putative childhood roots of OCD. Psychoanalytic theories of OCD lost favor in the last quarter of the 20th century as new, more effective behavioral and pharmacologic treatments were introduced.

Learning theory models of OCD gained influence as a result of the success of behavior therapy and the growth of cognitive neuroscience.[32,33] Conditioning models gave way to more sophisticated cognitive models[32,34] (see the articles by Stern and Steven Taylor and by Lewin and colleagues in this issue for additional details). The efficacy of a behavior therapy technique referred to as exposure and response prevention has been confirmed in numerous studies of patients with OCD.

## NEUROCHEMICAL HYPOTHESES
### Serotonin

The observation in 1975 that clomipramine was beneficial in patients with OCD ushered in a new era of neurobiological investigations.[35] Previously, OCD had been considered refractory to pharmacotherapy. In contrast with other tricyclic antidepressants, clomipramine is a potent inhibitor of serotonin reuptake. The serotonin hypothesis of OCD was born out of a series of case reports,[35] later confirmed by randomized clinical trials,[36,37] that serotonin reuptake inhibitors (SRIs) were effective in this disorder. These findings were buttressed by biochemical data from patients chronically treated with SRIs[38] and by early pharmacologic challenge studies.[39] With the introduction of selective serotonin reuptake inhibitors (SSRIs) like fluvoxamine, these drugs were also shown to be effective in OCD.[40] To date, more than 20 randomized clinical trials have established the efficacy of SRIs or SSRIs in OCD[41] These findings were buttressed by biochemical data from patients chronically treated by SRIs[38] and by early pharmacologic challenge studies.[39] With the introduction of SSRIs like fluvoxamine, these drugs were also shown to be effective in OCD.[40,42] To date, more than 20 randomized clinical trials have established the efficacy of SRIs or SSRIs in OCD[41] (see the article by Pittenger and Block for more details on pharmacologic treatment of OCD.)

The fact that SSRIs are effective in OCD is not a distinguishing feature, because these medications have a broad spectrum of action in psychiatric conditions, including depression and anxiety disorders. What stands out is that other antidepressant agents that lack potency for serotonin transporter binding are generally ineffective in OCD. In contrast, many antidepressants with other molecular targets are effective in the treatment of depression and other neuropsychiatric disorders but not in OCD. The preferential efficacy of SRIs and SSRIs in OCD is well established.[41] Initially, clomipramine was shown to be more effective than tricyclic antidepressants like desipramine, which were predominantly norepinephrine reuptake inhibitors.[43] Later, SSRIs such as fluvoxamine and sertraline were also shown to be superior to desipramine.[36,44]

These drug response data led researchers to hypothesize that dysfunction in brain serotonergic systems might be related to the etiology of OCD. However, interpretations about pathophysiology based on treatment response and the presumed mechanism of action of the intervention are fraught with problems that have plagued the field of psychiatry for decades. Whether it is the serendipitous discovery of neuroleptics improving positive symptoms of schizophrenia (leading to the dopamine hypothesis of schizophrenia) or SRIs reducing obsessive-compulsive symptoms, this reverse path to understanding etiology has yielded few new insights or novel treatments.

A number of neurobiological investigations into the role of serotonin in OCD were launched across multiple laboratories in the 1980s and 1990s. Many of these involved pharmacologic challenge paradigms with probes of serotonin function such as m-chlorophenylpiperazine.[39,45] These studies were designed to provoke obsessive-compulsive symptoms as well as induce a measurable, blood-based neurohumoral signal that could be compared with the response in healthy subjects. In addition, multiple drug trials of other serotonergic agents (eg, buspirone, tryptophan) were initiated, mostly as adjunctive agents to augment SSRIs in partial or nonresponders to SSRI monotherapy. Unfortunately, randomized clinical trials failed to identify serotonergic agents that could augment SSRI treatment in OCD.[46,47] By the same token, pharmacologic challenge studies were generally inconclusive and eventually abandoned.[45,48] One of the most surprising negative findings was the failure of acute tryptophan depletion to provoke a transient return of obsessive-compulsive symptoms in patients with OCD who had responded to SRIs.[49] In contrast, this paradigm induced worsening of depressive symptoms, as it had in studies of depressed patients taking SRIs.[50] The effectiveness of SRIs in OCD remains a tantalizing clue about a role for serotonin in OCD, but additional research, perhaps using new tools, is needed to identify whether a disturbance in serotonin function exists and if it has any etiologic significance. At present, the most parsimonious (but quite speculative) explanation for the preferential efficacy of SRIs in OCD is that these medications enhance the activity of a serotonergic system that compensates for a disturbance in a functionally coupled system that is more directly tied to the underlying neurobiology of OCD.[51]

### Glutamate

A role of the glutamatergic system in OCD has been gaining traction as a result of emerging imaging data,[52] genomic studies,[53] biochemical studies of cerebrospinal fluid,[54,55] and animal models of aberrant grooming behavior.[56] These findings have spurred interest in testing the efficacy of medications (eg, riluzole) that modulate glutamate function. (See the article by Pittenger and Block for a discussion of glutamatergic agents in OCD.) Pittenger and colleagues,[57] provide an excellent review of the glutamatergic theory of OCD elsewhere. A role for glutamate in OCD is highly compatible with circuit-based theories of OCD discussed briefly herein.

## NEUROCIRCUITRY HYPOTHESES

Functional brain imaging studies in OCD are remarkably consistent compared with findings in most other neuropsychiatric conditions.[58] Both positron emission tomography[59] and functional magnetic resonance imaging[60] have shown increased activation in regions of the orbitofrontal cortex, the anterior cingulate cortex, and parts of the basal ganglia (particularly the head of the caudate nucleus) in the symptomatic state compared with healthy controls.[61] These areas of abnormal activation tend to normalize with successful treatment upon repeated testing, whether with medications or behavioral approaches.[61,62] Additional evidence for a role of the basal ganglia in OCD are case reports of "accidents of nature," such as Sydenham chorea,[63] von Economo encephalitis,[64] and ischemic events,[65] in which insults to the basal ganglia, particularly the globus pallidus, produced obsessive-compulsive behaviors. (For further details on brain imaging in OCD see the article in this issue by Stern and Taylor as well as reviews published elsewhere[58]).

A confluence of data led to the hypothesis that frontal–striatal function is disrupted in OCD. In addition to the functional brain imaging findings mentioned, the seminal work by Alexander and colleagues[66] influenced OCD researchers to consider certain parallel segregated cortico-striato-thalamo-cortical loops as the neuroanatomic substrate for obsessive-compulsive behavior.[61] More recent revisions of these models offer a more complex picture,[58] with patterns of cortical and subcortical changes in OCD seeming to depend on the cognitive task under investigation (see the article by Stern and Taylor elsewhere in this issue). Another component of these circuit-based hypotheses has been the therapeutic benefit of neurosurgery in intractable OCD.[67] Both experience with ablative surgery and deep brain stimulation are compatible with dysfunction of white matter tracts implicated in network theories of OCD.[68]

One of the most important technical and conceptual developments in circuit-based theories of OCD has been the change in focus from static regions of interest to interrogation of functional networks subserving different cognitive or behavioral functions germane to the pathophysiology of OCD.[34,69–75] The investigation of network connectivity in OCD identifies changes in the functional organization of the brain, which could contribute to many of the observed alterations in brain activation and behavior.

## SUMMARY

In the DSM-5, OCD has transferred from anxiety disorders to a new grouping of obsessive-compulsive and related disorders. Ultimately, the diagnostic classification of OCD is less important than elucidation of its pathophysiology so that more effective treatments can be developed, especially for those many patients resistant to conventional therapies. The observation that SRIs are preferentially effective in OCD led to the so-called serotonin hypothesis of OCD. However, direct support for a role of serotonin in the pathophysiology (eg, biomarkers in pharmacologic challenge studies) of OCD remains elusive. A glutamatergic hypothesis of OCD has been gaining traction based on imaging data, genomic studies, biochemical studies, and animal models of aberrant grooming behavior. These findings have spurred interest in testing the efficacy of medications (eg, riluzole) that modulate glutamate function. Functional imaging studies (both functional magnetic resonance imaging and positron emission tomography) show fairly consistent evidence for increased activity in brain regions that form a cortico-striato-thalamo-cortical circuit. Furthermore, these abnormalities normalize during successful treatment of OC symptoms, whether with SRIs or cognitive–behavioral therapy. A common substrate of various interventions (whether drug, behavioral, or device) may be modulation (at different nodes) of the cortico-striato-thalamo-cortical circuit. Hypotheses that integrate knowledge over multiple levels of analysis (eg, genetics, neurochemical, and circuit networks) stand the best chance of advancing our understanding of OCD.[76]

## REFERENCES

1. American Psychiatric Association, DSM-5 Task Force. Diagnostic and statistical manual of mental disorders: DSM-5. 5th edition. Washington, DC: American Psychiatric Association; 2013.
2. Phillips KA, Stein DJ, Rauch SL, et al. Should an obsessive-compulsive spectrum grouping of disorders be included in DSM-V? Depress Anxiety 2010; 27(6):528–55.
3. Husted DS, Shapira NA, Goodman WK. The neurocircuitry of obsessive-compulsive disorder and disgust. Prog Neuropsychopharmacol Biol Psychiatry 2006;30(3):389–99.
4. Fiddick L. There is more than the amygdala: potential threat assessment in the cingulate cortex. Neurosci Biobehav Rev 2011;35(4):1007–18.
5. Cisler JM, Olatunji BO, Lohr JM. Disgust, fear, and the anxiety disorders: a critical review. Clin Psychol Rev 2009;29(1):34–46.
6. Via E, Cardoner N, Pujol J, et al. Amygdala activation and symptom dimensions in obsessive-compulsive disorder. Br J Psychiatry 2014;204(1):61–8.
7. Insel T, Cuthbert B, Garvey M, et al. Research domain criteria (RDoC): toward a new classification framework for research on mental disorders. Am J Psychiatry 2010;167(7):748–51.
8. Storch EA, Abramowitz J, Goodman WK. Where does obsessive-compulsive disorder belong in DSM-V? Depress Anxiety 2008;25(4):336–47.

9. Monzani B, Rijsdijk F, Harris J, et al. The structure of genetic and environmental risk factors for dimensional representations of DSM-5 obsessive-compulsive spectrum disorders. JAMA Psychiatry 2014;71(2):182–9.

10. Torres AR, Prince MJ, Bebbington PE, et al. Obsessive-compulsive disorder: prevalence, comorbidity, impact, and help-seeking in the British National Psychiatric Morbidity Survey of 2000. Am J Psychiatry 2006;163(11):1978–85.

11. Ruscio AM, Stein DJ, Chiu WT, et al. The epidemiology of obsessive-compulsive disorder in the National Comorbidity Survey Replication. Mol Psychiatry 2010; 15(1):53–63.

12. Whiteford HA, Degenhardt L, Rehm J, et al. Global burden of disease attributable to mental and substance use disorders: findings from the Global Burden of Disease Study 2010. Lancet 2013;382(9904):1575–86.

13. Karno M, Golding JM, Sorenson SB, et al. The epidemiology of obsessive-compulsive disorder in five US communities. Arch Gen Psychiatry 1988;45(12): 1094–9.

14. Rasmussen SA, Eisen JL. The epidemiology and clinical features of obsessive compulsive disorder. Psychiatr Clin North Am 1992;15(4):743–58.

15. Bloch MH, Green C, Kichuk SA, et al. Long-term outcome in adults with obsessive-compulsive disorder. Depress Anxiety 2013;30(8):716–22.

16. Eisen JL, Pinto A, Mancebo MC, et al. A 2-year prospective follow-up study of the course of obsessive-compulsive disorder. J Clin Psychiatry 2010;71(8): 1033–9.

17. Storch EA, Lack CW, Merlo LJ, et al. Clinical features of children and adolescents with obsessive-compulsive disorder and hoarding symptoms. Compr Psychiatry 2007;48(4):313–8.

18. Murphy TK, Storch EA, Lewin AB, et al. Clinical factors associated with pediatric autoimmune neuropsychiatric disorders associated with streptococcal infections. J Pediatr 2012;160(2):314–9.

19. Storch EA, Larson MJ, Price LH, et al. Psychometric analysis of the Yale-Brown Obsessive-Compulsive Scale Second Edition Symptom Checklist. J Anxiety Disord 2010;24(6):650–6.

20. Swets M, Dekker J, van Emmerik-van Oortmerssen K, et al. The obsessive compulsive spectrum in schizophrenia, a meta-analysis and meta-regression exploring prevalence rates. Schizophr Res 2014;152(2–3):458–68.

21. Storch EA, Milsom VA, Merlo LJ, et al. Insight in pediatric obsessive-compulsive disorder: associations with clinical presentation. Psychiatry Res 2008;160(2): 212–20.

22. Storch EA, Kaufman DA, Bagner D, et al. Florida obsessive-compulsive inventory: development, reliability, and validity. J Clin Psychol 2007;63(9):851–9.

23. Goodman WK, Price LH, Rasmussen SA, et al. The Yale-Brown Obsessive Compulsive Scale. I. development, use, and reliability. Arch Gen Psychiatry 1989;46(11):1006–11.

24. Eapen V, Robertson MM, Alsobrook JP 2nd, et al. Obsessive compulsive symptoms in Gilles de la Tourette syndrome and obsessive compulsive disorder: differences by diagnosis and family history. Am J Med Genet 1997;74(4):432–8.

25. Miguel EC, Baer L, Coffey BJ, et al. Phenomenological differences appearing with repetitive behaviours in obsessive-compulsive disorder and Gilles de la Tourette's syndrome. Br J Psychiatry 1997;170:140–5.

26. Holzer JC, Goodman WK, McDougle CJ, et al. Obsessive-compulsive disorder with and without a chronic tic disorder. A comparison of symptoms in 70 patients. Br J Psychiatry 1994;164(4):469–73.

27. Leckman JF, Walker DE, Goodman WK, et al. "Just right" perceptions associated with compulsive behavior in Tourette's syndrome. Am J Psychiatry 1994;151(5): 675–80.
28. Berrios GE. Obsessive-compulsive disorder: its conceptual history in France during the 19th century. Compr Psychiatry 1989;30(4):283–95.
29. Greenberg D, Huppert JD. Scrupulosity: a unique subtype of obsessive-compulsive disorder. Curr Psychiatry Rep 2010;12(4):282–9.
30. Burton R, Lichfield J, Short J, et al, English Printing Collection (Library of Congress), George Fabyan Collection (Library of Congress). The anatomy of melancholy, what it is: with all the kindes, causes, symptomes, prognostickes, and severall cures of it: in three maine partitions with their severall sections, members, and subsections, philosophically, medicinally, historically, opened and cut up. 1st edition. Oxford (United Kingdom): Printed by Iohn Lichfield and Iames Short for Henry Cripps; 1621.
31. May-Tolzmann U. Obsessional neurosis: a nosographic innovation by Freud. Hist Psychiatry 1998;9(35):335–53.
32. Abramowitz JS, McKay D, Taylor S. Clinical handbook of obsessive-compulsive disorder and related problems. Baltimore (MD): Johns Hopkins University Press; 2008.
33. Rachman SJ. Obsessions and compulsions. Englewood Cliffs (NJ): Prentice-Hall; 1980.
34. Stern ER, Welsh RC, Fitzgerald KD, et al. Hyperactive error responses and altered connectivity in ventromedial and frontoinsular cortices in obsessive-compulsive disorder. Biol Psychiatry 2011;69(6):583–91.
35. Yaryura-Tobias JA, Neziroglu F. The action of chlorimipramine in obsessive-compulsive neurosis: a pilot study. Curr Ther Res Clin Exp 1975;17(1):111–6.
36. Goodman WK, Price LH, Delgado PL, et al. Specificity of serotonin reuptake inhibitors in the treatment of obsessive-compulsive disorder. Comparison of fluvoxamine and desipramine. Arch Gen Psychiatry 1990;47(6):577–85.
37. Katz RJ, DeVeaugh-Geiss J, Landau P. Clomipramine in obsessive-compulsive disorder. Biol Psychiatry 1990;28(5):401–14.
38. Thoren P, Asberg M, Cronholm B, et al. Clomipramine treatment of obsessive-compulsive disorder. I. A controlled clinical trial. Arch Gen Psychiatry 1980; 37(11):1281–5.
39. Zohar J, Mueller EA, Insel TR, et al. Serotonergic responsivity in obsessive-compulsive disorder. Comparison of patients and healthy controls. Arch Gen Psychiatry 1987;44(11):946–51.
40. Goodman WK, Price LH, Rasmussen SA, et al. Efficacy of fluvoxamine in obsessive-compulsive disorder. A double-blind comparison with placebo. Arch Gen Psychiatry 1989;46(1):36–44.
41. Soomro GM. Obsessive compulsive disorder. Clin Evid (Online) 2012;1–28.
42. Perse TL, Greist JH, Jefferson JW, et al. Fluvoxamine treatment of obsessive-compulsive disorder. Am J Psychiatry 1987;144(12):1543–8.
43. Leonard HL, Swedo SE, Rapoport JL, et al. Treatment of obsessive-compulsive disorder with clomipramine and desipramine in children and adolescents. A double-blind crossover comparison. Arch Gen Psychiatry 1989;46(12):1088–92.
44. Hoehn-Saric R, Ninan P, Black DW, et al. Multicenter double-blind comparison of sertraline and desipramine for concurrent obsessive-compulsive and major depressive disorders. Arch Gen Psychiatry 2000;57(1):76–82.
45. Goodman WK, McDougle CJ, Price LH, et al. m-Chlorophenylpiperazine in patients with obsessive-compulsive disorder: absence of symptom exacerbation. Biol Psychiatry 1995;38(3):138–49.

46. McDougle CJ, Goodman WK, Leckman JF, et al. Limited therapeutic effect of addition of buspirone in fluvoxamine-refractory obsessive-compulsive disorder. Am J Psychiatry 1993;150(4):647–9.

47. McDougle CJ, Price LH, Goodman WK, et al. A controlled trial of lithium augmentation in fluvoxamine-refractory obsessive-compulsive disorder: lack of efficacy. J Clin Psychopharmacol 1991;11(3):175–84.

48. Charney DS, Goodman WK, Price LH, et al. Serotonin function in obsessive-compulsive disorder. A comparison of the effects of tryptophan and m-chlorophenylpiperazine in patients and healthy subjects. Arch Gen Psychiatry 1988; 45(2):177–85.

49. Barr LC, Goodman WK, McDougle CJ, et al. Tryptophan depletion in patients with obsessive-compulsive disorder who respond to serotonin reuptake inhibitors. Arch Gen Psychiatry 1994;51(4):309–17.

50. Delgado PL, Charney DS, Price LH, et al. Serotonin function and the mechanism of antidepressant action. Reversal of antidepressant-induced remission by rapid depletion of plasma tryptophan. Arch Gen Psychiatry 1990;47(5):411–8.

51. Goodman WK, McDougle CJ, Price LH, et al. Beyond the serotonin hypothesis: a role for dopamine in some forms of obsessive compulsive disorder? J Clin Psychiatry 1990;51(Suppl):36–43 [discussion: 55–8].

52. Brennan BP, Rauch SL, Jensen JE, et al. A critical review of magnetic resonance spectroscopy studies of obsessive-compulsive disorder. Biol Psychiatry 2013; 73(1):24–31.

53. Stewart SE, Mayerfeld C, Arnold PD, et al. Meta-analysis of association between obsessive-compulsive disorder and the 3' region of neuronal glutamate transporter gene SLC1A1. Am J Med Genet B Neuropsychiatr Genet 2013;162B(4):367–79.

54. Bhattacharyya S, Khanna S, Chakrabarty K, et al. Anti-brain autoantibodies and altered excitatory neurotransmitters in obsessive-compulsive disorder. Neuropsychopharmacology 2009;34(12):2489–96.

55. Chakrabarty K, Bhattacharyya S, Christopher R, et al. Glutamatergic dysfunction in OCD. Neuropsychopharmacology 2005;30(9):1735–40.

56. Bienvenu OJ, Wang Y, Shugart YY, et al. Sapap3 and pathological grooming in humans: Results from the OCD collaborative genetics study. Am J Med Genet B Neuropsychiatr Genet 2009;150B(5):710–20.

57. Pittenger C, Bloch MH, Williams K. Glutamate abnormalities in obsessive compulsive disorder: neurobiology, pathophysiology, and treatment. Pharmacol Ther 2011;132(3):314–32.

58. Milad MR, Rauch SL. Obsessive-compulsive disorder: beyond segregated cortico-striatal pathways. Trends Cogn Sci 2012;16(1):43–51.

59. Baxter LR Jr, Schwartz JM, Mazziotta JC, et al. Cerebral glucose metabolic rates in nondepressed patients with obsessive-compulsive disorder. Am J Psychiatry 1988;145(12):1560–3.

60. Breiter HC, Rauch SL, Kwong KK, et al. Functional magnetic resonance imaging of symptom provocation in obsessive-compulsive disorder. Arch Gen Psychiatry 1996;53(7):595–606.

61. Saxena S, Rauch SL. Functional neuroimaging and the neuroanatomy of obsessive-compulsive disorder. Psychiatr Clin North Am 2000;23(3):563–86.

62. Schwartz JM, Stoessel PW, Baxter LR Jr, et al. Systematic changes in cerebral glucose metabolic rate after successful behavior modification treatment of obsessive-compulsive disorder. Arch Gen Psychiatry 1996;53(2):109–13.

63. Asbahr FR, Garvey MA, Snider LA, et al. Obsessive-compulsive symptoms among patients with Sydenham chorea. Biol Psychiatry 2005;57(9):1073–6.

64. Cheyette SR, Cummings JL. Encephalitis lethargica: lessons for contemporary neuropsychiatry. J Neuropsychiatry Clin Neurosci 1995;7(2):125–34.
65. Thobois S, Jouanneau E, Bouvard M, et al. Obsessive-compulsive disorder after unilateral caudate nucleus bleeding. Acta Neurochir (Wien) 2004;146(9): 1027–31 [discussion: 1031].
66. Alexander GE, DeLong MR, Strick PL. Parallel organization of functionally segregated circuits linking basal ganglia and cortex. Annu Rev Neurosci 1986;9:357–81.
67. Greenberg BD, Gabriels LA, Malone DA Jr, et al. Deep brain stimulation of the ventral internal capsule/ventral striatum for obsessive-compulsive disorder: worldwide experience. Mol Psychiatry 2010;15(1):64–79.
68. Greenberg BD, Rauch SL, Haber SN. Invasive circuitry-based neurotherapeutics: stereotactic ablation and deep brain stimulation for OCD. Neuropsychopharmacology 2010;35(1):317–36.
69. Anticevic A, Hu S, Zhang S, et al. Global resting-state functional magnetic resonance imaging analysis identifies frontal cortex, striatal, and cerebellar dysconnectivity in obsessive-compulsive disorder. Biol Psychiatry 2014;75(8):595–605.
70. Beucke JC, Sepulcre J, Talukdar T, et al. Abnormally high degree connectivity of the orbitofrontal cortex in obsessive-compulsive disorder. JAMA Psychiatry 2013;70(6):619–29.
71. Cocchi L, Harrison BJ, Pujol J, et al. Functional alterations of large-scale brain networks related to cognitive control in obsessive-compulsive disorder. Hum Brain Mapp 2012;33(5):1089–106.
72. Fitzgerald KD, Welsh RC, Stern ER, et al. Developmental alterations of frontal-striatal-thalamic connectivity in obsessive-compulsive disorder. J Am Acad Child Adolesc Psychiatry 2011;50(9):938–48.e3.
73. Harrison BJ, Soriano-Mas C, Pujol J, et al. Altered corticostriatal functional connectivity in obsessive-compulsive disorder. Arch Gen Psychiatry 2009;66(11): 1189–200.
74. Jang JH, Kim JH, Jung WH, et al. Functional connectivity in fronto-subcortical circuitry during the resting state in obsessive-compulsive disorder. Neurosci Lett 2010;474(3):158–62.
75. Stern ER, Fitzgerald KD, Welsh RC, et al. Resting-state functional connectivity between fronto-parietal and default mode networks in obsessive-compulsive disorder. PLoS One 2012;7(5):e36356.
76. Pauls DL, Abramovitch A, Rauch SL, et al. Obsessive-compulsive disorder: an integrative genetic and neurobiological perspective. Nat Rev Neurosci 2014; 15(6):410–24.

# Tics and Tourette Syndrome

Zoey A. Shaw, BA, Barbara J. Coffey, MD, MS*

## KEYWORDS

- Tourette syndrome ● Tic disorder ● Tics ● Obsessive-compulsive disorder
- Comorbidity ● Treatment

## KEY POINTS

- Tourette syndrome (TS) is a childhood onset neurodevelopmental disorder characterized by multiple motor and vocal tics. Other tic disorders include persistent (chronic) motor or vocal tic disorder and provisional tic disorder.
- The prevalence of TS is estimated to be 1% of the world's population.
- The cause and pathophysiology of tic disorders remain largely unknown.
- Most patients have 1 or more psychiatric comorbid disorders, such as attention-deficit/hyperactivity disorder or obsessive-compulsive disorder.
- Treatment is multimodal, including both pharmacotherapy and cognitive-behavioral treatment, and requires disentanglement of tics and comorbid symptoms.

## INTRODUCTION

Tourette syndrome (TS), also known as Gilles de la Tourette syndrome or Tourette's disorder, is a childhood onset neurodevelopmental disorder with a prevalence estimated at 1% of the world's population.[1] TS is characterized by multiple motor tics and at least 1 vocal tic, both present for greater than 1 year, with onset before age 18 years.[2] Other tic disorders according to the *Diagnostic and Statistical Manual of Mental Disorders, Fifth Edition* (DSM-5) include persistent (chronic) motor or vocal tic disorder, in which exclusively motor or vocal tics are present for more than 1 year, and provisional tic disorder, in which motor or vocal tics have been present for less than 1 year.[2]

Disclosures: Z.A. Shaw has no conflicts of interest or financial ties to disclose. Dr B.J. Coffey has received research support from National Institute of Mental Health grants, NIMH R01 MH092292-01A1, NIH R01 RFA MH-02-002, NIMH 1K08MH01415-01, Tourette Syndrome Association, Otsuka and Shire. She serves on the advisory board for Genco Sciences, Quintiles, and the American Academy of Child and Adolescent Psychiatry.
Icahn School of Medicine at Mount Sinai, Department of Psychiatry, One Gustave L. Levy Place, Box 1230, New York, NY 10029, USA
* Corresponding author.
*E-mail address:* barbara.coffey@mssm.edu

Psychiatr Clin N Am 37 (2014) 269–286
http://dx.doi.org/10.1016/j.psc.2014.05.001
0193-953X/14/$ – see front matter © 2014 Elsevier Inc. All rights reserved.

| Abbreviations | |
|---|---|
| ADHD | Attention deficit hyperactivity disorder |
| CBIT | Comprehensive behavioral intervention for tics |
| ERP | Exposure and response prevention |
| HRT | Habit reversal therapy |
| OCD | Obsessive compulsive disorder |
| PANS | Pediatric acute-onset neuropsychiatric syndrome |
| PANDAS | Pediatric autoimmune neuropsychiatric disorders associated with streptococcus |
| RCTs | Randomized controlled trials |
| SSRIs | Selective serotonin reuptake inhibitors |
| TS | Tourette syndrome |
| YGTSS | Yale Global Tic Severity Scale |

A tic is defined as a sudden, rapid, involuntary, nonrhythmic movement or vocalization. Tics result from the movement of 1 muscle or group of muscles and are characterized by their anatomical location, number, frequency, duration, and complexity. They are classified as either simple or complex. Simple tics involve 1 muscle group or sound, whereas complex tics are slower and more purposeful, involving multiple muscle groups or multiple sounds, words, or phrases. Examples of simple and complex tics are listed in **Table 1**.

Simple motor tics are the most common presentation of tic disorders, and include eye blinking, shoulder shrugging, or head/neck jerking. Complex motor tics are characterized by coordinated and more purposeful movements involving multiple muscle groups; examples include tapping, stepping in a certain pattern, and circling. Simple vocal tics, also known as phonic tics, are characterized by the utterance of a brief sound, such as throat clearing, coughing, or sniffing. Complex vocal tics involve the production of multiple sounds and include repetition of syllables, words, or phrases; palilalia occurs with repeating one's own words or phrases and echolalia with the repetition of others' words or phrases. Coprolalia, the involuntary utterance of obscenities, is a less common complex vocal tic. In the typical course of TS, the onset of motor tics precedes vocal tics, and motor tics progress in a head to toe direction.[3]

**Table 1**
**Simple and complex motor and vocal tics**

| Tic Symptoms | Examples |
|---|---|
| Simple motor tics: sudden, brief, repetitive, and involuntary movements that involve a limited number of muscle groups | Eye blinking, eye movements, facial grimacing, shoulder shrugging, head or shoulder jerking, abdominal tensing, nose twitching, mouth movements, lip pouting, arm jerking |
| Complex motor tics: distinct, coordinated, and involuntary patterns of movements involving several muscle groups | Tapping, stepping in a certain pattern, circling, hopping, jumping, bending, twisting, sniffing or touching objects, biting |
| Simple vocal tics: sudden, brief, and involuntary utterance of meaningless sounds | Throat clearing, coughing, sniffling, grunting, spitting, screeching, barking, hissing, gurgling |
| Complex vocal tics: repetitive, purposeless and involuntary utterances of words, phrases, or statements | Palilalia (repeating one's own words/phrases), echolalia (repeating others' words/phrases), copralalia (involuntary utterance of obscenities) |

The onset of tics typically occurs between the ages of 4 and 6 years and, in most cases, reaches peak lifetime severity between the ages of 10 and 12 years.[4] Tics usually occur in bouts, and wax and wane in frequency and intensity over time. For most children with TS, tics begin to decline in adolescence; two-thirds of children with TS experience marked improvement or complete remission of tics by adulthood.[5] More than 90% of individuals with TS or chronic tic disorder report premonitory urges, which are frequent, uncomfortable sensory phenomena that immediately precede the tic and are relieved by its completion.[6]

Comorbid psychiatric disorders are frequent in individuals with TS. The most common are attention-deficit/hyperactivity disorder (ADHD) and obsessive-compulsive disorder (OCD). Although prevalence estimates of psychiatric comorbidities in TS vary, most studies report high prevalence rates, some as great as 90% in clinically referred samples.[7] ADHD symptoms typically develop before the age of 7 years but can occur up to age 12 years and often precede the development of tics. In contrast, OCD symptoms typically develop after the onset of tics. Comorbid ADHD and OCD generally interfere more with overall functioning than do the tics themselves.[8]

## EPIDEMIOLOGY

Although recent epidemiological studies have reported that TS and chronic tic disorders are more common than previously recognized, prevalence estimates vary. Current lifetime rate estimates vary from 1 to 30 per 1000 children in European and Asian populations. The most common international prevalence figure for TS is 1%.[1] A study conducted by the US Centers for Disease Control in 2007[9] reported a TS prevalence rate between 0.3% and 1.0% of children aged 6 to 17 years. TS is 3 to 4 times more frequent in males than females, and although it affects people of all racial and ethnic groups, a TS diagnosis is twice as likely among non-Hispanic white people than Hispanic and non-Hispanic black people.[9]

Other tic disorders are more common than TS, with reported prevalence figures ranging from 4% to 50% of school-age children.[10] Provisional (formerly, transient) tic disorder is the most common; prevalence rates indicate occurrence in up to 20% of school-age children.[11] In a study of 4479 Swedish school children aged 7 to 15 years,[11] TS was identified in 0.6% of the total population, another 0.8% had chronic motor tics, 0.5% chronic vocal tics, and 4.8% transient tics. In total, 6.6% of 7-year-old to 15-year-old children had experienced a tic disorder during the last year. These results are analogous to a more recent study[10] of more than 800 children in Spain aged 4 to 16 years, which reported a prevalence of approximately 6.5% for all tic disorders. Most tics were reported to be mild in severity and duration.

TS is highly comorbid with many other psychiatric disorders. A recent US Centers for Disease Control and Prevention epidemiological study[9] reported that nearly 80% of youth with TS had also been diagnosed with an internalizing or behavioral disorder. The most common comorbid diagnosis in children with TS is ADHD, which is reported in more than 60% of children aged 6 to 17 years.[9] A bidirectional relationship is reported, in that 50% to 75% of patients with TS also meet criteria for ADHD, and 20% to 30% of patients with ADHD meet criteria for a tic disorder.[12,13] Another frequently observed comorbid disorder is OCD, as approximately one-third of youth with TS meet full diagnostic criteria for OCD throughout their lifetime, and up to 90% may experience subthreshold OCD symptoms, such as aggressive obsessions, repetitive counting, touching, or symmetry needs.[5,14,15] Individuals with OCD have a 7% lifetime risk of TS and 20% risk of tics.[16] Children with TS are also reported to have higher rates of comorbid depressive and anxiety disorders, as well as disruptive behavior disorders, developmental disorders, and learning disabilities, although few studies have investigated the prevalence of these disorders.

## NEUROBIOLOGY/GENETICS

Despite significant investigation over the past several decades, the cause and pathophysiology of tic disorders remain largely unknown. Twin and family studies have repeatedly shown that TS is highly heritable. Monozygotic twin studies[17] show 50% to 70% concordance for TS and 70% to 95% for tic disorder, whereas dizygotic twins show 8% and 23% concordance, respectively.[18] Further, first-degree relatives of affected individuals have a 5-fold to 15-fold increased risk of TS compared with the general population, representing one of the highest familial recurrence rates among common neuropsychiatric diseases.[19] Although the mode of transmission is unknown, current data[20] suggest a bilineal model, with inheritance occurring from both maternal and paternal sides.

Results of the first TS genome-wide association study were recently published,[19] which included 1285 cases and 4964 ancestry-matched controls. Although no markers achieved a genome-wide threshold of significance, this study laid the groundwork for the identification of common TS susceptibility variants in the future, when larger sample sizes can be analyzed. The top signal was found in rs7868992 on chromosome 9q32 within COL27A. Chromosomal rearrangement, candidate gene, and genome-wide linkage studies have also been conducted, and although the search for a disease-causing mutation remains elusive, several other loci have been identified as candidate susceptibility regions.

Linkage studies in families have shown 3p21.3, 7q35-36, 8q21.4, 9pter, 18q22.3, and, most recently, SLITRK1 near 13q31 as areas of interest.[21] The SLITRK1 gene is believed to be involved in dendritic growth and is expressed in brain regions implicated in TS, such as the cortex, thalamic, subthalamic and globus pallidus nuclei, striatum, and cerebellum.[22] However, recent studies[23,24] have shown that SLITRK1, and more specifically SLITRK var321, is a rare mutation not necessarily associated with familial TS and seems to be a rare cause of TS.

Another possible genetic cause of TS is a rare mutation in L-histidine decarboxylase, an enzyme expressed in the central nervous system, which catalyzes the biosynthesis of histamine from histidine. This mutation, which decreases histamine production, was detected in 2 generations of a family with autosomal dominant inheritance of TS (1 father and 8 offspring with TS), and suggests the possibility of using pharmacological manipulation of histaminergic neurotransmission to treat TS.[25] Taken together and given the variety of findings, TS is believed to have a complex inheritance pattern. Moreover, environmental factors, such as psychosocial stressors, perinatal insults, maternal smoking, low birth weight, and exposure to sex hormone during brain development, are also believed to contribute to the onset and course of TS. The overall expression of TS is multifactorial[21]; an overview of risk factors is presented in **Box 1**.

TS is believed to involve aberrances in dopamine signaling, as shown by increased levels of dopaminergic innervation in the striatum of individuals with TS.[26] This finding supports the efficacy of neuroleptic drugs that block $D_2$ dopamine receptors in the treatment of tics. Increasing evidence also suggests that TS is caused by disinhibition in the corticostriatothalamocortical pathways in the basal ganglia, striatum, and frontal lobes, which is believed to lead to dysfunction of the motor and limbic systems. Magnetic resonance imaging (MRI) studies support a cause from within this circuit and have reported reduction in caudate volume, as well as asymmetry in the caudate and putamen compared with healthy control individuals.[27] Studies of patients with OCD[28,29] also show structural abnormalities in the caudate nucleus and thalamus

---

**Box 1**
**Risk factors for Tourette's disorder**

Family history (first-degree relatives have higher percentage of TS, chronic tics, and OCD)

Male

Comorbid psychiatric disorders

- ADHD: 50% to 75% of patients with TS meet criteria; up to 30% of patients with ADHD meet criteria for a tic disorder

- OCD: 20% to 40% of patients with TS meet full criteria and up to 90% have subthreshold symptoms; up to 30% of patients with OCD meet criteria for a tic disorder

- Other mood and anxiety disorders

Stress, anxiety, and excitement

Certain environmental risks (an individual with a tic disorder may observe and then repeat or mimic a gesture or sound made by another person)

Obstetrical complications, low birth weight, and maternal smoking during pregnancy

---

compared with control individuals, indicating overlapping neuroanatomical features of OCD and TS. Further studies[30] found that caudate nucleus volume correlated significantly and inversely with the severity of tic and OCD symptoms in early adulthood. Moreover, volumetric MRI studies in both TS and OCD[28,29] have shown abnormal volumes and asymmetry in prefrontal cortical regions, including thinning in the anterior cingulate gyrus and orbitofrontal cortex.

## CLINICAL FEATURES

Onset of TS typically occurs at age 4 to 6 years with simple motor tics such as eye blinking, facial grimacing, and head jerking. Motor tics usually progress in a rostrocaudal direction over time.[4] Vocal tics typically develop 1 to 2 years after the onset of motor tics and begin as simple vocalizations, such as throat clearing, coughing, sniffling, and utterance of brief sounds.[31]

Tics generally occur in bouts, and wax and wane in severity over time. An individual's repertoire of tics commonly changes. Tic symptoms generally peak in early adolescence, between the ages of 10 and 12 years, when both motor and vocal tics often become more complex. Motor tics tend to evolve into more complex movements, such as tapping, jumping, and stepping in a certain pattern, whereas vocal tics can develop into the repetition of words or phrases. Tics typically decline in late adolescence. One study[5] reported that in a group of 82 children followed from initial evaluation to adulthood, more than one-third were completely tic free at follow-up, around half had minimal to mild tics, and fewer than a quarter had moderate or severe tics.

More than 90% of individuals with TS or chronic tic disorders report premonitory urges, which are frequent, uncomfortable sensory phenomena that immediately precede the tic and are relieved by the completion of the tic.[6] Similar to the need to sneeze or itch, examples of premonitory urges include tightness in the neck relieved by neck stretching, or a feeling of needing to move or repeat behaviors until it feels "just right".[32] The urges are described as intrusive, and in many individuals cause more distress than the tics themselves.[33] Premonitory urges are believed to play an important role in maintenance of tics. Behavioral models suggest that tics are negatively reinforced every time they reduce or eliminate the discomfort associated with the premonitory urge.[6] Tics are believed to be actions performed to alleviate the discomfort associated with the premonitory sensation.[6] Awareness of premonitory urges increases with age, and such urges are believed to be associated with brain activity within the insular and cingulate motor areas of the cortex.[34]

Although strong evidence suggests that tics arise from neurobiological dysfunction, environmental events can also have an immediate and direct impact on tic occurrence. Factors such as fatigue, stress, anxiety, and social activities are commonly associated with tic exacerbations, whereas relaxation and focused concentration, especially involving fine motor movements such as dancing or sporting activities, are associated with tic attenuation.[35] Many individuals with TS are able to successfully suppress tics for a period, but suppression may be associated with more severe premonitory urges, discomfort, and exhaustion.[36]

Obsessive-compulsive symptoms, developmentally inappropriate motoric hyperactivity and inattention, depressed mood, worry and fears, and irritability and aggressive dyscontrol are among the most common psychiatric comorbidities in TS.[37] Although prevalence figures for psychiatric comorbidity vary, most studies report high prevalence rates, some as great as 90% in clinically referred samples.[7,8] The most common comorbid disorders are OCD and ADHD, which occur in about 20% to 60% and 50% to 75% of individuals with TS, respectively. Co-occurring OCD and ADHD often cause more distress and interfere with patients' overall functioning more often than do tics themselves. A recent study of functional impairment in children with TS[38] found that non–tic-related problems, most often OCD or ADHD symptoms, caused more dysfunction than the tics. Overall, individuals with TS and comorbid conditions are reported to experience a more severe course. In addition to ADHD and OCD, mood disorders, oppositional defiant disorders, and non-OCD anxiety disorders are reported in individuals with TS.[39] One study reported that comorbid mood disorders were the strongest predictors of psychiatric hospitalization and illness severity in a group of patients with TS.[40]

## OCD

OCD is characterized by the occurrence of obsessions, which are recurrent and intrusive thoughts, ideas, images, or impulses, and compulsions, which are repetitive behaviors or mental acts sought to prevent or reduce anxiety or distress. OCD is highly comorbid with TS. Twenty percent to 40% of patients with TS meet full criteria for OCD, and up to 90% have subthreshold symptoms, such as aggressive obsessions, repetitive counting, touching, or symmetry needs.[14] The association between TS and OCD has also been established in genetic studies, which have reported higher rates of OCD in relatives of patients with TS and higher rates of tics or TS in relatives of patients with OCD. Female first-degree relatives of TS probands were found to have a higher risk of OCD, whereas male relatives had a higher risk of tic disorders.[41]

Researchers have attempted to delineate the phenomenological differences between tics and compulsions on the grounds that compulsions are usually accompanied by autonomic anxiety and complex thinking processes, whereas tics are an involuntary response to short-lived sensory symptoms and not associated with autonomic arousal.[42] Although this distinction holds true for many symptoms, areas of overlap exist, especially between complex motor tics and compulsions. For example, repetitive behaviors, such as touching or eye blinking, may result from a need to relieve an urge or unpleasant sensation (tic) or to neutralize a superstitious fear (compulsion).[42] However, individuals who have OCD with and without tics differ in the subjective experiences that precede their repetitive behaviors. Patients with TS plus OCD often describe sensorimotor symptoms associated with their repetitive behaviors, whereas patients with OCD alone report more cognitive and autonomic anxiety.[43] Further distinctions in clinical features of OCD in patients with and without TS exist. Patients with TS and OCD often describe a need or feeling to get things just right and repeat behaviors to achieve a feeling of symmetry or exactness in touch or appearance. Conversely, in patients with OCD without TS, contamination or illness concerns are more common.[44]

Other clinical features that are shown to be more common among patients with tic-related OCD include intrusive, violent, and sexual images or thoughts,[45] hoarding and counting rituals, ticlike compulsions (such as the need to touch, tab, or rub items), and symmetry/ordering symptoms. Further, a higher comorbidity with trichotillomania, body dysmorphic disorder, bipolar disorder, ADHD, social phobia, and substance abuse disorder exist in the population with tic-related OCD. Comorbid OCD causes more impairment and greater disability than tic disorders alone.[8]

### ADHD

ADHD is characterized by an enduring pattern of developmentally inappropriate inattention or hyperactivity and impulsive behavior. ADHD is the most common comorbid disorder in children with TS, reported in 60% to 80% of cases.[46] As many as half of clinically referred patients with TS show signs of ADHD 2 to 3 years before tic onset.[13] Co-occurring TS and ADHD are often manifested by academic difficulties, peer rejection, family conflict, and disruptive behaviors. A consortium study of 6805 cases[12] reported that when compared with TS alone, TS plus ADHD was associated with earlier onset of TS and significantly higher rates of anger control problems, oppositional defiant disorder, learning disabilities, mood disorders, sleep difficulties, social skills deficits, sexually inappropriate behaviors, and self-injurious behaviors. Another study[47] reported that children with TS plus ADHD experienced more emotional and behavioral problems and had greater difficulty with social adaptation than control individuals and those with TS alone.

Learning and academic problems are also common in children with TS. In a database of 5450 patients with TS, 1235 (22.7%) had learning disabilities.[48] Patients with TS have been shown to have difficulties with executive function, social problem solving, procedural learning, fine motor control, motor inhibition, nonverbal memory, and visual motor integration.[49] Comorbid ADHD often intensifies these deficits.

Although the nature of the relationship between TS and ADHD is not firmly established, some studies[50] suggest that a dysregulation of dopamine neurotransmitter function underlies the pathophysiology of both disorders. Other studies[51] posit that 2 types of ADHD exist in patients with TS; 1 type precedes TS and is genetically independent, the other follows and is part of the syndrome. Regardless of cause, the presence of ADHD predicts greater functional impairment throughout the life course than TS alone. In 1 study,[52] adults with TS plus ADHD had significantly more depression, anxiety, obsessive-compulsive symptoms, and maladaptive behaviors than those with TS alone. Further, comorbid ADHD is shown to be more persistent than TS, as tics have been shown to have little impact on adult ADHD outcome.[53]

### Mood and Anxiety Disorders

Co-occurring mood and anxiety disorders are frequently observed in clinically referred youth and adults with TS.[40,54] One study,[55] which evaluated lifetime rates of non-OCD anxiety disorders in youth with TS in a TS specialized clinic and general pediatric psychopharmacology clinic, reported 40% and 35% prevalence, respectively. Numerous studies have shown increased rates of anxiety symptoms in individuals with TS compared with normal controls. A recent study reported that except for social and simple phobia, all other anxiety disorders, including panic disorder, agoraphobia, separation anxiety disorder, and generalized anxiety disorder, were overrepresented among individuals with TS with high tic severity. Separation anxiety disorder predicted highest tic severity.[38,55] Taken together, evidence suggests that non-OCD anxiety disorders are risk factors for TS and increased tic severity.

Mood disorders, including major depression and bipolar disorder, have also been described in clinically referred patients with TS.[56] Although patients with TS are reported to score higher on depression rating scales than normal controls,[54] it is not clear whether mood disorders are primary or secondary to the demoralization and impairment related to TS and having a chronic illness. One study that examined psychosocial functioning in adolescents with TS compared with age-matched peers[57] found that, when controlling for ADHD, TS youth still showed higher overall rates of major depression compared with healthy controls.

## DIAGNOSIS

Diagnostic evaluation of TS and chronic tic disorders begins with a comprehensive and detailed history from caregivers and a physical and mental status examination of the individual. Because tics wax and wane over time, they may not be observable during an individual's initial visits, but the absence of tics does not exclude a TS diagnosis. Detailed information about the development and course of tics, as well as documentation of tic type, frequency, and severity, should be obtained from the individual, family members, and teachers. Because there exists no formal diagnostic test for TS, this classic history informs diagnosis. The Yale Global Tic Severity Scale (YGTSS) is a validated clinician-administered dimensional rating scale used to rate the severity of motor and vocal tics over 5 domains, including number, frequency, intensity, complexity, and interference of tics with daily life; it also includes a tic-related impairment score reflecting impact on academic, occupational, social, and family functioning, as well as impact on self-esteem[58]. The YGTSS is used to quantitatively evaluate tic severity and impact over time.

Clinicians must consider the potential for other neurological and medical disorders in the differential diagnosis, as outlined in **Table 2**. Differential diagnoses include dystonia, myoclonus, pediatric acute onset neuropsychiatric syndrome (PANS), pediatric autoimmune neuropsychiatric disorders associated with *Streptococcus* (PANDAS), Sydenham chorea, allergies, cough variant asthma, stereotypic movements, compulsions, complex motor tics, and body-focused repetitive behaviors. If these conditions are suspected, radiological imaging, electroencephalography, and consultation with the appropriate medical specialist should be completed. Basic laboratory testing is a standard component of the initial evaluation to rule out other medical problems. Because TS is so highly comorbid with other psychiatric disorders, it is important to comprehensively evaluate each patient for the presence of these disorders and assess the role that each disorder plays in contributing to distress and functional impairment. A comprehensive family history should also be obtained, because tics often run in families.

## TREATMENT

Treatment of TS is based on a consideration of the impact of tics on social, emotional, family, and academic/occupational functioning. Mild tics that do not cause significant distress or interfere with daily functioning need not be treated and require only support and active monitoring. Education about TS and related comorbid disorders is important to alleviate distress and reduce stigma. Clarification that tics are involuntary and out of the child's control helps parents and teachers understand the diagnosis and strengthens the child's self-confidence and self-esteem. Referral to the Tourette Syndrome Association, a national resource for families, caregivers, and professionals, is helpful in providing information and referrals to specialists.

**Table 2**
**Differential diagnoses: motor and vocal tics**

| Differential Diagnosis | Features |
|---|---|
| Dystonia | Sustained contracture of both agonist and antagonist muscles; may follow neuroleptic use |
| Myoclonus | Sudden and involuntary movement, single or multiple muscle jerks, not suppressible; no premonitory urge |
| Choreiform movements | Rapid, random, continual, irregular, dancelike, nonstereotyped actions, which are usually bilateral and affect all parts of the body (ie, face, trunk, and limbs) Sydenham chorea develops weeks to months after *Streptococcus* infection |
| Compulsions in OCD | Complex behavior patterns that occur in response to an obsession or according to rigidly applied rules |
| Stereotypic movement disorder, or stereotypies in autism spectrum disorder | Nonfunctional, usually rhythmic, nonchanging, seemingly fixed driven behaviors, which are generally more complex than tics |
| Pediatric autoimmune neuropsychiatric disorders associated with *Streptococcus*/ pediatric acute onset neuropsychiatric syndrome | Tics or OCD symptoms with explosive, abrupt, or dramatic onset after group A streptococcal infection or other infectious agent; associated with other neuropsychiatric symptoms |
| Allergies | Allergic rhinitis and conjunctivitis may present with sniffing, eye blinking, and other facial ticlike symptoms |
| Cough variant asthma | Chronic cough associated with exposure to allergens or after resolution of an upper respiratory infection may have a similar presentation |

When tics are moderate or severe, cause significant distress, and interfere with functioning, treatment is indicated. According to Hartmann and Worbe,[59] treatment is recommended if tics cause (1) sustained social problems (eg, social isolation or bullying), (2) social or emotional problems (eg, reactive depressive symptoms), (3) functional impairment, or (4) subjective discomfort (eg, pain or injury). First-line treatment of children and adults currently is cognitive-behavioral therapy, specifically habit reversal therapy (HRT), a component of comprehensive behavioral intervention for tics (CBIT). If behavior therapy alone is unsuccessful and tics continue to cause distress and interference, pharmacotherapy is recommended.

### Nonpharmacological Treatments for Tics

Behavioral interventions have reported success in treating tics.[60] HRT is the most commonly used behavioral treatment of TS and has consistently shown efficacy in randomized controlled trials (RCTs) in children and adults.[60] HRT comprises components that include awareness training, competing response practice, habit control motivation, and generalization training. These techniques teach patients to become aware of their tic occurrence, often by recognition of premonitory urges, and to perform a voluntary competing behavior to interrupt or inhibit the tic.[60] Often the competing response engages antagonistic muscles to the muscles required to perform the tic, and is initiated for 1 to 3 minutes or until the urge to perform the tic disappears.[61] CBIT is another first-line behavioral treatment that uses HRT, in addition to functional assessment and function-based intervention procedures, to help reduce influences in daily life that exacerbate tics.[62] Research[63] has shown the superiority of HRT and CBIT over supportive therapy and psychoeducation alone in the tic management for children and adults.

Exposure and response prevention (ERP) is another behavioral therapy technique used to treat TS. ERP for tics is derived from its application in OCD and is based on the association between premonitory urges and tics. In ERP, patients are asked to suppress their tics for a prolonged period after experiencing a premonitory urge in order to interrupt the association between unpleasant premonitory sensation and tic, causing the urge to produce a reduction in tics.[61] ERP for tics has been studied in 1 RCT trial,[64] and when compared with HRT, both treatments resulted in significant reduction in tic frequency.

### Pharmacological Treatments for Tics

Once the decision is made to use pharmacotherapy, monotherapy should be initiated at the lowest possible dose with gradual titration. Recommended first-line pharmacotherapy for mild to moderate tics consists of off-label use of α-adrenergic agonists because of their proven efficacy for tics and low potential for adverse events. The 2 most commonly used $\alpha_2$ agonists for the treatment of TS are clonidine and guanfacine; both act via a presynaptic $\alpha_2$ adrenoceptor mechanism, thus promoting the release of norepinephrine. Several trials[65,66] have supported the efficacy of clonidine and guanfacine in reducing tics in patients with and without ADHD, as these agents are also often used for treatment of ADHD. Common adverse effects of the α-agonists include sedation, headache, hypotension, and upset stomach. Guanfacine is usually preferred, because it tends to cause less drowsiness and sedation. Benzodiazepines, such as clonazepam, may also be recommended as first-line treatment of tics, especially when the patient has significant comorbid anxiety.

If $\alpha_2$ agonists prove unsuccessful, patients with moderate to severe tics can be treated with neuroleptics.[67] Only 2 medications, haloperidol and pimozide, have been approved by the US Food and Drug Administration for the treatment of TS in the United States. Both are first-generation neuroleptic and antipsychotic drugs that work via dopamine $D_2$ receptor antagonism. However, adverse effects associated with these drugs are significant, and include sedation, depression, weight gain, hepatotoxicity, and drug-induced movement disorders.[7,68] Further, pimozide is associated with extrapyramidal symptoms, such as akathisia and acute dystonic reactions, parkinsonism, and tardive syndromes, such as tardive dyskinesia and tardive dystonia. Atypical second-generation antipsychotics, which have fewer side effects and less risk of tardive syndromes,[69] have replaced the typical antipsychotics for the treatment of tics. Atypical antipsychotics that have been studied for the treatment of TS include risperidone, aripiprazole, quetiapine, ziprasidone, and olanzapine. These medications work through dopamine $D_2$ receptor antagonism, as do typical antipsychotics, and also block serotonin receptors to varying degrees.

The most rigorously studied atypical antipsychotic for the treatment of TS is risperidone; its efficacy in tic reduction has been shown in RCTs when compared with pimozide[70] and placebo.[71] Similar trials showed significant tic reduction with olanzapine[72] and ziprasidone.[73] A large, industry-sponsored controlled trial of aripiprazole for the treatment of tics is currently under way.[74] The mechanism of action of aripiprazole differs from other atypical antipsychotics because it is a partial agonist at dopamine

$D_2$ and $D_3$ receptors and a partial agonist at serotonin 5-HT (1A) receptors. A previous open-label study[75–77] of children and adolescents with TS treated with aripiprazole over 8 weeks resulted in a significant reduction in YGTSS total tic score. Adverse effects of the atypical neuroleptics include sedation and metabolic effects, including weight gain and glucose intolerance. Onabotulinumtoxin A injections have also been reported to reduce tics and the associated uncomfortable premonitory urge,[78,79] and may be considered when medication fails to improve mild to moderate tics that are causing distress and impairment. Other pharmacotherapeutic agents that may reduce tics include atomoxetine,[80] tetrabenazine,[81] topiramate[82,83] baclofen,[84] and nicotine gum in combination with other medications.[85] An overview of treatment options is presented in **Table 3** and **Fig. 1**.

## Treatment of Tics and OCD

Treatment of tics and OCD is indicated if symptoms are causing distress or impairment to the individual, and aims to reduce impairment from OCD and control tic severity. A multimodal treatment approach is generally recommended, which includes psychosocial intervention and medication. For psychosocial treatment, ERP, a form of cognitive-behavioral therapy, has been shown to be effective in treating OCD without tic disorders and is just beginning to be studied in individuals with TS. The only RCT to date,[64] which included both children and adults with TS, compared 12 2-hour ERP sessions with 10 1-hour HRT sessions and reported no differences between conditions; both groups achieved significant reduction in tic frequency and severity. This study provides support for ERP for the treatment of OCD and TS, but indicates that further investigation is necessary.

Although selective serotonin reuptake inhibitors (SSRIs) are the first-line pharmacological treatment of OCD, no clinical trials have specifically evaluated the pharmacological treatment of OCD symptoms in patients with TS. However, data do exist from several clinical trials that evaluated SSRIs in individuals with OCD that have included patients with tics. These trials allowed for the retrospective comparison of the clinical effects of SSRIs in individuals with OCD with and without tics. In 1

| Table 3 Treatment of Tourette's disorder | |
|---|---|
| **Medication** | |
| α-Adrenergic agonists<br>Clonidine, 0.025–0.4 mg daily<br>Guanfacine, 0.25–4 mg daily | α-Adrenergic side effects include sedation, headache, hypotension, and stomach upset |
| Second-generation antipsychotics<br>Aripiprazole, 1–15 mg daily<br>Risperidone, 0.125–3 mg daily | Second-generation antipsychotics: monitor metabolic side effects; baseline height/weight, hemoglobin A1C, lipid panel |
| Pimozide or haloperidol<br>Haloperidol, 0.25–4.0 mg daily<br>Pimozide, 0.5–8.0 mg daily | Pimozide/haloperidol: monitor extrapyramidal symptoms, particularly dyskinesias |
| **Psychological** | |
| CBIT<br>HRT | Generally, first-line treatment, which uses premonitory urge/sensation awareness to develop competing response; evidence of durability |
| **Other** | |
| Botulinum toxin injection | May be beneficial for isolated motor tics (eye blinking) and decreases premonitory urge |

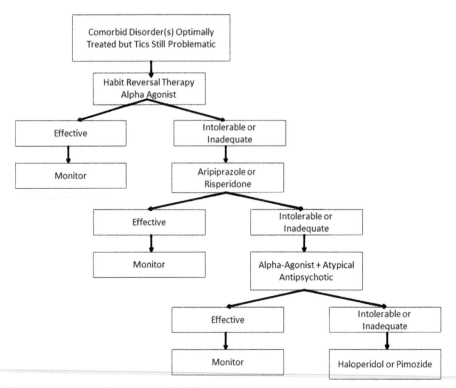

**Fig. 1.** Management/treatment algorithm.

study, McDougle and colleagues[86] compared 33 adult patients with OCD with and without tics who had undergone an 8-week trial of fluvoxamine. Although fluvox-amine treatment was associated with a statistically significant improvement in Yale-Brown Obsessive-Compulsive Scale (Y-BOCS) scores in both groups, significant differences in Y-BOCS change scores were found in patients with OCD with and without tics; a 32% decrease in Y-BOCS score occurred in patients with OCD only compared with a 17% decrease in patients with OCD and tics. Further, treatment responsiveness varied among groups, as 52% of patients with OCD without tics responded to fluvoxamine, whereas only 21% of patients with OCD with comorbid tics responded. Similar results were achieved in a study of pediatric OCD by Geller and colleagues,[87] which reported that coexisting chronic tic disorder is associated with a lower SSRI response rate compared with OCD alone; however, both the tic and OCD group and OCD only group improved significantly (53% vs 71%). March and colleagues[88] evaluated the difference between sertraline and placebo on OCD symptom severity in children and adolescents and found that in the presence of a tic disorder, sertraline did not differ from placebo, whereas in the absence of a tic disorder, sertraline proved significantly superior to placebo. Taken together, these studies show that patients with OCD with comorbid tics or TS show a lower response rate to SSRIs than those without tics, both in terms of percentage of responders and symptom reduction, but still result in some improvement in tic-related OCD.[88] Further study on the pharmacological treatment of OCD in patients with TS is necessary.

## Treatment of Tics and ADHD

Treatment of tics and ADHD is based on a consideration of the impact of tics, in the context of ADHD, on social, emotional, family, and academic/occupational functioning. ADHD symptoms are often more impairing than tics, and a multimodal treatment approach, including medication, individual therapy, and educational services, is recommended. Despite older case reports and warning labels surrounding the use of stimulants for ADHD symptoms in patients with tic disorder, recent studies[89–91] have shown that stimulants may be used safely and effectively for ADHD symptoms in patients with tics. Most often, the methylphenidate-derived stimulants are best tolerated, and it is recommended that treatment be initiated at the lowest dose with gradual titration, as some patients may experience a temporary increase in tics. If tic exacerbation endures, the stimulant dose may be adjusted or the patient should be switched to another agent.

For patients who cannot tolerate stimulants, treatment with an $\alpha$-adrenergic agonist may be helpful for ADHD symptoms, such as impulsivity and motor restlessness, as well as tics.[65] Atomoxetine has also proved helpful; a recent study[80] reported that in children with ADHD and tics, tics improved relative to placebo. Taken together, in a meta-analysis examining pharmacotherapy treatment of children with ADHD and tic disorders, Bloch and colleagues[92] found that methylphenidate, $\alpha_2$ agonists, desipramine, and atomoxetine were effective in improving ADHD symptoms in children with comorbid tics. $\alpha_2$ Agonists and atomoxetine significantly improved comorbid tic symptoms, and although supratherapeutic doses of dextroamphetamine reportedly worsened tics, therapeutic doses of dextroamphetamine and methylphenidate did not. In addition to these medications, HRT may also be helpful for children with co-occurring tics and ADHD.

## SUMMARY

Tics are common, early onset neurodevelopmental disorders. TS, the most complex of the tic disorders, is characterized by a high prevalence of psychiatric comorbidity. Bidirectional overlap of OCD, tics, and TS is manifest by common underlying genomics, phenomenology, and clinical course; although there is some similarity in response to cognitive-behavioral treatment, there are differences reported in response to pharmacotherapy. More research is needed to disentangle the common phenomenology of repetitive behaviors, which are observed in patients with both TS and OCD, so as to target treatment more specifically.

## REFERENCES

1. Robertson MM, Eapen V, Cavanna AE. The international prevalence, epidemiology, and clinical phenomenology of Tourette syndrome: a cross-cultural perspective. J Psychosom Res 2009;67(6):475–83.
2. American Psychiatric Association. Diagnostic and statistical manual of mental disorders. 5th edition. Arlington (VA): American Psychiatric Association; 2013.
3. Robertson MM. The Gilles de la Tourette syndrome: the current status. Arch Dis Child Educ Pract Ed 2012;97(5):166–75.
4. Bloch MH, Leckman JF. Clinical course of Tourette syndrome. J Psychosom Res 2009;67:497–501.
5. Bloch MH, Peterson BS, Scahill L, et al. Adulthood outcome of tic and obsessive-compulsive symptom severity in children with Tourette syndrome. Arch Pediatr Adolesc Med 2006;160(1):65–9.

6. Reese HE, Scahill L, Peterson AL, et al. The premonitory urge to tic: measurement, characteristics, and correlates in older adolescents and adults. Behav Ther 2014;45:177–86.

7. Robertson MM. Tourette syndrome, associated conditions and the complexities of treatment. Brain 2000;123:425–62.

8. Coffey B, Miguel E, Biederman J, et al. Tourette's disorder with and without obsessive compulsive disorder in adults: are they different? J Nerv Ment Dis 1998;186:201–15.

9. Centers for Disease Control and Prevention. Prevalence of diagnosed Tourette syndrome in persons aged 6-17 years–United States, 2007. MMWR Morb Mortal Wkly Rep 2009;58(21):581–5.

10. Linazasoro G, Van Blercom N, de Zarate CO. Prevalence of tic disorder in two schools in the Basque country: results and methodological caveats. Mov Disord 2006;21(12):106–9.

11. Khalifa N, Von Knorring AL. Prevalence of tic disorders and Tourette syndrome in a Swedish school population. Dev Med Child Neurol 2003;45:315–9.

12. Freeman RD, Tourette Syndrome International Database Consortium. Tic disorders and ADHD: answers from a world-wide clinical dataset on Tourette syndrome. Eur Child Adolesc Psychiatry 2007;16(1):15–23.

13. Spencer T, Biederman T, Wilens T. Attention-deficit/hyperactivity disorder and comorbidity. Pediatr Clin North Am 1999;46(5):915–27.

14. Grad LR, Pelcovits D, Olson M, et al. Obsessive-compulsive symptomatology in children with Tourette's syndrome. J Am Acad Child Adolesc Psychiatry 1987; 26:69–73.

15. Swedo S, Rapoport J, Leonard H, et al. Obsessive compulsive disorder in children and adolescents. Arch Gen Psychiatry 1989;46:335.

16. Robertson M, Banerjee S, Fox Hiley P, et al. Personality disorders and psychopathology in Tourette's syndrome: a controlled study. Br J Psychiatry 1997;171: 283–6.

17. Hyde TM, Aaronson BA, Randolph C, et al. Relationship of birth weight to the phenotypic expression of Gilles de la Tourette's syndrome in monozygotic twins. Br J Psychiatry 1994;164:811–7.

18. Price RA, Kidd KK, Cohen DJ, et al. A twin study of Tourette syndrome. Arch Gen Psychiatry 1985;42:815–20.

19. Scharf JM, Yu CA, Matthews BM, et al. Genome-wide association study of Tourette syndrome. Mol Psychiatry 2013;18(6):721–8.

20. Kurlan R, Eapen V, Stern J, et al. Bilineal transmission in Tourette's syndrome families. Neurology 1994;44(12):2336–42.

21. Swain JE, Scahill L, Lombroso PJ, et al. Tourette syndrome and tic disorders: a decade of progress. J Am Acad Child Adolesc Psychiatry 2007; 46:947–68.

22. Abelson JF, Kwan KY, O'Roak BJ, et al. Sequence variants in SLITRK1 are associated with Tourette's syndrome. Science 2005;310:317–20.

23. Fabbrini G, Pasquini M, Aurilia C, et al. Large Italian family with Gilles de la Tourette syndrome: clinical study and analysis of the SLITRK1 gene. Mov Disord 2007;22:2229–34.

24. Scharf JM, Moorjani P, Fagerness J, et al. Lack of association between SLITRK1-var321 and Tourette syndrome in a large family-based sample. Neurology 2008; 70:1495–6.

25. Ercan-Sencicek AG, Stillman AA, Ghosh AK, et al. L-histidine decarboxylase and Tourette's syndrome. N Engl J Med 2010;362:1901–8.

26. Wolf SS, Jones DW, Knable MB, et al. Tourette syndrome: prediction of phenotypic variation in monozygotic twins by caudate nucleus D2 receptor binding. Science 1996;273:1225–7.
27. Singer HS, Minzer K. Neurobiology of Tourette's syndrome: concepts of neuroanatomic localization and neurochemical abnormalities. Brain Dev 2003;25(1):70–84.
28. Rauch SL. Neuroimaging research and the neurobiology of obsessive compulsive disorder: where do we go from here? Biol Psychiatry 2000;47:168–70.
29. Whiteside SP, Port JD, Abramowitz JS. A meta-analysis of functional neuroimaging on obsessive-compulsive disorder. Psychiatry Res 2004;132:69–79.
30. Bloch MH, Leckman JF, Zhu H, et al. Caudate volumes in childhood predict symptom severity in adults with Tourette syndrome. Neurology 2005;65(8):1253–8.
31. Leckman JF, Zhang H, Vitale A, et al. Course of tic severity in Tourette syndrome: the first two decades. Pediatrics 1998;102(1):14–9.
32. Kwak C, Dat Voung K, Jankovic J. Premonitory sensory phenomenon in Tourette's syndrome. Mov Disord 2003;18(12):1530–3.
33. Cohen AJ, Leckman JF. Sensory phenomena associated with Gilles de la Tourette's syndrome. J Clin Psychiatry 1992;53(9):319–23.
34. Jackson SR, Parkinson A, Kim SY, et al. On the functional anatomy of the urge-for-action. Cogn Neurosci 2011;2(3–4):227–43.
35. Conelea CA, Woods DW. The influence of contextual factors on tic expression in Tourette's syndrome: a review. J Psychosom Res 2008;65:487–96.
36. Himle MB, Woods DW, Conelea CA, et al. Investigating the effects of tic suppression on premonitory urge ratings in children and adolescents with Tourette's syndrome. Behav Res Ther 2007;45(12):2964–76.
37. Coffey BJ, Jummani R. ADHD and Tourette's disorder. In: Adler L, editor. Attention-deficit hyperactivity disorder in adults and children. New York: Cambridge University Press; 2014.
38. Storch EA, Lack CW, Simons LE, et al. A measure of functional impairment in youth with Tourette's syndrome. J Pediatr Psychol 2007;32:950–9.
39. Kurlan R, Como PG, Miller B, et al. The behavioral spectrum of tic disorders: a community-based study. Neurology 2002;59(3):414–20.
40. Coffey B, Biederman J, Geller D, et al. Distinguishing illness severity from tic severity in children and adolescents with Tourette's disorder. J Am Acad Child Adolesc Psychiatry 2000;39:556–61.
41. Pauls DL. The genetics of obsessive compulsive disorder and Gilles de la Tourette's syndrome. Psychiatr Clin North Am 1992;15:759–66.
42. Miguel EC, Coffey BJ, Baer L, et al. Phenomenology of intentional repetitive behaviors in obsessive-compulsive disorder and Tourette's disorder. J Clin Psychiatry 1995;56(6):246–55.
43. Miguel EC, Baer L, Coffey BJ, et al. Phenomenological differences appearing with repetitive behaviours in obsessive-compulsive disorder and Gilles de la Tourette's syndrome. Br J Psychiatry 1997;170:140–5.
44. Leckman JF, Walker DE, Goodman WK, et al. "Just right" perceptions associated with compulsive behavior in Tourette's syndrome. Am J Psychiatry 1994;151:675–80.
45. Swerdlow RN, Zinner S, Farber HR, et al. Symptoms in obsessive-compulsive disorder and Tourette syndrome: a spectrum? CNS Spectr 1999;4(3):21–33.
46. Cavanna AE, Rickards H. The psychopathological spectrum of Gilles de la Tourette syndrome. Neurosci Biobehav Rev 2013;37:1008–15.

47. Carter AS, O'Donnell DA, Schultz RT, et al. Social and emotional adjustment in children affected with Gilles de la Tourette's syndrome: associations with ADHD and family functioning. J Child Psychol Psychiatry 2000;41(2):215–23.
48. Burd L, Freeman RD, Klug MG, et al. Tourette syndrome and learning disabilities. BMC Pediatr 2005;5:34.
49. Coffey BJ, Zwilling A. Psychiatric conditions associated with Tourette syndrome. In: Walkup JT, editor. A family's guide to Tourette syndrome. Bayside (NY): Tourette's Syndrome Association; 2012. p. 24–7.
50. Kerbeshian J, Burd L, Klug M. Comorbid Tourette's disorder and bipolar disorder: an etiologic perspective. Am J Psychiatry 1995;152:1646–51.
51. Pauls DL, Leckman JF, Cohen DJ. Familial relationship between Gilles de la Tourette's syndrome, attention deficit disorder, learning disabilities, speech disorders, and stuttering. J Am Acad Child Adolesc Psychiatry 1993;32: 1044–50.
52. Haddad AD, Umoh G, Bhatia V, et al. Adults with Tourette's syndrome with and without attention deficit hyperactivity disorder. Acta Psychiatr Scand 2009; 1240(4):299–307.
53. Spencer T, Biederman J, Coffey B, et al. The 4-year course of tic disorders in boys with attention-deficit/hyperactivity disorder. Arch Gen Psychiatry 1999; 56:842–7.
54. Robertson MM, Channon S, Baker J, et al. The psychopathology of Gilles de la Tourette's syndrome. A controlled study. Br J Psychiatry 1993;162:114–7.
55. Coffey B, Biederman J, Smoller J, et al. Anxiety disorders and Tic severity in juveniles with Tourette's disorder. J Am Acad Child Adolesc Psychiatry 2000;39: 562–8.
56. Comings BG, Comings DE. A controlled study of Tourette syndrome V. Depression and mania. Am J Hum Genet 1987;41:804–21.
57. Gorman DA, Thompson N, Plessen KJ, et al. Psychosocial outcome and psychiatric comorbidity in older adolescents with Tourette syndrome: controlled study. Br J Psychiatry 2010;99:39–60.
58. Leckman JF, Riddle MA, Hardin MT, et al. The Yale Global Tic Severity Scale: initial testing of a clinician-rated scale of tic severity. J Am Acad Child Adolesc Psychiatry 1989;28(4):566–73.
59. Hartmann A, Worbe Y. Pharmacological treatment of Gilles de la Tourette syndrome. Neurosci Biobehav Rev 2013;37:1157–61.
60. Verdellen C, van de Griendt J, Hartmann A, et al, ESSTS Guidelines Group. European clinical guidelines for Tourette syndrome and other tic disorders. Part III: behavioural and psychosocial interventions. Eur Child Adolesc Psychiatry 2011; 20:197–207.
61. Frank M, Cavanna AE. Behavioral treatments for Tourette syndrome: an evidence-based review. Behav Neurol 2013;27(1):105–17.
62. McGuire JF, Piacentini J, Brennan EA, et al. A meta-analysis of behavior therapy for Tourette syndrome. J Psychiatr Res 2014;50:106–12.
63. Piacentini J, Woods DW, Scahill L, et al. Behavior therapy for children with Tourette disorder: a randomized controlled trial. JAMA 2010;303(19):1929–37.
64. Verdellen CW, Keijsers GP, Cath DC, et al. Exposure with response prevention versus habit reversal in Tourette's syndrome: a controlled study. Behav Res Ther 2004;42:501–11.
65. Scahill L, Chappell PB, Kim YS, et al. A placebo-controlled study of guanfacine in the treatment of children with tic disorders and attention deficit hyperactivity disorder. Am J Psychiatry 2001;158:1067–74.

66. Leckman JF, Hardin MT, Riddle MA, et al. Clonidine treatment of Gilles de la Tourette syndrome. Arch Gen Psychiatry 1991;48:324–8.
67. Chen JJ, Ondo WG, Dashtipour K, et al. Tetrabenazine for the treatment of hyperkinetic movement disorders: a review of the literature. Clin Ther 2012;34: 1487–504.
68. Panagiotopoulos C, Ronsley R, Elbe D, et al. First do no harm: promoting an evidence-based approach to atypical antipsychotic use in children and adolescents. J Can Acad Child Adolesc Psychiatry 2010;19:124–37.
69. Correll CU, Kane JM. One-year incidence rates of tardive dyskinesia in children and adolescents treated with second-generation antipsychotics: a systematic review. J Child Adolesc Psychopharmacol 2007;17:647–56.
70. Gilbert DL, Batterson JR, Sethuraman G, et al. Tic reduction with risperidone versus pimozide in a randomized, double-blind, crossover trial. J Am Acad Child Adolesc Psychiatry 2004;43(2):206–14.
71. Dion Y, Annable L, Sandor P, et al. Risperidone in the treatment of Tourette syndrome: a double-blind, placebo-controlled trial. J Clin Psychopharmacol 2002; 22(1):31–9.
72. Onofrj M, Paci C, D'Andreamatteo G, et al. Olanzapine in severe Gilles de la Tourette syndrome: a 52-week double-blind cross-over study vs. low-dose pimozide. J Neurol 2000;247:443–6.
73. Sallee FR, Kurlan R, Goetz CG, et al. Ziprasidone treatment of children and adolescents with Tourette's syndrome: a pilot study. J Am Acad Child Adolesc Psychiatry 2000;39:292–9.
74. Otsuka Pharmaceutical Development & Commercialization. Safety and tolerability of once-daily oral aripiprazole in children and adolescents with Tourette's disorder. Bethesda (MD): National Library of Medicine (US); 2000. Available at: http://clinicaltrials.gov/show/NCT01727713. Accessed April 22, 2014.
75. Cui YH, Zheng Y, Yang YP, et al. Effectiveness and tolerability of aripiprazole in children and adolescents with Tourette's disorder: a pilot study in China. J Child Adolesc Psychopharmacol 2010;20(4):291–8.
76. Lyon GJ, Samar S, Jummani R, et al. Aripiprazole in children and adolescents with Tourette's disorder: an open-label safety and tolerability study. J Child Adolesc Psychopharmacol 2009;19(6):623–33.
77. Murphy TK, Bengtson MA, Soto O, et al. Case series on the use of aripiprazole for Tourette syndrome. Int J Neuropsychopharmacol 2005;83(3):489–90.
78. Jankovic J. Botulinum toxin in movement disorders. Curr Opin Neurol 1994;7: 358–66.
79. Kwak CH, Hanna PA, Jankovic J. Botulinum toxin in the treatment of tics. Arch Neurol 2000;57:1190–3.
80. Allen AJ, Kurlan RM, Gilbert DL, et al. Atomoxetine treatment in children and adolescents with ADHD and comorbid tic disorders. Neurology 2005;65:1941–9.
81. Porta M, Sassi M, Cavallazzi M, et al. Tourette's syndrome and role of tetrabenazine: review and personal experience. Clin Drug Investig 2008;28(7): 443–59.
82. Jankovic J, Jimenez-Shahed J, Brown LW. A randomized, double-blind, placebo-controlled study of topiramate in the treatment of Tourette syndrome. J Neurol Neurosurg Psychiatry 2010;81(1):70–3.
83. Yang CS, Zhang LL, Zeng LN, et al. Topiramate for Tourette's syndrome in children: a meta-analysis. Pediatr Neurol 2013;49(5):344–50.
84. Awaad Y. Tics in Tourette syndrome: new treatment options. J Child Neurol 1999; 14(5):316–9.

85. Silver AA, Shytle RD, Philipp MK, et al. Transdermal nicotine and haloperidol in Tourette's disorder: a double-blind placebo-controlled study. J Clin Psychiatry 2001;62(9):707–14.
86. McDougle CJ, Goodman WK, Leckman JF, et al. Haloperidol addition in fluvoxamine-refractory obsessive-compulsive disorder: a double-blind, placebo controlled study in patients with and without tics. Arch Gen Psychiatry 1994; 51(4):302–8.
87. Geller DA, Biederman J, Stewart SE, et al. Which SSRI? A meta-analysis of pharmacotherapy trials in pediatric obsessive-compulsive disorder. Am J Psychiatry 2003;160(11):1919–28.
88. March JS, Franklin ME, Leonard H, et al. Tics moderate treatment outcome with sertraline but not cognitive-behavior therapy in pediatric obsessive-compulsive disorder. Biol Psychiatry 2007;61(3):344–7.
89. Lowe TL, Cohen DJ, Detlor J, et al. Stimulant medications precipitate Tourette's syndrome. JAMA 1982;247(12):1729–31.
90. Gadow KD, Sverd J, Sprafkin J, et al. Efficacy of methylphenidate for attention-deficit hyperactivity disorder in children with tic disorder. Arch Gen Psychiatry 1995;52(6):444–55.
91. Tourette's Syndrome Study Group. Treatment of ADHD in children with tics: a randomized controlled trial. Neurology 2002;58(4):527–36.
92. Bloch MH, Panza KE, Landeros-Weisenberger A, et al. Meta-analysis: treatment of attention-deficit/hyperactivity disorder in children with comorbid tic disorders. J Am Acad Child Adolesc Psychiatry 2009;48(9):884–93.

# Body Dysmorphic Disorder

Angela Fang, MA, Natalie L. Matheny, BA, Sabine Wilhelm, PhD*

## KEYWORDS

- Body dysmorphic disorder • Obsessive-compulsive spectrum • Treatment
- Cognitive-behavioral therapy • Serotonin reuptake inhibitor

## KEY POINTS

- Body dysmorphic disorder (BDD) has garnered much research attention in the past decade. Pharmacologic and nonpharmacologic treatment options are available but limited.
- The first-line pharmacotherapies for BDD are serotonin reuptake inhibitors (SRIs) which seem to require relatively high doses and long trial durations.
- The most empirically supported nonpharmacologic intervention for BDD is cognitive-behavioral therapy (CBT), which is a time-limited, symptom-focused treatment that involves psychoeducation, cognitive restructuring, perceptual/mirror retraining, exposure and response prevention, and relapse prevention.
- Available data from medication and CBT trials are limiting as far as generalizability and lack of well-controlled designs. It remains unclear which modality is more efficacious and whether combination therapies offer additional advantages over monotherapies.
- Highly delusional patients may be more likely to seek treatment from nonpsychiatric professionals, such as cosmetic surgeons, dermatologists, and dentists, for their BDD concerns.

## OVERVIEW: NATURE OF THE PROBLEM

Characterized as a disorder of imagined ugliness, BDD has long been described in the psychiatric literature. BDD was introduced only in 1980 to the *Diagnostic and Statistical Manual of Mental Disorders (DSM)-III*[1] as an atypical somatoform disorder, called *dysmorphophobia*, and was given a separate diagnosis in *DSM* (Third Edition Revised)[2] in the somatoform disorders section. By the time the *DSM* (Fourth Edition,

Dr S. Wilhelm has received research support from National Institute of Mental Health grants 5 R01 MH091078-03, 5 R01 MH093402-03, the US Food and Drug Administration, the International OCD Foundation, and the Tourette Syndrome Association. Forest Laboratories provided her with medication and matching placebo for a National Institute of Mental Health–funded study. Dr S. Wilhelm has received royalties from Elsevier Publications, Guilford Publications, New Harbinger Publications, and Oxford University Press. She has also received speaking honoraria from various academic institutions.

OCD and Related Disorders Program, Department of Psychiatry, Massachusetts General Hospital, Harvard Medical School, 185 Cambridge Street, 2nd Floor, Boston, MA 02114, USA
* Corresponding author.
*E-mail address:* wilhelm@psych.mgh.harvard.edu

| Abbreviations | |
| --- | --- |
| AN | Anorexia nervosa |
| BDD | Body dysmorphic disorder |
| CBT | Cognitive-behavioral therapy |
| DSM | Diagnostic and Statistical Manual of Mental Disorders |
| OCD | Obsessive-compulsive disorder |
| SAD | Social anxiety disorder |
| SRI | Serotonin reuptake inhibitor |

Text Revision) was published,[3] the classification of BDD evolved to include a criterion that the disorder was not better accounted for by another mental disorder (such as anorexia nervosa [AN]); however, it was still classified as a somatoform disorder. Given the recent research attention on the strong relationship between BDD and obsessive-compulsive disorder (OCD),[4,5] the DSM (Fifth Edition) now includes BDD under a new section for OCD and related disorders.[6] Thus, the predominant view today is that BDD is an obsessive-compulsive spectrum disorder due to strong evidence of the overlap between BDD and OCD in terms of phenomenology, comorbidity, and treatment response.

Despite such revisions in the DSM, BDD has consistently been defined by an excessive preoccupation with imagined defects in physical appearance. BDD differs from normal appearance concerns because it is associated with significant distress and can lead to meaningful functional impairment in interpersonal relationships and occupational status. When real physical defects are present, BDD is marked by exaggerated concerns about the severity of the defect, as manifested by a strong frequency, duration, and intensity of preoccupation about the defect. Individuals with BDD exhibit ritualistic patterns of thoughts and behaviors associated with hiding, correcting, or fixing the perceived defect, such as intrusive thoughts about appearance, mirror checking, and camouflaging.[7–9] They may also engage in significant avoidance of people, places, or situations where they think that their appearance may be evaluated. An individual's preoccupation may become difficult for a person to control and could consume several hours of the day. Case studies have shown that individuals may become so preoccupied and distressed by their perceived defect or flaw that they may stop working or socializing and, in severe cases, may become housebound.[7]

In BDD, a person's focus of concern may center around 1 or many body parts, with the most common areas involving the skin, hair, and nose.[8,10] Preoccupation with several different aspects of appearance is not uncommon.[8,10] Individuals with BDD often experience low self-esteem as well as feelings of disgust or embarrassment. Due to the shame and secretive nature of the illness, BDD is often under-recognized or left untreated and represents an understudied research area in the literature.[7,9]

This review aims to provide an updated overview of BDD in terms of its psychopathology, etiology, epidemiology, and nosology, with an emphasis on current pharmacologic and nonpharmacologic treatment options for BDD. The authors also aim to integrate recent empirical data that inform these areas as well as identify areas of further research and provide suggestions for future directions.

## ASSOCIATED CLINICAL FEATURES
### Delusionality

Perhaps one of the most debilitating clinical characteristics of BDD is delusionality. Many individuals with BDD are completely convinced that their perceived defects are real, to the extent that others take special notice of their flaws.[11] In a study conducted by Phillips,[12] 129 patients with BDD were interviewed using the Brown Assessment of Beliefs Scale,[13] which is an instrument designed to assess delusionality. Of the 129 patients assessed, 108 (84%) were either delusional or had poor insight in their disorder. Furthermore, 60 participants (46.5%) were completely convinced that their appearance beliefs were true. Another study examining characteristics of 100 participants with BDD found that 52 had delusional BDD and 48 had a nondelusional form of BDD.[14] Few differences were found between groups demographically or clinically, and neither group responded to treatment with antipsychotic medication alone. These results indicate that patients with delusional versus nondelusional BDD are not different but rather patients with delusional BDD may be suffering from a more severe form of the disorder.[14] Moreover, increased rates of delusionality may be unique to BDD compared with other related disorders. For example, although BDD and OCD are thought to be similar disorders, research has shown that rates of delusionality and a lack of insight are higher in BDD than OCD.[15] These findings shed light on implications for further research as well as treatment strategies for BDD.

## Suicidality

Empirical research suggests that the rate of suicidal ideation and completed suicide is particularly high in BDD.[16,17] Studies have shown that the rates of suicidal ideation over a lifetime in patients with BDD is as high as 80%, with up to 25% of patients actually attempting suicide.[16] One particular study[18] found that of 185 subjects with BDD, the mean suicidal ideation rate was 10 to 25 times higher and the mean annual suicide attempt rate was 2 to 12 times higher than the average US population. Furthermore, in this study, the completed suicide rate was approximately 45 times higher than the general population. Clinical correlates of suicidal ideation and attempts include a more severe lifetime course of BDD as well as comorbid disorders, such as major depressive disorder, bipolar disorder, and borderline personality disorder.[18] Risk factors include psychiatric hospitalizations, unemployment, poor social support, poor self-esteem, and a history of abuse.[16]

## ETIOLOGY

BDD has a complex etiology, because multiple biological, psychological, and socio-environmental factors have been proposed as having a role in the development and maintenance of BDD.[19] For example, certain biological factors may be involved in the pathophysiology of BDD, such as volumetric brain abnormalities in the orbitofrontal cortex and anterior cingulate cortex[20] as well as asymmetry of the caudate nucleus and greater white matter volume compared with healthy control participants.[21] In addition, one study found that BDD symptom severity correlated significantly with the size of the left inferior frontal gyrus and the right amygdala, although volumetric differences in these brain regions were not found between BDD patients and healthy control participants.[22] Similarly, individuals with BDD showed hyperactivity of the left orbitofrontal cortex and bilateral head of the caudate nucleus during visual processing of their own face compared with a familiar face.[23] Although these studies vary widely in terms of sample characteristics and task demands, researchers have interpreted these findings as demonstrating pathophysiologic mechanisms similar to OCD. Furthermore, findings from family studies indicate that the prevalence of BDD is significantly higher among first-degree relatives of probands with OCD compared with other obsessive-compulsive spectrum disorders, such as hypochondriasis, eating disorders, and impulse control disorders,[24] which supports the conceptualization of BDD as an obsessive-compulsive spectrum disorder.

Extensive research has also examined the role of certain cognitive and socioenvironmental factors in the etiology of BDD.[25,26] Social learning models[26] postulate that early learning experiences in childhood reinforce maladaptive beliefs about appearance. Through classical or evaluative conditioning, individuals may begin to develop aversive reactions to appearance, leading to the development of core beliefs surrounding the value of attractiveness.

Cognitive-behavioral models are widely accepted psychological theories of BDD and have been proposed to explain some of the mechanisms involved in the development and maintenance of BDD. These models highlight the diathesis-stress model and integrate biological predispositions, cultural factors, early childhood experiences, and psychological vulnerabilities as factors that influence the etiology and maintenance of BDD.[27,28] For example, cognitive-behavioral models of BDD[27,28] emphasize the cognitive aspects underlying BDD, such as maladaptive beliefs about the importance of appearance. Veale[27] hypothesized that external events, such as looking at oneself in the mirror (which he called the view of oneself as an aesthetic object), combined with intrusive thoughts might trigger a process of excessive self-focused attention. This self-focused attention then leads to a negative appraisal of body image in which an individual may develop core beliefs linking failure or worthlessness to appearance, for example, "If I am defective, then I will be alone all my life." As a result, individuals often ruminate on their perceived ugliness and compare themselves to an impossibly ideal appearance. Because individuals with BDD are so self-focused on aversive imagery, they are unable to accurately observe the actions of others to discredit their own fears of negative evaluation. Reactions to their perceived image and maladaptive thoughts may invoke disgust and lead an individual to engage in ritualistic safety behaviors, such as camouflaging to alter appearance, avoiding social situations, skin-picking, reassurance seeking, or escaping uncomfortable situations. Although engagement in these ritualistic behaviors is meant to relieve anxiety, the behavior itself tends to decrease distress only briefly and instead increases self-consciousness and preoccupation over time.[27-29]

Empirical findings on cognitive biases in BDD are consistent with cognitive-behavioral models. Studies have demonstrated that patients with BDD show a selective attentional bias for emotional words (positive or negative in valence) compared with neutral words in an emotional Stroop paradigm.[30] Individuals with BDD are also more likely to make negative interpretations of ambiguous body-related and social scenarios than their OCD and healthy counterparts.[31] These attentional and interpretation tendencies support the notion that BDD may in part be maintained by cognitive factors.

## EPIDEMIOLOGY
### Prevalence

Population-based estimates of the point prevalence of BDD using nationwide, representative samples have ranged from 1.7% to 2.4%.[32-34] These studies have methodological differences and vary widely in terms of BDD symptom assessment, because some studies used self-report methods, and others used in-person structured clinical interviews. In college student populations, prevalence rates seem higher, at 5.3%.[35] A cross-cultural comparison study of body image concerns and probable BDD diagnosis among American and German college students found that body image preoccupation was higher among American students, but BDD diagnosis did not differ between groups.[36]

Prevalence estimates are generally higher in clinical samples. Among outpatients, the prevalence of BDD ranges between 1.8% and 6.7%,[37,38] and among inpatients, the prevalence ranges from 13.1% to 16.0%.[39,40] Evidence also indicates a prevalence rate of 7.7% and 24.5% among samples of patients who sought nonpsychiatric treatment options, such as cosmetic surgery and dermatologic treatments.[41–43]

## Gender Differences

A recent epidemiologic study of the prevalence of BDD in the United States showed a slight preponderance of BDD in women (2.5%) compared with men (2.2%).[33] Other evidence indicates that men with BDD are more likely single and living alone compared with women with BDD.[44] Furthermore, there seem to be gender differences in body parts of concern because men are more likely to obsess about their genitals, body build, and hair thinning/balding whereas women are more likely to obsess about their skin, stomach, weight, breasts, buttocks, thighs, legs, hips, toes, and excessive body hair.[44] Thus, gender may be an important moderator of BDD symptoms and clinical presentation.

## Course and Outcome

Retrospective data suggest that the typical age of onset of BDD is approximately 16.0 ± 6.9 years, with a mode of 13 years.[45] BDD tends to be a severe and chronic disorder, because recent data from a 4-year prospective naturalistic study indicate a low probability (20%) of full remission after 4 years, and a high probability (42%) of full relapse during 4 years after remission.[46] Furthermore, in this study, more severe BDD symptoms at intake predicted lower remission probability. Such evidence underscores the often unremitting course of BDD and the importance of conducting further research to enhance the detection and treatment of BDD.

## NOSOLOGIC ISSUES

Much available data support the ostensible link between OCD and BDD, and the conceptualization of BDD as an obsessive-compulsive spectrum disorder (for review, see Refs.[4,47]). For example, individuals with OCD and BDD share similarities in cognitive biases, such as high levels of perfectionism and preference for symmetry, as well as similarities in repetitive checking behaviors and avoidance of triggering situations.[4] Other studies demonstrate comorbidity rates as high as 30% between OCD and BDD samples, and preferential response to SRIs in both disorders.[5,48] There are important differences between the 2 disorders.[48–50] Individuals with BDD tend to be less likely to be married, are more likely to be unemployed, demonstrate a higher rate of suicidal ideation, exhibit poorer insight, and have a higher comorbidity with major depression and substance use disorders compared with individuals with OCD.[50,51]

Recent research attention has also examined the relationship between BDD and other related disorders, such as social anxiety disorder (SAD), because a core feature of both disorders is a pathologic concern of being negatively evaluated by others.[52–55] Empirical evidence suggests that BDD and SAD may have a similar gender distribution and history of suicide attempts, but SAD may be associated with an earlier age of onset, and BDD may be associated with greater psychiatric hospitalizations as well as a lesser likelihood of being married.[54] In addition, data indicate that individuals with BDD (but not SAD) are more likely to have OCD, an eating disorder, or a psychotic disorder compared with individuals with SAD (but not BDD),[54] which suggests that BDD and SAD may be less closely related than previously thought. Consistent with this view, a study examining the effect of an attention retraining cognitive intervention for SAD on BDD concerns in a sample of patients with primary SAD found that attention retraining significantly improved BDD but not SAD symptoms.[56] This finding supports the possibility that BDD and SAD may be maintained by separate and distinguishable cognitive mechanisms, such as selective attentional or visual processing of specific emotional stimuli. Future research on the relationship between BDD and SAD should test this hypothesis to clarify their nosology.

BDD also shares diagnostic and conceptual overlap with eating disorders, because a primary concern in both disorders involves a preoccupation with physical appearance and body dissatisfaction.[57] One study comparing individuals with AN and individuals with BDD found that those with AN reported more weight- and shape-related body image concerns, whereas those with BDD showed more diverse appearance concerns.[58] Moreover, a recent study showed that 12% of inpatients with eating disorders had comorbid BDD and displayed a high prevalence of dissatisfaction with non–weight-related body image concerns, which is consistent with the view that these 2 disorders are highly overlapping.[59]

Furthermore, most people with BDD have poor insight or delusional BDD beliefs, not recognizing that the appearance flaws they perceive are actually minimal or nonexistent. Individuals with BDD are often strongly convinced that they are physically flawed.[11] They often have delusions of reference that people are laughing at or taking special notice of their perceived appearance defect.[60] Few untreated patients have good insight. An insight specifier has been included in the DSM (Fifth Edition) to emphasize that individuals with BDD might present with a range of insight (eg, allowing individuals to be classified as having "absent insight/delusional beliefs").[6] BDD differs, however, from psychotic disorders in that BDD is more commonly associated with fluctuating insight,[60] whereas insight impairment in psychotic disorders is typically more stable. In addition, BDD is typically not associated with other psychotic symptoms, such as auditory hallucinations, or perceptual and motor disturbances, and, in contrast to individuals with a psychotic disorder, those with BDD tend to display only delusions that center around their appearance concerns. Data show that fewer than 3% of patients with either delusional or nondelusional variants of BDD also meet criteria for a psychotic disorder, which suggests a low rate of comorbidity.[61] Furthermore, researchers have observed that the degree of certainty about the perceived appearance defects may change over time and depend on situational context.[62] Thus, the conceptualization of BDD as a psychotic disorder does not seem a sufficient explanation of the range of insight that has been observed in BDD.

## TREATMENT APPROACHES

Studies have shown that some types of pharmacologic and nonpharmacologic interventions can be successful in the treatment of BDD.[63–65] Existing information on the relative efficacy of these approaches is, however, lacking. In addition, the treatment outcome studies on BDD are limiting as far as their generalizability, because they typically do not include suicidal individuals, as well as their methodological rigor, because few randomized controlled trials have been conducted. Although treatment outcome research has been promising, the efficacy of combination treatments as well as moderators of treatment response requires further investigation.

### Pharmacologic Treatment Options

Medication trials for BDD have focused primarily on SRIs through open-label and randomized controlled trials. These trials include treatment with fluoxetine,[66] fluvoxamine,[67,68] citalopram,[69] escitalopram,[70] and clomipramine versus desipramine.[71] In all of these studies, BDD symptoms improved and response rates ranged from 53% to 73%. A controlled double-blind crossover trial[71] that compared the SRI clomipramine to the non-SRI antidepressant desipramine found that clomipramine was more efficacious for BDD, which suggests that antidepressants are not universally effective for BDD and underscores the importance of testing strategies to specifically treat BDD symptoms.[64] This finding is consistent with previous studies showing that SRI trials led to improvements in BDD symptoms compared with non-SRI tricyclic antidepressants.[72,73] Thus, given that the use of non-SRI medications as a monotherapy for BDD has not been well studied, the first-line pharmacotherapy for BDD is SRI medication.

Although randomized controlled trials of SRIs for BDD are limited, available evidence indicates that BDD may require higher SRI doses and longer trial durations.[64] For example, previous studies have shown a mean time to SRI response of 6 to 9 weeks.[66,68] In addition, the mean fluoxetine dose in one study[66] was high (77.7 $\pm$ 8.0 mg/d). Studies show that citalopram[69] and escitalopram[70] have faster response times, with significant improvement within 4.6 and 4.7 weeks, respectively. Studies have yet to directly compare dosing structures and trial durations across different SRIs, however. Based on clinical expertise, experts recommend using higher doses of SRIs with patients who tolerate the medication well and have only partially responded to the highest recommended dose.[64] In addition, tailoring SRI titration and dosing to each patient is recommended, based on factors, such as severity of illness and patient preference.[64] Further research is needed to determine the optimal dose and timing of SRIs for BDD. Moreover, studies examining augmentation of SRIs for BDD with other pharmacologic agents are even fewer, with existing data available from case studies, small open-label trials, and chart review studies, which suggest that the use of certain SRI augmentation strategies may be beneficial, such as buspirone or clomipramine.[74] The lack of data on SRI augmentation is problematic, given the substantial percentage of patients who do not respond or only partially respond to SRIs. Thus, future research should systematically examine optimal use of SRIs as well as SRI augmentation in larger, controlled trials.

A point of contention exists in the exploration of treatment of delusional BDD. Although delusional symptoms arising in other disorders have typically been treated by antipsychotic medications, several studies have shown that delusional patients with BDD are just as likely as nondelusional patients with BDD to respond to SSRIs.[64,66,71] For example, treatment with fluoxetine was shown just as efficacious for individuals with delusional BDD as it was for those with nondelusional BDD.[66] Furthermore, Hollander and colleagues[71] found that clomipramine was more effective than desipramine regardless of whether or not the patient was delusional. Additionally, retrospective studies have shown that antipsychotics alone were rarely effective for delusional BDD.[12] As such, experts recommend that delusional BDD be treated with an SRI rather than an antipsychotic alone.[64]

### Nonpharmacologic Treatment Options

CBT, the most studied and empirically supported form of psychological treatment, has been found effective for BDD.[65] A typical course of CBT for BDD involves several core treatment components, such as psychoeducation, motivational enhancement, cognitive restructuring, in vivo exposures and response prevention, perceptual mirror retraining, and relapse prevention.[28,75,76] During psychoeducation, a therapist explains the CBT model to a patient and develops an individualized model for the patient, which includes factors that may have contributed to the development and maintenance of the disorder. The therapist and patient then work together to evaluate the accuracy of maladaptive thoughts and work toward developing more adaptive beliefs, which is a technique used in cognitive therapy. Furthermore, treatment also includes techniques used in behavior therapy, such as exposure and response prevention. During exposure and response prevention, patients are asked to confront situations that typically make them nervous without engaging in ritualistic responses, such as mirror checking or avoidance, and to allow the anxiety to subside on its own. Similarly, during perceptual and mirror retraining, patients are trained to describe their appearance in an objective, nonjudgmental manner while standing at least an arm's length away from the mirror. Consistent with the goals of cognitive therapy, this technique promotes more objective ways of describing appearance and disrupts the typical manner in which patients relate to the mirror. In the last few sessions of CBT, the therapist and patient work on relapse prevention to help the patient maintain achievements in therapy over the long term.[28,75,76]

Recently, Wilhelm and colleagues[76] pilot tested a new form of modular CBT for BDD, which represented a more flexible, individualized treatment approach that would be ideal for treating the heterogeneous nature of BDD. Twelve adults with primary BDD were delivered treatment in 18 to 22 sessions. Core CBT treatment components were supplemented with modular interventions, including a skin picking and hair plucking module, a muscularity and shape/weight module, and a cosmetic treatment module. Eighty percent of the study completers were responders to the treatment—scores on the BDD modification of the Yale-Brown Obsessive Compulsive Scale,[77] which is a measure of BDD symptom severity, decreased significantly at posttreatment. Furthermore, these effects were still present at the 3-month and 6-month follow-up sessions. Results from this study suggested that a flexible, modular approach to CBT may be efficacious for individuals with BDD by targeting individual psychopathology and symptomatology. Although most CBT treatment approaches include a combination of cognitive and behavioral techniques, research has shown that behavior therapy alone (without explicit cognitive interventions) can be effective.[78] Furthermore, these treatments have shown effective in both individual and group treatment settings.[29,79–82]

### Combination Therapies

To date, no studies have directly compared the efficacy of CBT versus pharmacotherapy for BDD nor have studies directly compared the efficacy of monotherapies with CBT or medications versus combination therapies. It remains unknown, therefore, whether combination therapies offer an incremental advantage over monotherapy alone.

A meta-analysis examined waitlist control studies and case studies involving psychological or pharmacologic treatments.[78] Psychological treatment was typically short term, ranging from 7 to 30 sessions. Results showed that psychological treatments (cognitive therapy, behavior therapy, and CBT) were all successful in treating BDD. Furthermore, although pharmacologic treatments were also found effective, researchers found a significantly greater effect size for CBT compared with medication treatments. These results should be interpreted with caution, because many participants included in the psychological intervention trials were on a stabilized regimen of medication, which may confound the true effect size of psychological interventions when used as a monotherapy.

### Surgical and Nonpsychiatric Treatments

Due to strong delusional convictions that appearance flaws are a physical rather than psychological problem, individuals with BDD may seek cosmetic or dermatologic treatment rather than psychological or pharmacologic treatment. One study found that among 289 individuals with BDD, nonpsychiatric medical treatment and surgery were sought by 76.4% and received by 66.0% of adults, with men and women equally likely to seek nonpsychiatric treatment.[83] A recent study showed that among a sample of 200 BDD patients, rhinoplasty and breast augmentation were the most commonly received surgical treatment of BDD concerns, constituting 37.7% and 8.2% of received surgical procedures in the sample, respectively.[84] As for minimally invasive procedures, collagen injections and microdermabrasion were the most commonly received procedures, constituting 50% and 19.2% of received minimally invasive procedures, respectively. Although an individual may be temporarily relieved after these cosmetic procedures, the effects are typically not long lasting. Data indicate that only 2.3% of surgical or minimally invasive procedures led to longer-term improvement in overall BDD symptoms.[84]

### Other Treatments

Case reports suggest that ECT is rarely efficacious for BDD symptoms,[85] with transient improvement most notably in depressive symptoms. Neurosurgery is another treatment option that has not been well-studied for BDD, although some researchers point to available case reports, which suggest that certain procedures (such as a modified leucotomy, capsulotomy, bilateral anterior cingulotomy and subcaudate tractotomy, and anterior capsulotomy) have been performed and may lead to substantial improvement in BDD symptoms, especially for patients who are severely ill or treatment refractory.[64]

### Treatment Resistance

Although some pharmacologic and nonpharmacologic treatments may be effective for BDD, barriers to treatment continue to pose difficulties. For instance, as discussed previously, delusional beliefs that appearance flaws are real may lead BDD patients to seek nonpsychiatric treatment options for their appearance concerns. Barriers to treatment might also include an individual's reluctance to talk about appearance concerns due to feelings of shame or the lack of awareness of BDD and its clinical characteristics and significance.[86]

Only a few studies have examined barriers to seeking treatment in BDD. Using an Internet survey, Buhlmann[87] examined a sample of 172 individuals with self-reported BDD. In this sample, researchers found that only 23.3% had been diagnosed by a mental health care provider, and fewer than 20% were receiving psychosocial or psychotropic treatment. Among the reasons cited for not seeking treatment, participants listed shame, not being able to find a treatment provider nearby, and the belief that only cosmetic surgery or other dermatologic treatments could help. Another Internet study conducted by Marques and colleagues[88] found similar results. A total of 401 participants with symptoms consistent with a diagnosis of BDD completed questionnaires measuring treatment utilization and treatment barriers. Consistent with past research, individuals sought cosmetic or dermatologic treatment of their concerns. Additionally, individuals experienced barriers to treatment, such as stigma, shame, and treatment skepticism. Researchers also found barriers to treatment related to ethnicity. In particular, Latinos with BDD symptoms endorsed higher rates of treatment barriers than white patients. Further research is necessary to examine how treatment barriers can be minimized in general and for minority groups in particular.

### Long-Term Recommendations

Evidence points to the long-term benefit of continuing an effective SRI, because the risk of relapse seems to increase significantly after discontinuation.[74] A chart review study found that approximately 87% of patients who discontinued an effective SRI relapsed within the next 6 months compared with only 8% of patients who continued an effective SRI.[89] It remains unknown whether receiving CBT while taking an SRI reduces the risk of relapse if the SRI is discontinued, but this should not be assumed and is important to study in future research.[64]

Long-term follow-up data on pharmacotherapy and CBT treatment trials are limited. Preliminary data suggest, however, that treatment gains from CBT are maintained at 3- and 6-month follow-up periods,[76] and in one study, gains were maintained after an intensive behavioral therapy program for up to 2 years.[79] Given the chronicity and severity of BDD, more research is needed to examine predictors of treatment outcome and factors influencing relapse.

## SUMMARY

BDD is a severe and chronic psychiatric disorder that has been largely underrecognized and underdiagnosed. Although research on BDD has increased over the past several decades, the disorder is still understudied. Specialized educational training for mental health care professionals as well as providers in medical settings, such as primary care providers, surgeons, dermatologists, and dentists, will be necessary for the proper diagnosis and subsequent treatment of this disorder. Future studies should examine the comparative efficacy of CBT versus pharmacotherapy in placebo-controlled studies as well as ways of enhancing treatment outcome either via combination therapies, SRI augmentation, or augmentation of other novel pharmacologic agents.

## REFERENCES

1. American Psychiatric Association. Diagnostic and statistical manual of mental disorders. 3rd edition. Washington, DC: Author; 1980.
2. American Psychiatric Association. Diagnostic and statistical manual of mental disorders. 3rd edition- revised. Washington, DC: Author; 1987.
3. American Psychiatric Association. Diagnostic and statistical manual of mental disorders. 4th edition- text revision. Washington, DC: Author; 2000.
4. Chosak A, Marques L, Greenberg JL, et al. Body dysmorphic disorder and obsessive-compulsive disorder: similarities, differences and the classification debate. Expert Rev Neurother 2008;8:1209–18.
5. Storch EA, Abramowitz J, Goodman WK. Where does obsessive-compulsive disorder belong in DSM-V? Depress Anxiety 2008;25:336–47.
6. American Psychiatric Association. Diagnostic and statistical manual of mental disorders. 5th edition. Washington, DC: Author; 2013.
7. Phillips KA. The broken mirror: understanding and treating body dysmorphic disorder (revised and expanded edition). New York: Oxford University Press; 2005.
8. Phillips KA, Menard W, Fay C, et al. Demographic characteristics, phenomenology, comorbidity, and family history in 200 individuals with body dysmorphic disorder. Psychosomatics 2005;46:317–25.
9. Wilhelm S. Feeling good about the way you look: a program for overcoming body image problems. New York: Guilford Press; 2006.
10. Phillips KA, Diaz SF. Gender differences in body dysmorphic disorder. J Nerv Ment Dis 1997;185:570–7.
11. Eisen JL, Phillips KA, Coles ME, et al. Insight in obsessive compulsive disorder and body dysmorphic disorder. Compr Psychiatry 2004;45:10–5.

12. Phillips KA. Psychosis in body dysmorphic disorder. J Psychiatr Res 2004;38: 63–72.
13. Eisen JL, Phillips KA, Baer L, et al. The brown assessment of beliefs scale: reliability and validity. Am J Psychiatry 1998;155:102–8.
14. Phillips KA, McElroy SL, Keck PE, et al. A comparison of delusional and nondelusionalbody dysmorphic disorder in 100 cases. Psychopharmacol Bull 1994; 30:179–86.
15. Phillips KA, Pinto A, Hart AS, et al. A comparison of insight in body dysmorphic disorder and obsessive–compulsive disorder. J Psychiatr Res 2012;46:1293–9. http://dx.doi.org/10.1016/j.jpsychires.2012.05.016.
16. Phillips KA. Suicidality in body dysmorphic disorder. Prim psychiatry 2007;14: 58–66.
17. Phillips KA, Coles ME, Menard W, et al. Suicidal ideation and suicide attempts in body dysmorphic disorder. J Clin Psychiatry 2005;66:717–25.
18. Phillips KA, Menard W. Suicidality in body dysmorphic disorder: a prospective study. Am J Psychiatry 2006;163:1280–2.
19. Feusner JD, Neziroglu F, Wilhelm S, et al. What causes BDD: research findings and a proposed model. Psychiatr Ann 2010;40:349–55.
20. Atmaca M, Bingol I, Aydin A, et al. Brain morphology of patients with body dysmorphic disorder. J Affect Disord 2010;123:258–63.
21. Rauch SL, Phillips KA, Segal E, et al. A preliminary morphometric magnetic resonance imaging study of regional brain volumes in body dysmorphic disorder. Psychiatry Res Neuroimaging 2003;122:13–9.
22. Feusner JD, Townsend J, Bystritsky A, et al. Regional brain volumes and symptom severity in body dysmorphic disorder. Psychiatry Res Neuroimaging 2009; 172:161–7.
23. Feusner JD, Moody T, Hembacher E, et al. Abnormalities of visual processing and frontostriatal systems in body dysmorphic disorder. Arch Gen Psychiatry 2010;67:197–205.
24. Bienvenu OJ, Samuels JF, Riddle MA, et al. The relationship of obsessive-compulsive disorder to possible spectrum disorders: results from a family study. Biol Psychiatry 2000;48:287–93.
25. Buhlmann U, Wilhelm S. Cognitive factors in body dysmorphic disorder. Psychiatr Ann 2004;34:922–6.
26. Neziroglu F, Khemlani-Patel S, Veale D. Social learning theory and cognitive behavioral models of body dysmorphic disorder. Body Image 2008;5:28–38.
27. Veale D. Advances in a cognitive behavioural model of body dysmorphic disorder. Body Image 2004;1:113–25.
28. Wilhelm S, Phillips KA, Steketee G. Cognitive-behavioral therapy for body dysmorphic disorder: a treatment manual. New York: Guilford Press; 2013.
29. Veale D, Gournay K, Dryden W, et al. Body dysmorphic disorder: a cognitive behavioural model and pilot randomised controlled trial. Behav Res Ther 1996;34: 717–29.
30. Buhlmann U, McNally RJ, Wilhelm S, et al. Selective processing of emotional information in body dysmorphic disorder. J Anxiety Disord 2002;16:289–98.
31. Buhlmann U, Wilhelm S, McNally RJ, et al. Interpretive biases for ambiguous information in body dysmorphic disorder. CNS Spectr 2002;7:435–6, 441–3.
32. Buhlmann U, Glaesmer H, Mewes R, et al. Updates on the prevalence of body dysmorphic disorder: a population-based survey. Psychiatry Res 2010;178: 171–5.

33. Koran LM, Abujaoude E, Large MD, et al. The prevalence of body dysmorphic disorder in the United States adult population. CNS Spectrums 2008;13:316–22.
34. Rief W, Buhlmann U, Wilhelm S, et al. The prevalence of body dysmorphic disorder: a population-based survey. Psychol Med 2006;36:877–85.
35. Bohne A, Wilhelm S, Keuthen NJ, et al. Prevalence of body dysmorphic disorder in a German college student sample. Psychiatry Res 2002;109:101–4.
36. Bohne A, Keuthen NJ, Wilhelm S, et al. Prevalence of symptoms of body dysmorphic disorder and its correlates: a cross-cultural comparison. Psychosomatics 2002;43:486–90.
37. Wilhelm S, Otto MW, Zucker BG, et al. Prevalence of body dysmorphic disorder in patients with anxiety disorders. J Anxiety Disord 1997;11:499–502.
38. van der Meer J, van Rood YR, van der Wee NJ, et al. Prevalence, demographic and clinical characteristics of body dysmorphic disorder among psychiatric outpatients with mood, anxiety or somatoform disorders. Nord J Psychiatry 2012; 66:232–8.
39. Conroy M, Menard W, Fleming-Ives K, et al. Prevalence and clinical characteristics of body dysmorphic disorder in an adult inpatient setting. Gen Hosp Psychiatry 2008;30:67–72.
40. Grant JE, Kim SW, Crow SJ. Prevalence and clinical features of body dysmorphic disorder in adolescent and adult psychiatric inpatients. J Clin Psychiatry 2001;62:517–22.
41. Alavi M, Kalafi Y, Dehbozorgi GR, et al. Body dysmorphic disorder and other psychiatric morbidity in aesthetic rhinoplasty candidates. J Plast Reconstr Aesthet Surg 2011;64:738–41.
42. Conrado LA, Hounie AG, Diniz JB, et al. Body dysmorphic disorder among dermatologic patients: prevalence and clinical features. J Am Acad Dermatol 2010;63:235–43.
43. Lai CS, Lee SS, Yeh YC, et al. Body dysmorphic disorder in patients with cosmetic surgery. Kaohsiung J Med Sci 2010;26:478–82.
44. Phillips KA, Menard W, Fay C. Gender similarities and differences in 200 individuals with body dysmorphic disorder. Compr Psychiatry 2006;47:77–87.
45. Gunstad J, Phillips KA. Axis I comorbidity in body dysmorphic disorder. Compr Psychiatry 2003;44:270–6.
46. Phillips KA, Menard W, Quinn E, et al. A four-year prospective observational follow-up study of course and predictors of course in body dysmorphic disorder. Psychol Med 2013;43:1109–17.
47. Phillips KA, Wilhelm S, Koran LM, et al. Body dysmorphic disorder: some key issues for DSM-V. Depress Anxiety 2010;27:573–91.
48. Phillips KA, McElroy SL, Hudson JI, et al. Body dysmorphic disorder: an obsessive-compulsive spectrum disorder, a form of affective spectrum disorder, or both? J Clin Psychiatry 1995;56:41–51.
49. Cororve MB, Gleaves DH. Body dysmorphic disorder: a review of conceptualizations, assessment, and treatment strategies. Clin Psychol Rev 2001;21:949–70.
50. Frare F, Perugi G, Ruffolo G, et al. Obsessive-compulsive disorder and body dysmorphic disorder: a comparison of clinical features. Eur Psychiatry 2004; 19:292–8.
51. Phillips KA, Pinto A, Menard W, et al. Obsessive-compulsive disorder versus body dysmorphic disorder: a comparison study of two possibly related disorders. Depress Anxiety 2007;24:399–409.
52. Coles ME, Phillips KA, Menard W, et al. Body dysmorphic disorder and social phobia: cross-sectional and prospective data. Depress Anxiety 2006;23:26–33.

53. Fang A, Asnaani A, Gutner CA, et al. Rejection sensitivity mediates the relationship between social anxiety and bodydysmorphic concerns. J Anxiety Disord 2011;25:946–9.

54. Kelly MM, Dalrymple K, Zimmerman M, et al. A comparison study of body dysmorphic disorder versus social phobia. Psychiatry Res 2013;205:109–16.

55. Kelly MM, Walters C, Phillips KA. Social anxiety and its relationship to functional impairment in body dysmorphic disorder. Behav Ther 2010;41:143–53.

56. Fang A, Sawyer AT, Aderka I, et al. Psychological treatment of social anxiety disorder improves body dysmorphic concerns. J Anxiety Disord 2013;27(7): 684–91.

57. Rosen JC. Body dysmorphic disorder: assessment and treatment. In: body image, eating disorders, and obesity: an integrative guide for assessment and treatment. Washington, DC: American Psychological Association; 2001. p. 149–70.

58. Rosen JC, Ramirez E. A comparison of eating disorders and body dysmorphic disorder on body image and psychological adjustment. J Psychosom Res 1998; 44:441–9.

59. Kollei I, Schieber K, de Zwaan M, et al. Body dysmorphic disorder and nonweight-related body image concerns in individuals with eating disorders. Int J Eat Disord 2013;46:52–9.

60. Phillips KA, McElroy SL. Insight, overvalued ideation, and delusional thinking in body dysmorphic disorder: theoretical and treatment implications. J Nerv Ment Dis 1993;181:699–702.

61. Phillips KA, Menard W, Pagano ME, et al. Delusional versus nondelusional body dysmorphic disorder: clinical features and course of illness. J Psychiatr Res 2006;40:95–104.

62. Phillips KA, Kim JM, Hudson JI. Body image disturbance in body dysmorphic disorder and eating disorders: obsessions or delusions? Psychiatr Clin North Am 1995;18:317–34.

63. Phillips KA. Pharmacologic treatment of body dysmorphic disorder: review of the evidence and a recommended treatment approach. CNS Spectrums 2002;7:453–60, 463.

64. Phillips KA, Hollander E. Treating body dysmorphic disorder with medication: evidence, misconceptions, and a suggested approach. Body Image 2008;5: 13–27.

65. Veale D. Cognitive behavioral therapy for body dysmorphic disorder. Psychiatr Ann 2010;40:333–40.

66. Phillips KA, Albertini RS, Rasmussen SA. A randomized placebo-controlled trial of fluoxetine in body dysmorphic disorder. Arch Gen Psychiatry 2002;59:381–8.

67. Perugi G, Giannotti D, Di Vaio S, et al. Fluvoxamine in the treatment of body dysmorphic disorder (dysmorphophobia). Int Clin Psychopharmacol 1996;11: 247–54.

68. Phillips KA, Dwight MM, McElroy SL. Efficacy and safety of fluvoxamine in body dysmorphic disorder. J Clin Psychiatry 1998;59:165–71.

69. Phillips KA, Najjar F. An open-label study of citalopram in body dysmorphic disorder. J Clin Psychiatry 2003;64:715–20.

70. Phillips KA. An open-label study of escitalopram in body dysmorphic disorder. Int Clin Psychopharmacol 2006;21:177–9.

71. Hollander E, Allen A, Kwon J, et al. Clomipramine vs. desipramine crossover trial in body dysmorphic disorder: selective efficacy of a serotonin reuptake inhibitor in imagined ugliness. Arch Gen Psychiatry 1999;56:1033–9.

72. Hollander E, Cohen L, Simeon D, et al. Fluvoxamine treatment of body dysmorphic disorder. J Clin Psychopharmacol 1994;14:75–7.
73. Phillips KA. Pharmacologic treatment of body dysmorphic disorder. Psychopharmacol Bull 1996;32:597–605.
74. Phillips KA, Albertini RS, Siniscalchi JM, et al. Effectiveness of pharmacotherapy for body dysmorphic disorder: a chart-review study. J Clin Psychiatry 2001;62: 721–7.
75. Veale D. Cognitive behaviour therapy for body dysmorphic disorder. In: Castle DJ, Phillips KA, editors. Disorders of body image. Petersfield (England): Wrightson Biomedical Publishing; 2002. p. 121–38.
76. Wilhelm S, Phillips KA, Fama JM, et al. Modular cognitive behavioral therapy for body dysmorphic disorder. Behav Ther 2011;42:624–33.
77. Phillips KA, Hollander E, Rasmussen SA, et al. A severity rating scale for body dysmorphic disorder: development, reliability, and validity of a modified version of the Yale-Brown Obsessive Compulsive Scale. Psychopharmacol Bull 1997; 33:17–22.
78. Williams J, Hadjistavropoulos T, Sharpe D. A meta-analysis of psychological and pharmacological treatments for body dysmorphic disorder. Behav Res Ther 2006;44:99–111.
79. McKay D. Two-year follow-up of behavioral treatment and maintenance for body dysmorphic disorder. Behav Modif 1999;23:620–9.
80. McKay D, Todaro J, Neziroglu F, et al. Body dysmorphic disorder: a preliminary evaluation of treatment and maintenance using exposure with response prevention. Behav Res Ther 1997;35:67–70.
81. Rosen JC, Reiter J, Orosan P. Cognitive-behavioral body image therapy for body dysmorphic disorder. J Consult Clin Psychol 1995;63:263–9.
82. Wilhelm S, Otto MW, Lohr B, et al. Cognitive behavior group therapy for body dysmorphic disorder: a case series. Behav Res Ther 1999;37:71–5.
83. Phillips KA, Grant J, Siniscalchi J, et al. Surgical and nonpsychiatric medical treatment of patients with body dysmorphic disorder. Psychosomatics 2001; 42:504–10.
84. Crerand CE, Menard M, Phillips KA. Surgical and minimally invasive cosmetic procedures among persons with body dysmorphic disorder. Ann Plast Surg 2010;65:11–6.
85. Carroll BJ, Yendrek R, Degroot C, et al. Response of major depression with psychosis and body dysmorphic disorder to ECT. Am J Psychiatry 1994;151:288–9.
86. Buhlmann U, Winter A. Perceived ugliness: an update on treatment-relevant aspects of body dysmorphic disorder. Curr Psychiatry Rep 2011;13:283–8.
87. Buhlmann U. Treatment barriers for individuals with body dysmorphic disorder: an Internet survey. J Nerv Ment Dis 2011;199:268–71.
88. Marques L, Weingarden HM, LeBlanc NJ, et al. Treatment utilization and barriers to treatment engagement among people with body dysmorphic symptoms. J Psychosom Res 2011;70:286–93.
89. Jain S, Grant JE, Menard W, et al. A chart-review study of SRI continuation treatment versus discontinuation in body dysmorphic disorder. Abstracts, National Institute of Mental Health NCDEU 44th Annual Meeting; Phoenix (AZ), June, 2004. p. 231.

# Diagnosis, Evaluation, and Management of Trichotillomania

Douglas W. Woods, PhD*, David C. Houghton, MS

## KEYWORDS

- Trichotillomania • Diagnosis • Obsessive-compulsive spectrum disorders
- Body-focused repetitive behaviors

## KEY POINTS

- Trichotillomania (TTM) is a fairly common condition that primarily affects women.
- TTM has multiple possible causes.
- A multimodal, multi-informant strategy should be used in the assessment of TTM.
- Effective pharmacologic treatments exist for adults with TTM, but more evidence is needed.
- Effective behavior therapies exist for those with TTM, but long-term maintenance is unclear.

## NATURE OF THE PROBLEM

TTM, or hairpulling disorder, is characterized by the repeated removal (or pulling) of hair from the body, resulting in significant hair loss. Estimates of the prevalence and gender distribution of this disorder vary due to changing diagnostic criteria, but recent prevalence studies suggest that TTM occurs in 0.6% to 3.6% of adults.[1] Furthermore, up to 11.03% of college-aged individuals pull their hair at least occasionally,[2] and many young children display hairpulling, although the behavior usually spontaneously remits by the time a child reaches 4 or 5 years of age.

TTM is generally more common in women than in men, but there are some discrepancies. Most research has shown that the gender ratio is skewed towards women at a 9:1 ratio,[3] but other studies have shown little or no gender difference.[4,5] A significant

Funding: The writing of this paper was supported by the National Institute of Mental Health of the National Institutes of Health under award number R01MH080966 to Dr. Woods. The content is solely the responsibility of the authors and does not necessarily represent the official views of the National Institutes of Health.
Disclosures: D.W. Woods receives royalties from Oxford University Press, Guilford Press, and Springer Press.
Department of Psychology, Texas A&M University, 4235 TAMU, College Station, TX 77843, USA
* Corresponding author.
E-mail address: dowoods@tamu.edu

| Abbreviations | |
|---|---|
| BDD | Body dysmorphic disorder |
| BFRB | Body-focused repetitive behavior |
| DSM | Diagnostic and Statistical Manual of Mental Disorders |
| HRT | Habit reversal training |
| MIST-A | Milwaukee Inventory for Styles of Trichotillomania–Adult Version |
| MIST-C | Milwaukee Inventory for Styles of Trichotillomania–Child Version |
| NAC | N-acetylcysteine |
| NIMH | National Institute of Mental Health |
| OCD | Obsessive-compulsive disorder |
| SCID | Structured Clinical Interview for DSM-IV |
| SPECT | Single-photon emission CT |
| SSRI | Selective serotonin reuptake inhibitor |
| TIS | Trichotillomania Impairment Scale |
| TSS | Trichotillomania Severity Scale |
| TTM | Trichotillomania |
| Y-BOCS-TM | Yale-Brown Obsessive Compulsive Scale–Trichotillomania |

number of people struggle with hairpulling at some point in their lifetime, with not all developing full-fledged TTM. In clinical samples, TTM most commonly manifests at approximately 13 years of age,[6] and a majority of individuals display a chronic but fluctuating course.[7] Community samples show similar epidemiology, but some have suggested that previous diagnostic criteria (eg, Diagnostic and Statistical Manual of Mental Disorders [Fourth Edition, Text Revision] [DSM-IV-TR]) excluded many individuals with hairpulling problems.[5]

Many who suffer from TTM experience shame, struggle with low self-esteem, and report repeated efforts to conceal hair loss. Individuals with TTM often avoid pulling in social situations and prefer to pull when alone or when engaged in sedentary activities, illustrating the ability to suppress pulling to avoid stigma. Creating a vicious circle, negative affective experiences, such as stress and anxiety, often exacerbate pulling.

Beyond the obvious cosmetic and social consequences of hairpulling,[5] the disorder is frequently associated with functional deficits. For example, a large Internet-based survey (N = 1697) on the effects of TTM found that persons with TTM suffered mild to moderate life impairment in many functional domains.[8] Compounding this problem, many medical and psychological practitioners possess inadequate knowledge about the disorder and its effective treatment,[9] resulting in clients reporting they often receive uninformed and ineffective care.[8] Significant portions of people with TTM avoid social and recreational activities, and TTM interferes with occupational duties at least once a month (eg, failing to pursue promotions or avoiding job interviews). Likewise, mild to moderate difficulties in academic functioning are evident, including school absences, difficulties in performing school responsibilities, and difficulty studying. Finally, psychological interference from TTM is evident in 3 domains: alcohol and substance abuse to cope with the effects of the disorder, TTM symptoms leading to the development of other emotional problems, and elevated levels of anxiety, depression, and stress. Overall, adults with TTM[8] report mild to moderate perceived functional disability across work, social, and family domains.

### Clinical Features

Early conceptualizations portrayed TTM as highly mechanistic and simple,[10–16] but more recent accounts differ by highlighting the behavioral heterogeneity and diverse phenomenology found in clinical cases.[7,17]

The method by which individuals remove hair differs between individuals. Most commonly, the hands, in particular, the thumb and forefinger, are used to remove the hair. Tweezers and other cosmetic devices however, are sometimes used. Typically, 1 or 2 hairs are pulled at a time, and multiple hairs can be pulled out during a pulling episode. The most common site from which pulling occurs is the scalp, followed by the eyebrows/eyelashes. Pubic hair, once believed a rare site of pulling, is now understood to be common in those with TTM.[8]

Rituals and behavioral patterns often precede pulling, such as combing through the hair, feeling individual hairs, tugging at hairs, and visually searching the scalp and hairline. Hairs may not be pulled at random but can be chosen based on specific characteristics (eg, hairs with certain lengths, colors, or textures or placement on the hairline).

Postpulling behavior is also clinically relevant and idiosyncratic. Although some individuals simply discard pulled hairs, others may play with the hair between their fingers, inspect the hair, bite the hair between the teeth, or ingest all or parts of the hair. Ingesting hairs can result in undigested masses of hair, called trichobezoars, which can potentially cause gastrointestinal injuries.[18] Clinicians should carefully assess whether clients eat pulled hairs and seek referral to a gastroenterologist if symptoms, such as abdominal pain, nausea, vomiting, and constipation, are present. If left untreated, trichobezoars can cause bowel obstruction, intestinal bleeding, acute pacreatitis, obstructive jaundice, or a perforated bowel.[18,19]

The environmental and affective context surrounding pulling should also be noted. Situational variables that often increase pulling include watching television, reading a book, doing homework, and grooming in front of the mirror.[20] Many people report specific emotional states (eg, stress or anxiety), a sense of tension, or an urge to pull that precedes an episode, which in turn is alleviated after pulling.[8]

Recent research has illuminated several distinct pulling styles of TTM, which may correspond to specific triggering factors. Christenson and colleagues[6] showed that a small percentage of people with TTM pulled only either completely outside of their awareness or when completely focused on pulling, but most (80%) engaged in both styles of pulling at different times. Christenson and Mackenzie[21] designated these 2 pulling styles as "automatic" and "focused." Automatic pulling is performed out of conscious awareness, often when engaged in a sedentary task. Individuals engaged in automatic pulling sometimes do not become aware of it until they later notice the consequences (eg, a pile of hairs on the ground or a new bald spot). Conversely, focused pulling seems to be a purposeful process. Examples of focused pulling include doing so because pulling feels pleasurable, reduces stress, removes hairs that look "out of place," or removes hairs deemed by some physical characteristic to be good for pulling. It has been suggested that focused pulling may constitute an attempt to regulate affect and/or aversive cognitions.[22,23] As discussed previously, most individuals with TTM display both styles in separate contexts.

### Diagnostic Criteria

TTM (hairpulling disorder) is listed in the *DSM* (Fifth Edition) (*DSM-5*)[24] under the new category of obsessive-compulsive disorders (OCDs) and related disorders. Additionally, 2 criteria were removed in the new edition. *DSM-IV-TR* required that those with TTM experience a preceding urge to pull hair that is subsequently relieved after pulling or have increased tension when attempting to refrain from pulling.[25] In the *DSM-5* revision process, however, it was argued that these criteria excluded many with significant hairpulling-related issues.[26] The current diagnostic system for TTM requires 5 criteria.

Criterion A requires that the person purposefully remove hair from any region of the body. Pulling may be associated with 1 or multiple sites. Although some may pull hairs in a concentrated area, resulting in easily identifiable bald spots, others may distribute their pulling over a larger area, causing thinning of the hair. The latter is more difficult to identify, and sometimes a distributed pattern of pulling is done purposefully to conceal hair loss.

Criteria B and C require an individual to have attempted to decrease or stop pulling and that the pulling causes significant distress or impairment in at least 1 important area of functioning. Many individuals pluck hair for cosmetic purposes, so TTM should not be diagnosed if attempts to stop have not been made and if the behavior does not cause significant distress or functional problems.

Criteria D and E are used to differentiate the main features of TTM with other medical and psychological conditions that might explain hairpulling or alopecia. These are discussed later.

### Comorbidities

Although TTM alone can cause problems, those with the disorder tend to have at least 1 comorbid diagnosis, which most often involves mood or anxiety disorders.[1,23,27] A clinical sample within a treatment study reported common co-occurring major depression (28.6%) and OCD (10.7%).[23] One study reported that more than one-third of adults with TTM sought treatment of another psychological disorder, with mood and anxiety disorders the most frequent of those complaints.[8] In children with TTM, it has been shown that 38.3% to 39.1% of treatment seekers had at least 1 comorbid diagnosis, with the most common being generalized anxiety, depression, social phobia, OCD, attention-deficit/hyperactivity disorder, and oppositional defiant disorder.[28,29] In another study, 23.6% of young children with TTM endorsed at least 1 diagnosis of an anxiety disorder, attention-deficit/hyperactivity disorder, OCD, a mood disorder, and a tic disorder,[30] whereas another found frequent co-occurring developmental problems, chronic pediatric concerns, and family stressors.[31]

Other common comorbidities include skin picking (excoriation) and other body-focused repetitive behaviors (BFRBs) (eg, nail and cheek biting). Skin picking and hairpulling share many phenomenological characteristics and have higher than expected comorbidity rates.[32] Additionally, Stein and colleagues[26] reported that 70% of persons with TTM have another BFRB, most frequently skin picking and nail biting. Excoriation disorder is located within the same category as TTM in the *DSM-5*, but nail and cheek biting are currently only diagnosable under the "Other Specified Obsessive-Compulsive and Related Disorder" category followed by the specifier of "body-focused repetitive behavior disorder."[24] These other BFRBs seem to have the same clinical features as TTM apart from the locus of the behavior being another physical target.

### ETIOLOGY

Various etiologic factors are believed to have an impact on the emergence and/or maintenance of TTM. Animal models and findings from fields of human neuroimaging, neurochemistry, and neuropsychology are discussed.

### Animal Models

Animal analogues to TTM have been used to try to understand the underlying pathology of the disorder. Many of these have focused on the neuroscience of habits and stereotypies as correlated constructs to hairpulling.[33,34] Several animal grooming behaviors have been put forth at models of TTM, including fur pulling,[35] barbering,[36,37] and feather picking.[38–42] Although animal models may eventually provide useful data regarding the pathologic processes discussed previously, there is still a large gap between these speculations and what is actually known about TTM.

## Imaging

Neuroimaging studies investigating the structure and function of TTM pathology have targeted areas that are known to be involved in OCD.[43] Although the literature on the neuroanatomic structure and function of TTM is sparse and does not offer clear conclusions about the disorder's etiology, what is known from imaging research about TTM is reviewed.

Several imaging studies have focused on structures known to be related to motor control, motor learning, and reward learning. One study, using MR imaging, found no differences in caudate volumes between TTM cases and controls.[44] Other studies found reduced left inferior frontal gyrus and left putamen volumes and increased right cuneal cortex volumes in those with TTM versus controls (n = 10 per group).[45,46] Another study found that TTM patients (n = 14) had smaller cerebellar volumes than controls (n = 12).[47]

More recently, several studies have examined whether there are abnormalities in neural circuitry in those with TTM. In a sample of comorbidity-free patients, Chamberlain and colleagues[48] found increased gray matter densities in brain regions involving affect regulation, motor habits, and top-down cognition in those with TTM (n = 18) compared with controls (n = 19). Furthermore, another study using diffusion tensor imaging found reduced integrity in white matter density within the anterior cingulate, presupplementary motor area, and temporal cortices in those with TTM (n = 18) versus controls (n = 19).[49] Such results are consistent with findings in OCD, where white matter density was abnormal in the frontal-striatal-thalamic pathways.[50] In the study done by Chamberlain and colleagues, fractional anisotrophy did not, however, predict TTM severity. Only recently have researchers demonstrated that mean diffusivity of white matter in the frontal-striatal-thalamic pathway was significantly correlated with longer TTM duration and increased TTM severity.[51] These results provide initial support for functional abnormalities in the brains of those with TTM regarding the processing and learning of sensorimotor functions.

Studies on possible functional deficits have used positron emission tomography, single-photon emission CT (SPECT), and functional MR imaging methods.[43] Using positron emission tomography, Swedo and colleagues[52] found that patients with TTM (n = 10) had higher resting cerebral glucose metabolic rates in the bilateral cerebellum and right parietal cortex relative to controls (n = 20). Additionally, a qualitative study on identical twins with TTM (n = 2) showed decreased perfusion of the temporal lobes during SPECT, with the more severely affected twin displaying more extensive temporal involvement.[53] Another study found that serotonin reuptake inhibitor treatment of TTM (n = 10) was associated with significant decreases in symptom severity and reduced activity in frontal cortical regions, the left putamen, and right anterior temporal lobe as measured by SPECT.[54] Finally, one study used functional MR imaging to measure brain activity during an implicit sequence-learning task and found no differences between those with TTM and controls.[55]

## Neurochemistry

Several neurotransmitter and neuropeptide systems have been thought to contribute to TTM pathology. Unfortunately, most of this evidence has been informed by looking at treatment response to medications designed to have an impact on these symptoms. Nonetheless, the literature on several molecular systems that have been implicated in the disorder is reviewed.

Much of the molecular research on TTM has focused on the monoaminergic systems (eg, the serotonin, dopamine, and norepinephrine systems). Swedo and colleagues[56] showed that clomipramine significantly reduced symptoms of TTM relative to desipramine, providing support for involvement of the serotonergic system. There is evidence in animal models that the dopamine system plays a significant role in stereotypic and grooming behaviors,[33,34,57,58] and stereotypic behaviors, such as hairpulling, have been shown to increase after a dosage of dopaminergic agonists[59] and decrease in response to dopamine blockers.[60–63] The norepinephrine system is understudied in TTM, but some investigators have suggested that the stop-signal response deficiency in patients with TTM is demonstrative of norepinephrine system involvement.[43] There is currently no study to the authors' knowledge that shows a treatment response for norepinephrine agents in TTM.

The limited research on the glutamate system has resulted in reports of TTM responding to N-acetylcysteine (NAC).[64,65] A placebo-controlled trial of this amino acid for adults with TTM yielded significant reductions in hairpulling symptoms,[66] although it was found ineffective in children.[67] The investigators of the adult trial suggested that NAC affects glutamate interactions in the nucleus accumbens, thereby reducing repetitive behaviors.

### Neuropsychological and Cognitive-Affective Variables

Some investigators have proposed that neuropsychological deficits play a role in the pathology of TTM. Little evidence has been shown for increased neurologic soft signs in TTM patients,[68] but Chamberlain and colleagues[43] noted several specific impairments seen in certain neuropsychological tasks in persons with TTM. For example, TTM patients performed poorly on a stop-signal task, which is thought to measure motor inhibitory control, yet displayed no abnormalities on a task assessing cognitive flexibility compared with persons with OCD.[69]

Cognitive-affective neuroscience has proposed relevant processes in the pathology of TTM, particularly those involved in the interaction with aversive stimuli (both internal and external), reward-driven repetitive behaviors, and disrupted control of behavior. Hairpulling behavior can be driven by different types of negative affect, such as high negative arousal (eg, stress) and insufficient levels of arousal (eg, boredom).[70] In TTM, hairpulling can be performed in response to negative affect, leading to emotional relief in the short term at the expense of strengthening pulling in the long term.

In addition to the pulling that is reinforced by the relief of negative affect, a process common in obsessive-compulsive–related disorders, Lochner and colleagues[71] noted that hairpulling is often pleasurable and showed that OCD and comorbid TTM often cluster together with pathologic gambling and hypersexual behavior. As such, TTM may involve a pathologic response to reward from both simple motor and complex stereotypic behaviors.

Disruption of control has also been proposed as a causal mechanism in disorders with varying degrees of motor dysfunction (eg, Tourette syndome, OCD, and TTM). There has been a growing interest in control mechanisms involved in both simple motor acts and executive decision making, leading some to the notion that disorders of unwanted repetitive behaviors constitute a compulsive-impulsive spectrum of disorders.[72]

### PATIENT EVALUATION OVERVIEW

Because TTM often occurs in private, is concealable, and could have numerous etiologies, a comprehensive, multimodal, multi-informant assessment is important. The various forms of TTM assessment are discussed.

## Physical Examination

Hairpulling usually results in patches of hair loss that are irregularly shaped and contain many broken hairs with different lengths. In some cases, TTM patients also pick at the skin around the hair follicles, resulting in inflammation and erythema. Dermatologic assessment begins with examining the type of hair loss to determine whether it is scarring or nonscarring. If the hair follicles are not permanently damaged and the follicular openings can be seen, the loss is nonscarring and the hair grows back once pulling remits.[73] Scarring occurs when the follicles are permanently damaged from constant stress and removal. In this case, the follicle openings are covered in scar tissue and the hair will not resume normal growth.[73] Mostaghimi[73] offers a detailed description of other conditions causing hair loss that should be differentiated from TTM.

## Diagnostic Interview

During the clinical interview, TTM can be assessed using a semistructured diagnostic interview. Major interviews, such as the Structured Clinical Interview for *DSM-IV* (SCID[74]) do not assess for TTM, but the Trichotillomania Diagnostic Interview[75] is a semistructured diagnostic inventory that corresponds to *DSM-IV-TR* criteria. Currently, there is no validated measure that aligns with *DSM-5* criteria. Lochner and colleagues,[76] however, used a questionnaire adapted from the SCID-I/P[77] that included additional questions addressing *DSM-5* criteria.

## Behavioral Assessment

TTM severity can be assessed by measuring hair loss (eg, photograph ratings, measuring bald spots, and collecting pulled hair), but this approach has challenges.[78] First, patients sometimes are reluctant to allow a clinician to examine or photograph areas from which they pull. Second, the process of collecting these types of data may increase the sense of shame already experienced by the patient. Third, the reliability and validity of these types of measures for TTM have not been extensively evaluated aside from inter-rater reliability, which has been found strong.[79] For these reasons, product measures are not often used in favor of self- or clinician-completed measures.

Another key approach to assessing TTM involves conducting a functional assessment of hairpulling. A functional assessment assumes that all behavior is tied to its antecedents (ie, the events preceding a behavior) and consequences (ie, the events following the behavior). Antecedents to hairpulling can be external (eg, settings or events that become temporally associated with pulling) or internal (eg, cognitions, emotions, or physical sensations that precede pulling). Consequences of pulling can be punishing (eg, the loss of hair and/or feeling of ugliness) or reinforcing (eg, the pleasurable physical sensation of pulling or control over negative emotions or aversive cognitions). Although not used as a measure of symptom improvement, the functional assessment aids in understanding factors that influence how and when a person pulls and ultimately guides treatment planning.

## Clinician Rating Scales

### National Institute of Mental Health Trichotillomania Scales

This semistructured clinical interview is composed of 2 separate clinical indices: the National Institute of Mental Health Trichotillomania Severity Scale (NIMH-TSS) and Trichotillomania Impairment Scale (NIMH-TIS).[56] The NIMH-TSS asks 5 questions regarding several key features of TTM: time spent pulling in the past week, time spent pulling the previous day, degree of resistance to pulling urges, distress associated with pulling, and functional impairment. Each question has scores ranging from 0 to 5, resulting in a total score of 0 to 25, with greater scores reflecting a greater level of symptom severity. The NIMH-TSS has demonstrated adequate psychometric properties in adults[79] and acceptable reliability in children.[80] The NIMH-TIS consists of 1 item and has scores ranging from 0 to 10, with greater scores reflecting greater impairment. It has demonstrated good inter-rater reliability and convergent validity in adult samples.[56,79,81]

### Yale-Brown Obsessive-Compulsive Scale–Trichotillomania

The Yale-Brown Obsessive-Compulsive Scale–Trichotillomania (Y-BOCS-TM) is a 10-item clinician-rated scale that is based on the Y-BOCS and measures hairpulling severity.[81,82] Scores on the individual items range from 0 to 5, resulting in a total severity score ranging from 0 to 50. There are 2 subscales: intrusive thoughts regarding hairpulling and actual pulling behaviors. The Y-BOCS-TM has demonstrated variable psychometrics in adult samples, as evidenced by low internal consistency, fair to excellent inter-rater reliability, adequate test-retest reliability, and mixed convergent validity.[81,82] Despite the moderately acceptable psychometric properties, the Y-BOCS-TM has been successfully used to assess progress in treatment outcome studies.[63,83]

### The Psychiatric Institute Trichotillomania Scale

The Psychiatric Institute Trichotillomania Scale is a semistructured clinician-administered scale that measures the number of body sites used for pulling, extent of hair loss, time spent pulling hair, resistance to urges, negative affect, and functional impairment.[84] It has 6 items that are scored on a 0 to 7 scale, resulting in possible scores from 0 to 42. The psychometric data are mixed, with low internal consistency, good inter-rater reliability, and acceptable convergent validity.[79,81,84] There are no published data on test-retest reliability or discriminant validity.

### Patient Rating Scales

### Massachusetts General Hospital Hairpulling Scale

The Massachusetts General Hospital Hairpulling Scale is one of the most widely used self-report measures of TTM, possessing satisfactory psychometric properties.[79,85,86] It consists of 2 factors: *Severity* and *Resistance and Control*.[87] The Massachusetts General Hospital Hairpulling Scale consists of 7 items that are scored on 5-point Likert scale, with higher scores indicating greater symptom severity. The scale is particularly useful in documenting change in symptoms throughout treatment.

### Trichotillomania Scale for Children

The Trichotillomania Scale for Children is a self-report questionnaire that measures clinical features of hairpulling in children and adolescents.[88] There are child and parent versions, both containing 15 items that are evenly divided into 3 subscales: severity, distress, and impairment. Items are scored on a 0 to 2 scale, with higher numbers reflecting more severe symptoms. Two independent studies have shown promising psychometric properties.[88,89]

### The Milwaukee Inventory for Styles of Trichotillomania–Adult Version and Child Version

The Milwaukee Inventory for Styles of Trichotillomania–Adult Version (MIST-A) and Child Version (MIST-C) were developed to assess different pulling styles in both adults and children.[20,90] The investigators labeled these pulling styles, *focused* and *automatic*. Exploratory factor analysis on the MIST-A revealed a 2-factor solution, including a focused factor and an automatic factor. Similar analyses on the MIST-C showed the same factor structure. Both scales demonstrated adequate internal consistency and good construct and discriminant validity. Further research revealed significant differences between pulling styles, such as high automatic pulling associated with greater stress and high focused pulling associated with higher TTM severity, depression, and functional impact.[91]

## DIAGNOSTIC DILEMMAS

It is important to understand other psychological conditions that can be confused with TTM. At first glance, some of these conditions have similar behavioral patterns but differ in terms of the function of hairpulling and appropriate treatment.

TTM, OCD, and other problematic repetitive behaviors have been conceptualized under the umbrella of obsessive-compulsive spectrum disorders. Thus, it will not come as a surprise that TTM and OCD can be difficult to distinguish. There are several differences, however, between TTM and OCD. First, persons with TTM often derive pleasure from hairpulling whereas those with OCD do not usually find pleasure during the performance of ritualistic behaviors. Second, TTM typically lacks the unwanted, intrusive, and repetitive thoughts preceding the behavior that are characteristic of OCD.[82,92] Third, there is a tendency for individuals with TTM to only perform 1 repetitive behavior as opposed to the multiple and complex rituals that are characteristic of OCD.[92] Finally, TTM and OCD tend to differ in their responsiveness to selective serotonin reuptake inhibitors (SSRIs),[93] with OCD showing positive response and TTM showing no response.

Body dysmorphic disorder (BDD) can also be difficult to differentiate from TTM. People with BDD tend to pull exclusively to "fix" a perceived physical defect (eg, hairline symmetry), whereas those with TTM tend to lack a cognitive fixation on hair-related cosmetic issues (except in advanced cases of TTM, where the concern is on the hair loss). Although individuals with TTM may report pulling hairs that they believe are "out of place" or "don't look right," this type of pulling is subsumed under a larger pattern of pulling that is reinforced by physical gratification rather than a cognitive fixation.[8] Another easily identifiable difference is that individuals with BDD pull because they believe doing so will make them more physically attractive, whereas those with TTM are frequently embarrassed or ashamed at the results of their hairpulling.

Neurodevelopmental disorders, such as autism spectrum disorder and stereotypic movement disorder, can also include repetitive hairpulling. In TTM, however, hairpulling may seem driven, but unlike stereotypies, it is not purposeless, and the movements are not always rhythmic. Also, neurodevelopmental disorders manifest during early childhood, whereas TTM often emerges later.[24]

Some investigators have noted that disorders involving affect regulation and self-injurious behaviors (eg, borderline personality disorder [BPD]) can have features similar to TTM.[78] Although there are surface similarities, in that self-injury and pulling may regulate emotion and lead to noticeable physical damage, there are important differences between the two conditions. First, individuals engaging in self-injurious behavior often do so to purposely experience pain,[94] whereas individuals with TTM do not generally experience this phenomenon. Second, self-injury tends to be more episodic compared with pulling, which is more habitual in nature.[95]

## TREATMENT
### Management Goals

The goals of treatment of TTM are left to individual patients. For some, complete abstinence from pulling is the goal, whereas for others, a significant reduction in the frequency of pulling combined with significant hair growth is an acceptable outcome. In any case, patients should understand that the focus of treatment, both biological and behavioral, is that the disorder is effectively managed but not necessarily cured.

Multiple reviews of treatment efficacy in TTM have been published in the past decade.[96–98] As a result, a thorough review is not conducted in this article, but a summary of the evidence supporting the efficacy of various treatments for TTM is presented.

### Pharmacologic Treatments

The most commonly prescribed class of medication for adults with TTM is the SSRIs.[8] In a meta-analysis of pharmacologic treatment studies, however, SSRIs failed to beat the pill placebo condition.[96] Clomipramine has demonstrated some moderate effectiveness over placebo, but the pharmacologic agent with the strongest empirical support in adults with TTM is the amino acid NAC. Grant and colleagues[66] found that 56% of those receiving NAC were treatment responders compared with 16% in the placebo condition. In addition, the data showed that NAC had few side effects. Unfortunately, a recent replication of the study in children was negative.[67] Overall, despite the high utilization rate as a treatment of TTM, evidence supporting the use of pharmacotherapy to treat TTM is scarce.

### Nonpharmacologic Treatments

Nearly all treatments for TTM with strong empirical support for their efficacy contain 2 primary elements: habit reversal training (HRT) and stimulus control. Although these elements are described in detail elsewhere,[99] a brief description of each is provided.

Stimulus control involves identifying situational factors that trigger pulling or sensory factors that maintain pulling and then teaching the patient to eliminate, reduce contact with, or otherwise modify these factors in a way that reduces pulling. For example, many people with TTM pull in front of mirrors or when bright lights are on in their bathroom. Stimulus control interventions include covering or removing mirrors and replacing bright bulbs with dimmer lights. Likewise, pulling may occur when sitting on a couch with an arm on the armrest. A simple stimulus control intervention may involve teaching a patient to sit in the middle of a couch so the hand is not as close to the head. Stimulus control interventions also include the modification of sensory stimuli. For example, people with TTM often receive tactile reinforcement by rolling the recently pulled hair between the fingers. As a way to modify this sensory input, the person with TTM may be encouraged to put bandages on the fingers they use to pull. By engaging in these stimulus control interventions, the response effort used to pull becomes greater, triggers to pull are reduced, and the sensory reinforcement for pulling is attenuated. All these factors can help reduce the pulling.

HRT is a behavioral treatment of several repetitive behaviors.[13,100] HRT involves 3 primary elements: awareness training, competing response training, and social support. Awareness training involves developing, with the patient, a detailed description of the pulling episode. After response description takes place, the patient is taught, in session, to acknowledge every time his or her hand begins to move toward the location of the pulling. If the patient correctly acknowledges this, he or she is praised by the therapist, and if the patient fails to notice, the therapist points it out. This awareness exercise continues until the patient is highly aware of the pulling activity.

After awareness is enhanced, the patient is taught to do a behavior that physically prevents the pulling from occurring. This is called the competing response, and the patient is asked to do the competing response whenever he or she notices pulling has started or when it is about to start. Patients are encouraged to do the competing response for 1 minute whenever either of these two events occurs. A typical competing response for hairpulling is to make a fist.

To provide encouragement to use the competing response, a social support person is typically identified and asked to help the patient in two ways. First, the support person is asked to remind the patient to use the competing response, when the patient fails to use the competing response correctly. Second, the support person is asked to genuinely praise the patient if he or she sees the patient use the competing response correctly.

There is strong evidence that the combination of stimulus control and HRT is an effective treatment of TTM.[101] There are also notable limitations. First, evidence suggests that although pulling can be reduced, the negative emotional experiences that often trigger pulling are not necessarily reduced,[8] thus leaving patients potentially vulnerable to a focused style of pulling. Second, and perhaps related, there is growing evidence that long-term maintenance of treatment gains is less than ideal. For these reasons, and because of a growing understanding that TTM often involves both automatic and focused styles, researchers have begun to incorporate additional treatment components addressing the aspects of pulling that deal with emotion regulation.

Twohig and Woods[102] and Woods and colleagues[23] incorporated stimulus control and HRT components into an acceptance-based treatment designed to teach patients to mindfully accept unpleasant urges, emotions, cognitions, and sensory experiences rather than react to them in a controlling fashion. Evidence from these initial studies were promising and showed that this acceptance-enhanced behavior therapy for TTM reduced both pulling severity and co-ocurring psychiatric symptoms while generally maintaining treatment gains at the 3-month follow-up. Similarly, Keuthen and colleagues[103] used dialectical behavior therapy, a treatment focused on teaching patients to regulate their emotion more effectively and demonstrated the superiority of dialectical behavior therapy over a minimal attention control condition.[103] In a review of all treatments of TTM, Bloch and colleagues[96] found that behavior therapy was the most effective intervention for TTM.

## SUMMARY

TTM is a poorly understood disorder that requires extensive empirical investigation. Despite what is known about TTM, those with the disorder report not receiving adequate treatment from medical professionals.[8] The information presented in this review, however, can help provide the tools to accurately diagnose and educate people about the causes and treatments for TTM.

Diagnosis starts with a thorough clinical interview and functional assessment. Building a comprehensive understanding of how hairpulling functions for an individual is paramount, particularly in consideration of the diverse phenomenology and behavioral heterogeneity of the disorder. Additionally, a physical examination of pulling sites and alopecia is recommended to differentiate TTM with unrelated dermatologic and medical conditions. As discussed previously, there are several useful measures for diagnosing the disorder, determining the severity of the symptoms, assessing functioning impairment, and tracking treatment progress.

Research has given preliminary insights to the neuroanatomical underpinnings of TTM. Such structures include the basal ganglia, prefrontal cortex, and midbrain. Existing neuroimaging data on TTM do not provide systematic conclusions regarding etiology, but the burgeoning research could eventually lead to innovative early diagnostic modalities and detection systems for all obsessive-compulsive spectrum disorders.

Several pathologic mechanisms have been implicated for their role in TTM, including cognitive-affective processes, neuropsychological deficits, and neurotransmitter systems. It seems that sensorimotor skill deficits exist in TTM patients, but the extent of understanding is still limited. Some investigators have used psychoactive medications to treat TTM with success, but research provides little more than speculative offerings toward the efficacy of these approaches.

Diagnostic approaches to TTM must consider the phenomenological similarity of other psychological disorders, in particular OCD and BDD. Careful inquiries regarding the cognitions and environmental contexts associated with pulling should allow clinicians to determine a proper diagnosis. Additionally, they should be careful to screen for other disorders that can either rule out or complicate a TTM diagnosis. The physical examination of hair loss should rule out any medical explanations and confirm TTM to be the cause. Finally, TTM often co-occurs with other BFRBs (eg, skin picking and nail biting). Assessing for these common comorbidities may prevent a harmful behavior from going unnoticed (as one may be more salient than the other) and allow for simultaneous treatment to be considered.

Although evidence exists for the use of NAC as a pharmacologic treatment of TTM, effective management should also involve some form of behavior therapy, incorporating the elements of HRT and stimulus control. In adults with the condition, it is likely beneficial to add components designed to help patients learn effective emotion regulation skills.

## REFERENCES

1. Christenson GA, Pyle RL, Mitchell JE. Estimate lifetime prevalence of trichotillomania in college students. J Clin Psychiatry 1991;52(10):415–7.
2. Hajcak G, Franklin ME, Simon RF, et al. Hairpulling and skin picking in relation to affective distress and obsessive-compulsive symptoms. J Psychopathol Behav Assess 2006;28:177–85.
3. Christenson GA. Trichotillomania: from prevalence to comorbidity. Psychiatry Times 1995;12:44–8.
4. Reeve E. Hair pulling in children and adolescents. In: Stein DJ, Christenson GA, Hollander E, editors. Trichotillomania. Washington, DC: American Psychiatric Press; 1999. p. 201–24.
5. Duke DC, Bozdin DK, Tavares P, et al. The phenomenology of hairpulling in a community sample. J Anxiety Disord 2009;23(8):1118–25.
6. Christenson GA, Mackenzie TB, Mitchell JE. Characteristics of 60 adults chronic hair pullers. Am J Psychiatry 1991;148:365–70.
7. Flessner CA, Woods DW, Franklin ME, et al. Cross-sectional study of women with trichotillomania: a preliminary examination of pulling styles, severity, phenomenology, and functional impact. Child Psychiatry Hum Dev 2009;40:153–67.
8. Woods DW, Flessner CA, Franklin ME, et al. The trichotillomania impact project (tip): exploring phenomenology, functional impairment, and treatment utilization. J Clin Psychiatry 2006;67:1877–88.
9. Marcks BA, Wetterneck CT, Woods DW. Investigating healthcare providers' knowledge of trichotillomania and its treatment. Cogn Behav Ther 2006;35(1):19–27.
10. Greenberg HR, Sarner CA. Trichotillomania: symptom and syndrome. Arch Gen Psychiatry 1965;12(5):482–9.
11. Delgado RA, Mannino FV. Some observations on trichotillomania in children. J Am Acad Child Psychiatry 1969;8(2):229–46.

12. Jonas AD. The importance of counterirritation in trichotillomania. Am J Psychiatry 1970;126(8):1184–5.
13. Azrin NH, Nunn RG. Habit control: stuttering, nailbiting, hairpulling, and tics. New York: Simon & Schuster; 1977.
14. Chauhan S, Jain RK, Dhir GG. Trichotillomania: a phenomenological study. Indian J Clin Psychol 1985;12(2):47–50.
15. Dawber R. Self-inflicted hair loss. Semin Dermatol 1985;4:53–7.
16. Muller SA. Trichotillomania: a histopathologic study in sixty-six patients. J Am Acad Dermatol 1990;23(1):56–62.
17. O'Sullivan RL, Mansueto CS, Lerner EA, et al. Characterization of trichotillomania: a phenomenological model with clinical relevance to obsessive-compulsive spectrum disorders. Psychiatr Clin North Am 2000;23(3):587–604.
18. Bouwer C, Stein DJ. Trichobezoars in trichotillomania: case report and literature overview. Psychosom Med 1998;60:658–60.
19. Muller SA. Trichotillomania. Dermatol Clin 1987;5:595–601.
20. Flessner CA, Woods DW, Franklin ME, et al. The Milwaukee inventory for styles of trichotillomania-child version (MIST-C): initial development and psychometric properties. Behav Modif 2007;31:896–918.
21. Christenson GA, Mackenzie TB. Trichotillomania. In: Hersen M, Ammerman RT, editors. Handbook of prescriptive treatment for adults. New York: Plenum Press; 1994. p. 217–35.
22. Begotka AM, Woods DW, Wetterneck CT. The relationship between experiential avoidance and the severity of trichotillomania in a nonreferred sample. J Behav Ther Exp Psychiatry 2004;35:17–24.
23. Woods DW, Wetterneck CT, Flessner CA. A controlled evaluation of acceptance and commitment therapy plus habit reversal as a treatment for trichotillomania. Behav Res Ther 2006;44:639–56.
24. American Psychiatric Association. Diagnostic and statistical manual of mental disorders. 5th edition. Washington, DC: American Psychiatric Publishing; 2013.
25. American Psychiatric Association. Diagnostic and statistical manual of mental disorders. 4th edition. Washington, DC: American Psychiatric Publishing; 2000.
26. Stein DJ, Grant JE, Frankling ME, et al. Trichotillomania (hair pulling disorder), skin picking disorder, and stereotypic movement disorder: toward DSM-V. Depress Anxiety 2010;27:611–26.
27. Diefenbach GJ, Mouton-Odum S, Stanley MA. Affective correlates of trichotillomania. Behav Res Ther 2002;40:1305–15.
28. Franklin ME, Flessner CA, Woods DW, et al. The child and adolescent trichotillomania impact project: descriptive psychopathology, comorbidity, functional impairment, and treatment utilization. J Dev Behav Pediatr 2008;29:493–500.
29. Tolin DF, Franklin ME, Diefenbach GJ, et al. Pediatric trichotillomania: descriptive psychopathology and an open trial of cognitive behavior therapy. Cogn Behav Ther 2007;36:129–44.
30. Walther MR, Snorrason I, Flessner CA, et al. The trichotillomania impact project in young children (TIP-YC): clinical characteristics, comorbidity, functional impairment and treatment utilization. Child Psychiatry Hum Dev 2014;45(1): 24–31. http://dx.doi.org/10.1007/s10578-013-0373-y.
31. Wright HH, Holmes GR. Trichotillomania (hair pulling) in toddlers. Psychol Rep 2003;92:228–30.
32. Snorrason I, Belleau EL, Woods DW. How related are hair pulling disorder (trichotillomania) and skin picking disorder? a review of evidence for comorbidity, similarities and shared etiology. Clin Psychol Rev 2012;32(7):618–29.

33. Berridge KC, Aldridge JW, Houchard KR, et al. Sequential super-stereotypy of an instinctive fixed action pattern in hyper- dopaminergic mutant mice: a model of obsessive compulsive disorder and Tourette's. BMC Biol 2005; 3(1):4.
34. Korff S, Stein DJ, Harvey BH. Stereotypic behaviour in the deer mouse: pharmacological validation and relevance for obsessive compulsive disorder. Progr Neuro Psychopharmacol Biol Psychiatr 2008;32(2):348–55.
35. Reinhardt V. Hair pulling: a review. Lab Anim 2005;39(4):361–9.
36. Garner JP, Weisker SM, Dufour B, et al. Barbering (fur and whisker trimming) by laboratory mice as a model of human trichotillomania and obsessive-compulsive spectrum disorders. Comp Med 2004;54:216–24.
37. Kalueff AV, Minasyan A, Keisala T, et al. Hair barbering in mice: implications for neurobehavioural research. Behav Processes 2006;71(1):8–15.
38. Bordnick PS, Thyer BA, Ritchie BW. Feather picking disorder and trichotillomania: an avian model of human psychopathology. J Behav Ther Exp Psychiatry 1994;25:189–96.
39. Garner JP, Meehan CL, Mench JA. Stereotypies in caged parrots, schizophrenia and autism: evidence for a common mechanism. Behav Brain Res 2003;145: 125–34.
40. Grindlinger HM, Ramsay E. Compulsive feather picking in birds. Arch Gen Psychiatry 1991;48:857.
41. Jenkins JR. Feather picking and self-mutilation in psittacine birds. Veterinary Clin North Am Exot Anim Pract 2001;4:651–67.
42. Seibert LM, Crowell-Davis SL, Wilson GH, et al. Placebo- controlled clomipramine trial for the treatment of feather picking disorder in cockatoos. J Am Anim Hosp Assoc 2004;40(4):261–9.
43. Chamberlain SR, Odlaug BL, Boulougouris V, et al. Trichotillomania: neurobiology and treatment. Neurosci Biobehav Rev 2009;33:831–42.
44. Stein DJ, Coetzer R, Lee M, et al. Magnetic resonance imaging in women with obsessive-compulsive disorder and trichotillomania. Psychiatr Res Neuroimaging 1997;74(3):177–82.
45. Grachev ID. MRI-based morphometric topographic parcellation of human neocortex in trichotillomania. Psychiatry Clin Neurosci 1997;51(5):315–21.
46. O'Sullivan RL, Rauch SL, Breiter HC, et al. Reduced basal ganglia volumes in trichotillomania measured via morphometric magnetic resonance imaging. Biol Psychiatry 1997;42(1):39–45.
47. Keuthen NJ, Makris N, Schlerf JE, et al. Evidence for reduced cerebellar volumes in trichotillomania. Biol Psychiatry 2007;61(3):374–81.
48. Chamberlain SR, Menzies LA, Fineberg NA, et al. Grey matter abnormalities in trichotillomania: morphometric magnetic resonance imaging study. Br J Psychiatry 2008;193(3):216–21.
49. Chamberlain SR, Hampshire A, Menzies LA, et al. Reduced brain white matter integrity in trichotillomania: a diffusion tensor imaging study. Arch Gen Psychiatry 2010;67(9):965–71.
50. Menzies L, Williams GB, Chamberlain SR, et al. White matter abnormalities in patients with obsessive-compulsive disorder and their first-degree relatives. Am J Psychiatry 2008;165:1308–15.
51. Roos A, Fouche JP, Stein DJ, et al. White matter integrity in hair-pulling disorder (trichotillomania). Psychiatr Res Neuroimaging 2013;211:246–50.
52. Swedo SE, Rapoport JL, Leonard HL, et al. Regional cerebral glucose metabolism of women with trichotillomania. Arch Gen Psychiatry 1991;48(9):828–33.

53. Vythilingum B, Warwick J, van Kradenburg J, et al. SPECT scans in identical twins with trichotillomania. J Neuropsychiatry Clin Neurosci 2002;14(3):340–2.
54. Stein DJ, van Heerden B, Hugo C, et al. Functional brain imaging and pharmacotherapy in trichotillomania: single photon emission computed tomography before and after treatment with selective serotonin reuptake inhibitor cilopram. Progr Neuro Psychopharmacol Biol Psychiatr 2002;26(5):885–90.
55. Rauch SL, Wright CI, Savage CR, et al. Brain activation during implicit sequence learning in individuals with trichotillomania. Psychiatr Res Neuroimaging 2007; 154(3):233–40.
56. Swedo SE, Leonard HL, Rapoport JL, et al. A double-blind comparison of clomipramine and desipramine in in the treatment of trichotillomania (hair pulling). N Engl J Med 1989;321:497–501.
57. Cooper SJ, Dourish CT. Neurobiology of stereotyped behavior. Oxford (United Kingdom): Clarendon Press/Oxford University Press; 1990.
58. Iglauer F, Rasim R. Treatment of psychogenic leather picking in psittacine birds with a dopamine antagonist. J Small Anim Pract 1993;34(11):564–6.
59. Martin A, Scahill L, Vitulano L, et al. Stimulant use and trichotillomania. J Am Acad Child Adolesc Psychiatry 1998;37(4):349–50.
60. Stein DJ, Hollander E. Low-dose pimozide augmentation of serotonin reuptake blockers in the treatment of trichotillomania. J Clin Psychiatry 1992;53(4): 123–6.
61. Stein DJ, Mendelsohn I, Potocnik F, et al. Use of the selective serotonin reuptake inhibitor citalopram in a possible animal analogue of obsessive-compulsive disorder. Depress Anxiety 1998;8(1):39–42.
62. Van Ameringen M, Mancini C, Oakman JM, et al. The potential role of haloperidol in the treatment of trichotillomania. J Affect Disord 1999;56(2):219–26.
63. Van Ameringen M, Mancini C, Patterson B, et al. A randomized, double-blind, placebo-controlled trial of olanzapine in the treatment of trichotillomania. J Clin Psychiatry 2010;71(10):1336–43.
64. Odlaug BL, Grant JE. N-acetylcysteine treatment of grooming disorders. J Clin Psychopharmacol 2007;27(2):227–9.
65. Coric V, Kelmendi B, Pittenger C, et al. Beneficial effects of the antiglutamatergic agent riluzole in a patient diagnosed with trichotillomania. J Clin Psychiatry 2007;68(1):170–1.
66. Grant JE, Odlaug BL, Kim SW. N-acetylcysteine, a glutamate modulator, in the treatment of trichotillomania: a double-blind, placebo- controlled study. Arch Gen Psychiatry 2009;66(7):756.
67. Bloch MH, Panza KE, Grant JE, et al. N- acetylcysteine in the treatment of pediatric trichotillomania: a randomized, double-blind, placebo-controlled add-on trial. J Am Acad Child Adolesc Psychiatry 2013;52(3):231–40.
68. Stein DJ, Hollander E, Simeon D, et al. Neurological soft signs in female trichotillomania patients, obsessive- compulsive disorder patients, and healthy control patients. J Neuropsychiatry Clin Neurosci 1994;6:184–7.
69. Chamberlain SR, Fineberg NA, Blackwell AD, et al. Motor inhibition and cognitive flexibility in obsessive-compulsive disorder and trichotillomania. Am J Psychiatry 2006;163(7):1282–4.
70. Christenson GA, Ristvedt SL, Mackenzie TB. Identification of trichotillomania cue profiles. Behav Res Ther 1993;31(3):315–20.
71. Lochner C, Hemmings SM, Kinnear CJ, et al. Cluster analysis of obsessive-compulsive spectrum disorders in patients with obsessive-compulsive disorder: clinical and genetic correlates. Compr Psychiatry 2005;46(1):14–9.

72. Stein DJ. Neurobiology of the obsessive-compulsive spectrum disorders. Biological Psychiatry 2000;47:296–304.
73. Mostaghimi L. Dermatological assessment of hair pulling and skin picking. In: Grant JE, Stein DJ, Woods DW, et al, editors. Trichotillomania, skin picking, & other body-focused repetitive behaviors. Arlington (VA): American Psychiatric Publishing; 2012. p. 97–112.
74. First MB, Spitzer RL, Gibbon M, et al. Structured clinical interview for DSM-IV axis I disorders. Patient edition (SCID I/P, version 2.0). New York: Biometrics Research Department; 1995.
75. Rothbaum BO, Ninan PT. The assessment of trichotillomania. Behav Res Ther 1994;32(6):651–62.
76. Lochner C, Grant JE, Odlaug BL, et al. DSM-5 field survey: hair-pulling disorder. Depress Anxiety 2012;29:1025–31.
77. First MB, Spitzer RL, Gibbon M, et al. Structured clinical interview for DSM-IV axis I disorders. Patient edition (SCID-I/P, Version 2.0, 8/98 Revision). New York: New York State Psychiatric Institute, Biometrics Research Department; 1998.
78. Franklin ME, Tolin DF. Treating trichotillomania. New York: Springer; 2007.
79. Diefenbach GJ, Tolin DF, Crocetto JS, et al. Assessment of trichotillomania: a psychometric evaluation of hair pulling scales. J Psychopathol Behav Assess 2005;27:169–78.
80. Franklin ME, Edson AL, Ledley DA, et al. Behavior therapy for adolescent trichotillomania: a randomized controlled trial. J Am Acad Child Adolesc Psychiatry 2011;50:763–71.
81. Stanley MA, Breckenridge JK, Snyder AG, et al. Clinician-rated measures of hair pulling: a preliminary psychometric evaluation. J Psychopathol Behav Assess 1999;21:157–82.
82. Stanley MA, Prather RC, Wagner AL, et al. Can the yale-brown obsessive-compulsive scale be used to assess trichotillomania? a preliminary report. Behav Res Ther 1993;31:171–7.
83. Stanley MA, Breckenridge JK, Swann AC, et al. Fluvoxamine treatment of trichotillomania. J Clin Psychopharmacol 1997;17:278–83.
84. Winchel RM, Jones JS, Molcho A, et al. The Psychiatric Institute Trichotillomania Scale (PITS). Psychopharmacol Bull 1992;28:463–76.
85. Keuthen NJ, O'Sullivan RL, Ricciardi JN, et al. The Massachusetts general hospital (MGH) hairpulling scale: 1. development and factor analysis. Psychother Psychosom 1995;64:141–5.
86. O'Sullivan RL, Keuthen NJ, Hayday CF, et al. The Massachusetts general hospital (MGH) hairpulling scale: 2. reliability and validity. Psychother Psychosom 1995;64(3–4):146–8.
87. Keuthen NJ, Flessner CA, Woods DW, et al. Factor analysis of the Massachusetts general hospital hairpulling scale. J Psychosom Res 2007;62:707–9.
88. Diefenbach GJ, Tolin DF, Franklin ME, et al. The trichotillomania scale for children (TSC): a new self-report measure to assess pediatric hair pulling. Paper presented at the Annual Meeting of the Association for Advancement of Behavior Therapy. Boston, November 2003.
89. Tolin DF, Diefenbach GJ, Flessner CA, et al. The trichotillomania scale for children: development and validation. Child Psychiatry Hum Dev 2008; 39:331–49.
90. Flessner CA, Woods DW, Franklin ME, et al. The Milwaukee inventory for subtypes of trichotillomania-adult version (MIST-A): development of an instrument

for assessment of "focused" and "automatic" hair pulling. J Psychopathol Behav Assess 2008;30:20–30.

91. Flessner CA, Conelea CA, Woods DW, et al. Styles of pulling in trichotillomania: exploring differences in symptom severity, phenomenology, and functional impact. Behav Res Ther 2008;46(3):345–57.

92. Stanley MA, Swann AC, Bowers TC, et al. A comparison of clinical features in trichotillomania and obsessive-compulsive disorder. Behav Res Ther 1992;30: 39–44.

93. Hale AS. Dopamine and the use of SSRIs for conditions other than depression. Hum Psychopharmacol 1996;11:103–8.

94. Linehan MM. Skills manual for treating borderline personality disorder. New York: Guilford Press; 1993.

95. Simeon D, Cohen LJ, Stein DJ, et al. Comorbid self-injurious behaviors in 71 female hair-pullers: a survey study. J Nerv Ment Dis 1997;185(2):117–9.

96. Bloch MH, Landeros-Weisenberger A, Dombrowski P, et al. Systematic review: pharmacological and behavioral treatment for trichotillomania. Biol Psychiatry 2007;62:839–46.

97. Duke DC, Keeley ML, Geffken GR, et al. Trichotillomania: a current review. Clin Psychol Rev 2010;30:181–93.

98. Franklin ME, Zagrabbe K, Benavides KL. Trichotillomania and its treatment a review and recommendations. Expert Rev Neurother 2011;11:1165–74.

99. Woods DW, Twohig MT. Trichotillomania: an ACT-enhanced behavior therapy approach therapist guide, vol. 1. Oxford University Press; 2008.

100. Woods DW, Miltenberger RG. Habit reversal: a review of applications and variations. J Behav Ther Exp Psychiatry 1995;26(2):123–31.

101. Bate KS, Malouff JM, Thorsteinsson ET, et al. The efficacy of habit reversal therapy for tics, habit disorders, and stuttering: a meta-analytic review. Clin Psychol Rev 2011;31:865–71.

102. Twohig MP, Woods DW. A preliminary investigation of acceptance and commitment therapy and habit reversal as a treatment for trichotillomania. Behavior Therapy 2004;35:803–20.

103. Keuthen NJ, Rothbaum BO, Fama J, et al. DBT-enhanced cognitive-behavioral treatment for trichotillomania; a randomized controlled trial. J Behav Addict 2012;1:106–14.

# Genetics of Obsessive-Compulsive Disorder and Related Disorders

Heidi A. Browne, BSc[a,b], Shannon L. Gair, BA[a],
Jeremiah M. Scharf, MD, PhD[c,d],*, Dorothy E. Grice, MD[a,b],*

## KEYWORDS

- OCD • Genetics • Heritability • Twin study • Familial recurrence • GWAS
- Candidate gene • Model system

## KEY POINTS

- Although most genetic studies focus primarily on obsessive-compulsive disorder (OCD) and Tourette Syndrome (TS), twin and family studies support a significant genetic contribution to OCD and also to related disorders (eg, Tourette syndrome), including chronic tic disorders, trichotillomania, skin-picking disorder, body dysmorphic disorder, and hoarding disorder.
- Recently, population-based studies and novel laboratory-based methods have confirmed substantial heritability in OCD and TS.
- Genomewide association studies and candidate gene studies have provided information on specific genes that may be involved in the pathobiology of OCD and related disorders, and for some genes studies using model systems have supported a likely role in OCD.
- A substantial portion of the genetic contribution to OCD is still unknown.

Disclosures: J.M. Scharf has received research support from the National Institutes of Health, grants U01 NS40024 and K02 NS085048 and the Tourette Syndrome Association (TSA) and serves on the TSA Scientific Advisory Board. He has received travel support from the TSA and from the European Commission (COST Action BM0905). D. E. Grice has received research support from the National Institutes of Health, grant R01 MH092516, the Tourette Syndrome Association (TSA), and the Tourette Syndrome Association of New Jersey. The other authors have no relevant financial or nonfinancial disclosures.
[a] OCD and Related Disorders Program, Division of Tics, OCD, and Related Disorders, Department of Psychiatry, Icahn School of Medicine at Mount Sinai, One Gustave L. Levy Place, Box 1230, New York, NY 10029, USA; [b] Friedman Brain Institute, Icahn School of Medicine at Mount Sinai, One Gustave L. Levy Place, New York, NY 10029, USA; [c] Movement Disorders Unit, Department of Neurology, Massachusetts General Hospital, Harvard Medical School, 185 Cambridge Street, 6254, Boston, MA 02114, USA; [d] Psychiatric and Neurodevelopmental Genetics Unit, Department of Psychiatry, Massachusetts General Hospital, Harvard Medical School, 185 Cambridge Street, 6254, Boston, MA 02114, USA
* Corresponding authors.
E-mail addresses: jscharf@partners.org; dorothy.grice@mssm.edu

| Abbreviations | |
|---|---|
| BDD | Body dysmorphic disorder |
| CI | Confidence interval |
| CNVs | Copy number variants |
| COMT | Catechol-O-methyltransferase |
| CT | Chronic tic disorder |
| DD | Developmental delay |
| GCTA | Genome wide complex trait analysis |
| GWAS | Genome wide association study |
| ID | Intellectual disability |
| IOCDFGC | International OCD Foundation Genetics Consortium |
| OC | Obsessive-compulsive |
| OCD | Obsessive-compulsive disorder |
| OCGAS | OCD Collaborative Genetic Association Study |
| RRR | Relative recurrence risk |
| SNP | Single nucleotide polymorphism |
| TS | Tourette syndrome |
| TTM | Trichotillomania |

## OVERVIEW

Obsessive-compulsive disorder (OCD) is a disorder that can onset during childhood or during adult life. As a result, OCD is a disorder of interest to both child and adult psychiatrists. There are several other disorders that either commonly co-occur with OCD or have overlapping or similar features and symptoms. Tourette syndrome (TS) is characterized the presence of both motor and vocal tics that onset in childhood and last at least 12 months. A related condition, chronic tic disorder (CT), (CT; defined by the presence of motor tics or vocal tics, but not both and also lasting more than one year) is thought to be an alternate phenotype to TS and shares genetic and biological underpinnings with TS. There is a substantial body of literature focused on the twin, familial, and genetic aspects of TS and CT, a summary of which is presented elsewhere in this issue in the article, "Tics and Tourette's Disorder" by Shaw and Coffey. Of relevance here is that chronic tic disorders (TS and CT) are often seen in conjunction with childhood-onset OCD, reflected in the recent addition of a *tic-related* specifier for OCD in DSM-5. Other OCD-related disorders beyond TS and CT, namely trichotillomania (TTM), skin picking disorder, body dysmorphic disorder (BDD), and hoarding disorder, occur across the lifespan. Although compared with TS and CT there is less specific genetic evidence that these other related disorders share pathobiology with OCD, there is growing evidence that overlapping genetic risk factors may exist across OCD, TTM, skin picking disorder, BDD, and hoarding disorder.

The earliest studies to support a role for genetic factors in OCD demonstrated a higher concordance rate for OCD among monozygotic twins compared with dizygotic twins. Although fewer studies have focused on TTM, skin picking disorder, BDD, and hoarding disorder, there is emergent evidence that some portion of risk for these related disorders is also rooted in genetic factors. These twin studies and subsequent family studies provide estimates of heritability in OCD and related disorders as high as 50%. Recently, powerful population-based epidemiologic studies and new molecular methods have confirmed significant heritability, indicating that genetics contribute substantially to risk for these disorders. Because OCD and related disorders show substantial heritability, familial recurrence risk is high. Over the past several years, several genomewide association studies (GWAS), candidate gene association studies and other studies have identified specific gene variants that seem to contribute to risk for OCD and related disorders. Each variant likely contributes only a small percentage of total risk, indicating that many different gene variations compose the genetic risk architecture for these disorders. Much of the specific genetic risk for OCD remains unknown. Nevertheless, there are examples of genes for which perturbations produce OCD-like phenotypes in animal model systems, allowing a laboratory platform to study the pathobiology and treatment of OCD and related disorders. Future work promises to continue to clarify the specific genes involved in risk for OCD as well as their interaction with environmental risk architecture.

## TWIN STUDIES AND HERITABILITY OF OCD

Although the familial nature of many core features of OCD is apparent to most seasoned clinicians, the first formal evidence for a genetic contribution to OCD came in 1965 from a case series that found monozygotic twins had a higher concordance for OCD than dizygotic twins.[1] Earlier studies had examined concordance rates in twins, but this was first to compare the concordance rates between monozygotic twins, so-called identical twins, who share all their genes, and dizygotic twins, so-called fraternal twins, who share on average about 50% of their genes. A higher concordance rate among monozygotic twins compared with dizygotic twins thus indicates a significant genetic basis for the disorder under study.

Follow-up studies have consistently found monozygotic twins to have higher concordance rates for OCD and obsessive-compulsive (OC) symptoms than dizygotic twins, confirming an important genetic contribution to OCD **(Table 1)**.[2–8] Beyond formal OCD diagnoses, a recent study determined that monozygotic twins have higher concordance than dizygotic twins on five OC symptom dimensions.[9] From these studies, heritability estimates have ranged from 27% to 65%.[10] Early twin studies on OCD typically had small sample sizes, were likely adversely influenced by ascertainment bias, and often used suboptimal statistical analysis. A more robust approach, structural equation modeling, is a newly developed multivariate approach that allows for more conclusive evidence about heritability rates.[9] To date, the largest and most statistically robust twin study found a monozygotic twin concordance rate of 0.52 and a dizygotic concordance rate of 0.21, with overall heritability for OCD estimated to be 48%.[8]

## TWIN STUDIES AND HERITABILITY OF RELATED DISORDERS

There are few twin studies of TTM, skin-picking disorder, BDD, and hoarding disorder. With such a limited body of evidence, it is difficult to draw substantial conclusions about heritability, genetic architecture, and risk for these disorders. The field awaits larger and thus more decisive studies. Renewed interest in transdiagnostic symptoms/phenotypes may be an innovative way to understand genetic risk factors. Available studies are summarized here.

### *TTM*

To date, only two studies have compared TTM concordance rates between monozygotic and dizygotic twins.[8,11] Both studies found a significant difference in concordance rates based on DSM-IV criteria for TTM. One study estimated heritability to be 76%.[11] Interestingly, there were no significant differences between monozygotic and dizygotic twin pairs for either skin-picking or hair manipulation, suggesting that different genetic mechanisms may underlie those two behaviors compared with

**Table 1**
**Twin studies of OCD comparing monozygotic and dizygotic concordance rates**

| Authors, Year | Number of Twin Pairs | MZ Concordance Rate | DZ Concordance Rate | Heritability Estimate |
|---|---|---|---|---|
| Innouye,[1] 1965 | 14 | 0.80 | 0.25 | — |
| Torgersen,[93] 1980 | 99 | — | — | 18% (male) 23% (female) |
| Carey & Gottesman,[94] 1981 | 30 | 0.87 | 0.47 | — |
| Clifford et al,[2] 1984 | 419 | 0.50 (male) 0.44 (female) | 0.22 (male) 0.11 (female) | 47% |
| Jonnal et al,[3] 2000 | 527 | 0.34 (female) | 0.14 (female) | 33% (compulsiveness) 26% (obsessiveness) |
| Eley et al,[4] 2003 | 4564 | 0.59 (male) 0.58 (female) | 0.19 (male) 0.28 (female) | 54% |
| Hudziak et al,[5] 2004 | 4246 | 0.51–0.59 (male) 0.46–0.57 (female) | 0.30–0.35 (male) 0.10–0.40 (female) | 45%–58% |
| Iervolino et al,[9] 2011 | 2053 | 0.47 | 0.28 | 38%–47% (OCS) |
| Monzani et al,[6] 2012 | 1474 | 0.51 | 0.25 | 51% |
| Mataix-Cols et al,[7] 2013 | 16,383 | 0.4 (male) 0.5 (female) | 0.2 (male) 0.15 (female) | 47% |
| Monzani et al,[8] 2014 | 5409 | 0.52 | 0.21 | 48% |

Summary of results from twin studies that compared rates of OCD or obsessive-compulsive symptoms (OCS) in monozygotic and dizygotic twins.
*Abbreviations:* DZ, dizygotic; MZ, monozygotic.

TTM. Another study estimated heritability to be only 32%[8] and did find TTM and skin-picking disorder to be clustered in cross-trait correlations.

### Skin-Picking Disorder

One group has shown skin-picking disorder concordance rates to be higher in monozygotic than dizygotic twin pairs.[6,8] In a population-based study comparing concordance rates of persistent skin picking disorder in female monozygotic and dizygotic twin pairs, the heritability estimate was 40%.[6] A follow-up study found a slightly higher heritability with an estimate of 47%.[8]

### Hoarding Disorder

The Twins UK registry was used to assess the genetic correlation of hoarding disorder.[8,12] There was a greater correlation between monozygotic than between dizygotic twins for two of the main features of hoarding: difficulty discarding and excessive acquisition. The estimated heritability for these traits was 45% and 49%, respectively.[12] The overall heritability for hoarding disorder was estimated to be 51%.[8] In contrast, another study found that hoarding had the least amount of genetic liability compared with other OC symptom dimensions.[9] Interestingly, a Swedish study of 1987 twin pairs found a greater correlation of hoarding in male monozygotic pairs than male dizygotic pairs (0.44 vs 0.17), but no difference in concordance between female monozygotic and female dizygotic twin pairs, suggesting a gender effect may impact risk.[13]

## BDD

Only one study compared monozygotic and dizygotic twin concordance rates for BDD. This study found higher concordance rates for monozygotic twins than dizygotic twins and estimated heritability at 43%.[8] Another study compared the genetic and environmental covariance between BDD and OCD traits.[14] In a sample of 1074 twin pairs, recruited from the Twins UK adult twin registry, 64% of the phenotypic correlation between OCD and BDD was explained by shared genetic factors. When examining specific OCD symptom dimensions (using the Obsessive-Compulsive Inventory - Revised), 82% of the correlation between symmetry/ordering symptoms and the obsessing dimensions were explained by common genetic factors. Modeling in a follow-up study suggests that OCD, hoarding disorder, and BDD are clustered together.[8] These results suggest a partial genetic overlap for OCD and BDD.

## FAMILIAL RECURRENCE RISK IN OCD AND RELATED DISORDERS

The likelihood that a biologically related family member, such as a child, will be affected with a disorder that is already present in a family is captured in recurrence risk. Although recurrence risk is derived from the study of families and not the study of genes or DNA, it is not uncommon to interpret recurrence risk as a proxy for genetic risk for a disorder. If substantial familial recurrence risk is documented in conjunction with twin and/or other family studies, this provides a solid rationale for follow-up molecular genetic analyses. For OCD, a large number of studies have included first-degree family members of individuals with OCD or related disorders to estimate the recurrence rates, typically by administering structured interviews, such as the Structured Clinical Interview for DSM or the Schedule for Affective Disorders and Schizophrenia, and assigning diagnoses by best-estimate diagnostic procedures.[15] These studies, which range in size from about 30 probands with OCD to over 300 probands with OCD and all available first-degree relatives, have estimated recurrence risk among first-degree relatives for lifetime OCD as low as 6% to as high as 55%, with most estimates falling between about 10% and 20%.[16–22] These estimates are significantly higher than the lifetime prevalence for OCD in the general population, which is estimated to be 0.7% to 3%,[23,24] and in each study the familial recurrence risk in affected families was significantly higher than the risk for OCD among relatives of controls. One previous and smaller study failed to find an increased risk among first-degree family members, although when the authors considered a broader definition of OCD (including individuals who had obsessions and/or compulsions but did not meet formal criteria for OCD), family members of probands with OCD were at increased risk, with 15.6% of relatives of probands with OCD affected versus 2.9% of relatives of controls.[25] Indeed, when OC symptoms and behaviors are considered as a broader phenotype, familial recurrence risk estimates are even higher among first-degree family members of probands with OCD.[16,18,20,21] Taken together, the increased risk for OCD and OC behaviors among first-degree relatives of individuals with OCD strongly supports a significant genetic contribution to both subdiagnostic OC symptoms and OCD itself.

In addition, there is evidence that pediatric-onset OCD may have a higher degree of familial aggregation compared with adult-onset OCD. Several studies have found that first-degree relatives of individuals with pediatric-onset OCD have higher rates of OCD compared with first-degree relatives of those with adult-onset OCD[16,17] or that age of onset in probands is correlated with age of onset in relatives.[18] A recent review examined 12 prior studies that compared familial recurrence risk between pediatric-onset and adult-onset probands and found a mean odds ratio of greater than one, in support of higher risk among relatives of pediatric-onset probands.[26] Of note, each of the studies except for one had confidence intervals (CIs) for the odds ratio that included one, and indeed not all studies have agreed that age of onset of OCD is associated with familiality.[20] Thus, is it possible that genetic factors play a greater role in pediatric-onset OCD compared with late-onset OCD, but more research needs to be done to clarify this possibility.

Multiple studies have also supported the familial relationship between OCD and several related disorders including BDD, TTM, and other grooming disorders, such as pathologic nail biting and pathologic skin picking. For example, it has been reported that first-degree relatives of probands with OCD are more likely than relatives of controls to have each of these disorders, with estimates of risk among relatives of probands with OCD as high as 6% for BDD, 4% for TTM, 15% for pathologic nail biting, and 17% for pathologic skin picking.[22,27,28] Moreover, it has been shown in two studies that first-degree relatives of individuals with chronic hair pulling have not only an increased risk for hair pulling disorders but also an increased risk for OCD, with recurrence risk estimates of 6.4% and 17%.[29,30] One study showed that some relatives of probands with hair pulling and OCD also had both disorders, but no relatives of probands with only hair pulling had both disorders. The authors thus suggest that there may be familial subtypes of OCD that are particularly associated with certain other related disorders.[30] Finally, there is also evidence that tic disorders, specifically TS and CT, are more common among first-degree relatives of individuals with OCD compared with relatives of controls, with recurrence risk estimates ranging from approximately 4% to 14%.[17–19,22,28] Taken together, these results support the possibility of overlapping genetic risk between OCD and several related disorders.

Although the family studies described herein are valuable and have moved the field ahead in important ways, most of these studies have used clinic-based and other convenience (i.e., non-population-based) samples, rendering them vulnerable to ascertainment bias and questionable generalizability. Moreover, the relatively small sample sizes result in low precision with associated wide CIs and variability between studies. An approach that has become available only in recent years to circumvent these issues is to use national health registries, available in several countries, such as Denmark and Sweden. These national registries provide a wealth of data for epidemiologic analyses including refined examination of familiality with high precision and very low ascertainment bias. One recent such study, for example, accessed Swedish registries to identify more than 24,000 individuals with OCD with matched controls from a total population of more than 13 million, as well as all first-degree, second-degree, and third-degree relatives. The authors showed with high precision that recurrence risk for OCD was higher for first-degree, second-degree, and third-degree relatives of probands with OCD compared with risk in the family members of controls. Moreover, risk was higher in first-degree relatives than second-degree relatives, and higher in second-degree relatives than third-degree relatives. Recurrence risk estimates were on the lower end of previous reports, as seen from the family studies described above, with odds ratios of approximately 4.5 to 5 for first-degree relatives. The authors also assessed risk in family members of pediatric-onset probands compared with adult-onset probands, reporting that relatives of pediatric-onset probands had slightly but nonsignificantly higher familial risk, lower than what has been reported in previous studies.[7] A similar population-based study performed using Danish national registries also confirmed that having a first-degree relative (mother, father, sibling, or offspring) was a risk factor for OCD.[31] A second research group also using the Danish registries focused on relative recurrence risk (RRR), which takes into account any fluctuations in population prevalence during the study period.

Averaged over all birth years, the sibling RRR of OCD was 4.9 and the sibling RRR for tic disorders (TD; including TS and CT) was 18.6. When examining risk to offspring of affected parents, even greater risk was documented with a parent-offspring RRR for OCD at 6.3 and for TD at 61.0 (Browne H, Hansen S, Buxbaum J, et al, manuscript submitted, 2014). These large, unbiased studies have thus supported the familial nature of OCD and rendered strong yet indirect evidence indicating a substantial genetic contribution to this disorder.

## HERITABILITY OF OCD AND RELATED DISORDERS VIA NOVEL METHODS

In recent years, genetic researchers have developed methods for estimating disease heritability directly from genomewide genotyping data through the use of linear mixed models.[32,33] Using these methods, as implemented in the statistical genetics package genomewide complex trait analysis (GCTA), one can estimate narrow-sense heritability ($h^2$) (i.e., the proportion of the disease phenotype that can be explained by additive genetic factors).[34] Conceptually, the method determines the amount of genomewide shared genetic variation between case-case and control-control pairs compared with case-control pairs. Of note, this estimate represents a lower bound of the true heritability of the disorder, because it does not capture gene-gene or gene-environment interactions well and can only detect common variation of the type found in single nucleotide polymorphism (SNP) genotyping arrays (commonly known as GWAS arrays); these estimates therefore do not capture heritability attributable to (1) genomic copy number variation (see later discussion), (2) rare to very rare genetic variation, or (3) *de novo* genetic variation. Nonetheless, it is an extremely powerful tool for complex genetic traits (such as psychiatric disorders in general and, of relevance here, OCD and related disorders), as it provides direct genetic evidence of disease heritability, which can be compared with traditional heritability estimates based on phenotypic concordance in twin or family studies.

Recently, the International OCD Foundation Genetics Consortium (IOCDFGC) and Tourette Syndrome Association International Consortium for Genetics used linear mixed models to estimate the additive heritability of OCD and TS derived from GWAS data.[35] Encouragingly, both disorders were confirmed to be highly heritable (OCD: $h^2 = 0.37$, SE = 0.07; TS: $h^2 = 0.58$, SE = 0.08). In addition, these direct heritability estimates were in the same range as the twin-based heritability estimates of OCD and TS, suggesting that most OCD and TS heritability may be explained by genetic variants captured by GWAS arrays. Davis and colleagues[35] subsequently partitioned the genome both by chromosome and by variant frequency to further dissect the underlying genetic architecture. For TS, the genetic variation contributing to heritability appeared to be nearly equally distributed across all autosomal chromosomes, with ~80% of variation explained by "common" genetic variants that are present in at least 5% of the general population, and ~20% explained by rare variants (<5% minor allele frequency). In contrast, OCD had a marked proportion of heritability present on chromosome 15, with the remaining genetic variation equally distributed across the rest of the genome. Surprisingly, the OCD heritability appeared to be limited to common variants present in greater than 30% of the general population. If verified in independent samples, these data together suggest that OCD and TS are both "polygenic" disorders, in that they arise due to the combination of many genetic variants (possibly hundreds or thousands), each of small to modest effect and individually present in a large proportion of the general population, but when combined, likely in combination with rarer, large effect variation and/or nongenetic/environmental risk factors, surpass a threshold and result in disease. An extrapolation of these observations would be the prediction that individuals in the general population with noninterfering OC symptoms may carry a small number of OCD risk variants and represent one end of a continuous OC phenotypic spectrum, while individuals with clinically significant OCD lie at the other end and harbor a large number of OCD risk alleles. Future analyses in population-based cohorts will be needed to examine this hypothesis directly.[10]

## GENOMEWIDE ASSOCIATION STUDIES IN OCD AND RELATED DISORDERS

To date, two GWAS of OCD have been conducted (1465 cases, 5557 controls, 400 parent-proband trios in the IOCDFGC study, and 1406 cases in 1065 families in the OCD Collaborative Genetic Association Study [OCGAS] GWAS) and one GWAS of TS (1285 cases, 4964 controls).[36–38] None of these studies identified a specific genetic variant in the final analysis surpassing the stringent threshold needed to achieve genomewide significance ($P \leq 5 \times 10^{-8}$).[39,40] Scharf and colleagues identified supportive evidence for the top TS GWAS SNP variant within an intron of the collagen type XXVIIa gene (COL27A1) in an additional 211 TS cases and 285 matched controls from 2 Latin American population isolates (combined P value $3.6 \times 10^{-7}$).[36] Stewart and colleagues detected a genomewide significant variant in SNP rs6131295 near BTBD3 ($P = 3.8 \times 10^{-8}$) in the subset of 400 parent-proband trios within the IOCDFGC OCD study, although this signal decreased to $P = 3.6 \times 10^{-5}$ in the final meta-analysis of all samples.[37] Mattheisen and colleagues[38] reported a top signal from the OCGAS study ($P = 4.1 \times 10^{-7}$) upstream of PTPRD, a tyrosine phosphatase that has been shown previously to be involved in regulation of both glutamatergic and GABAergic synapse formation. Interestingly, the top signals from the initial IOCDFGC OCD GWAS were enriched in the OCGAS GWAS ($P = .018$), suggesting that a subset of these variants may represent true OCD susceptibility loci.

Given the sample sizes needed to discover definitive common disease variants in other neuropsychiatric disorders, the absence of genomewide significant results in the initial OCD, and TS, GWAS is not surprising in retrospect.[41] However, the GCTA heritability study described above provides strong evidence that additional GWAS of OCD and TS with larger sample numbers should identify definitive OCD and TS genes. The current OCD/TS results parallel early GWAS of bipolar disorder and schizophrenia in which initial experiments did not produce genomewide significant results, yet the first definitive susceptibility genes were detected in GWAS of approximately 4000 to 5000 cases.[42–45] Furthermore, as a result of worldwide collaborative efforts in the Psychiatric Genomics Consortium, the most recent schizophrenia GWAS with 35,000 cases has identified 108 independent associations in 97 genes, including known drug targets (dopamine D2 receptor, DRD2), syndromic causes of psychosis (TCF4, previously known to cause Pitt-Hopkins syndrome), and novel druggable targets (T-type calcium channel genes, CACNA1C).[46,47]

GWAS data have also been used to examine the genetic relationship between OCD and TS/CT. As noted above, numerous family studies have suggested that OCD and TS/CT are genetically related,[48,49] although this relationship has never been verified at the molecular level. Using linear mixed models, Davis and colleagues[35] identified a significant genetic correlation between OCD and TS cases ($r = 0.41$), although they could not exclude within-subject comorbidity as the source of this shared signal. A subsequent combined OCD/TS analysis also supported the presence of overlapping genetic signals between the two disorders (Yu D, Mathews CA, Scharf JM, et al, Am J Psychiatry, in press.). In addition, using a second technique to examine the aggregated, polygenic signal within and across GWAS, Yu and colleagues demonstrated that while a polygenic risk score derived from a "discovery sample" of 1154 OCD cases without known tics could predict OCD case/control status in a second "target" sample, the addition of 345 OCD cases with co-occurring TS/CT (increasing the total discovery sample to 1499 OCD cases) significantly decreased the ability of the OCD discovery sample to predict OCD case/control status in the target sample. These data suggest that OCD with co-occurring TS/CT may have a subset of distinct genetic loci compared with OCD without tics and offers biological support for the "tic-related" specifier for OCD discussed above.

## CNV STUDIES IN OCD AND RELATED DISORDERS

Submicroscopic deletions and duplications of DNA segments throughout the genome, collectively known as copy number variants (CNVs), have emerged in recent years as another major component of the genetic architecture of a wide range of developmental neuropsychiatric disorders.[50] In particular, these studies have reported the presence of recurrent, large (>500 kb), rare (often de novo) CNVs in multiple regions of the genome in which the same deletions and duplications can be found in individuals with different neurodevelopmental disorders, including schizophrenia, autism, intellectual disability (ID), developmental delay (DD), epilepsy, bipolar disorder, and attention deficit hyperactivity disorder.[50–52] Two CNV studies of specific chromosomal regions have been conducted in OCD[53,54] as well as 3 moderately sized (each <500 cases) genomewide CNV analyses of TS.[55–57] Although none of the studies identified a genomic region statistically associated with either OCD or TS, exonic NRXN1 deletions were found in two of the TS studies,[55,57] and Fernandez and colleagues[56] identified an enrichment of CNVs in histamine-signaling pathway genes in the other TS study.

A recent joint CNV analysis of OCD and TS (2699 subjects with either disorder) found a 3.3-fold increased burden of large (>500 kb) deletions within the subset of neurodevelopmental loci previously reported to harbor large, recurrent pathogenic CNVs.[58] Five of the 10 neurodevelopmental deletions were located within the 16p13.11 locus previously associated with ID/DD, seizures, and autism; four of five deletions were in OCD cases, whereas one subject had TS. Three of the OCD/TS 16p13.11 deletions were found to be de novo events: one in an OCD subject without tics, one with TS without OCD, and one with OCD and CT. These results support the hypothesis that OCD and TS/CT have some shared genetic susceptibility, although these observations require replication given the small number of observed events. In addition, McGrath and colleagues[58] found three 22q11 duplications and one de novo 22q11 deletion in subjects with OCD. Given prior reports of three TS subjects with 22q11 duplications, this region may also prove to be a shared genetic locus for both disorders.[56,57,59,60]

## CANDIDATE GENE STUDIES IN OCD AND RELATED DISORDERS

Although a large number of candidate genes have been reported to be associated with OCD and related disorders, no single gene has acquired the stringent level of statistical evidence to be considered a definitive risk gene. The strongest OCD candidate gene to date is the neuronal glutamate transporter gene, SLC1A1, although a recent meta-analysis of existing genetic association data did not find nominal significance following correction for multiple hypothesis testing.[61] A separate meta-analysis reported significant associations for three loci: the serotonin transporter promoter variant (5-HTTLPR) $L_a$ versus ($L_g$+S) alleles; COMT Met/Val; and the serotonin 2A receptor (HTR2A).[62] Although these 3 loci met the prespecified corrected significance threshold of $\alpha < 0.05$, it is important to note that these three signals are still below the standard genomewide significant threshold of $5 \times 10^{-8}$ for conclusive evidence of a disease susceptibility gene. Whether a candidate gene study should meet genome-wide evidence is a matter of debate; however, the history of psychiatric genetics has made it clear that many candidate gene studies of nominal significance are not readily replicated.

Rare variation has been studied first in TS and this led to interesting follow-up findings in OCD and related disorders. In TS, rare variation in 2 genes, *SLITRK1* and *HDC*, have been identified in individual TS families.[63,64] A frameshift mutation in *SLITRK1* was initially found in one TS proband and his mother, who had TTM, as well as 2 individuals with a rare variation in an miRNA-binding site in the 3'UTR of the gene that was not found in 3600 control chromosomes. Based on these findings, subsequent association studies looking at common variation have produced conflicting results,[65–71] and the recent TS GWAS found no association with *SLITRK1*, although one of the top statistical signals was located in the 2-Mb region between *SLITRK1* and the adjacent gene *SLITRK6*.[36] Of note, preliminary sequencing studies of *SLITRK1* in patients with OCD and TTM have suggested that rare variation may also be associated with these 2 related disorders.[72–74] With the advent of genome and exome sequencing, new appreciation of the high frequency of amino-acid altering variations in the general population now supports the need for follow-up studies in larger case-control samples and/or studies of *de novo* variation in parent-proband trios to determine the significance of these results.[75]

A frameshift mutation in the histidine carboxylase gene, *HDC*, the rate-limiting enzyme in histamine biosynthesis, has been identified in one family consisting of a father and 8 offspring with TS.[64] Although rare variants in *HDC* have not been identified in additional TS cases, Fernandez and colleagues[56] found an enrichment of histamine signaling pathway genes in their TS CNV analysis, and a recent association study in 520 TS nuclear families reported a significant association of 2 *HDC* SNPs with TS ($P = .0018$).[76] Future analyses in additional samples will be needed to examine both common and rare *HDC* variation in TS, OCD, and related disorders.

## MODEL SYSTEMS IN OCD AND RELATED DISORDERS

Genetic manipulations that produce compulsive-like behaviors in animals provide a valuable model system for understanding the neurobiological underpinnings of OCD and related disorders, as well as a platform in which to generate and test novel treatments. Because of the paucity of information on specific genes that contribute to risk for OCD in humans, these models tend to rely on genetic manipulations that produce behavioral phenotypes in animals that appear analogous to human compulsions; in some instances, the specific genetic manipulation has been found to confer risk for human OCD, and in other examples, the specific gene has not been validated in human OCD. Frequently these genes are highly expressed in corticostriatal circuits, dysfunction in which is thought to mediate compulsive behaviors and tics.[77–80] In their review on animal models of OC spectrum disorders, Camilla d'Angelo and colleagues[81] describe standard criteria used to assess these models, including face validity (phenotypic similarity between the model and the human condition), predictive validity (how well the animal model predicts efficacy of treatment of the disorder being modeled), and construct validity (how close the underlying mechanism of the model mimics the underlying mechanism of the disorder).

One such animal model is the *Sapap3* knockout mouse. Interestingly, *Sapap3* is expressed highly in striatum, and electrophysiological and biochemical studies of these animals reveal abnormalities in corticostriatal synapses. An in-depth characterization of these mice show that they reliably exhibit both increased anxiety in behavioral testing as well as excessive self-grooming behaviors that lead to facial hair loss and skin lesions. The self-grooming is considered reminiscent of the compulsive behaviors seen in OCD and also bears commonalities with features seen in human grooming disorders such as TTM and pathologic skin picking, giving the model face validity. Moreover, the abnormal self-grooming and anxiety behaviors are reduced by subchronic treatment (6 days) with fluoxetine (an empirically based treatment of OCD in humans) but not by a single dose of fluoxetine, making the model even more reminiscent of human OCD[82] and giving the model predictive validity. Not only does the Sapap3 knockout mouse thus provide a useful model for potentially characterizing the neuropathology of and evaluating novel treatments for OCD and related disorders, but SAPAP3 has also been shown to be a promising candidate for these disorders in humans, thus giving the model construct validity. Studies have now shown that SNPs and other variants in SAPAP3 appear to be enriched in individuals with grooming disorders (pathologic nail biting, pathologic skin picking, or TTM) compared with controls,[83] and in at least one study variants in SAPAP3 were enriched in individuals with OCD as well.[84] Distinct variants in SAPAP3 have also been reported in TS.[85]

A similar animal model, with face, predictive, and construct validity, exists with the Slitrk5 knockout mouse (Slitrk1-6 is a family of related proteins; see Candidate gene studies in OCD and related disorders, above). Similar to the SAPAP3 knockout mice, these animals exhibit increased anxiety in behavioral testing. In addition, they exhibit excessive self-grooming, which leads to facial hair loss and skin lesions, akin to pathologic grooming behavior specifically and perhaps compulsive behavior more generally. These behaviors also improve with fluoxetine treatment. Moreover, the knockout mice show selective overactivation of the orbitofrontal cortex, much like what has been shown in human imaging studies of OCD, and neuronal electrophysiological recordings from these animals reveal abnormal corticostriatal neurotransmission.[86] The Slitrk5 knockout mouse thus provides a useful model for OCD and related disorders in terms of both neuropathophysiology and behavioral abnormalities. It is notable that variations in the related protein, Slitrk1, have been found in cases of human OCD and TS.[63,74] However, the Slitrk5 knockout mouse seems to be a more useful model for studying OCD and related disorders; while the Slitrk1 knockout mouse has been shown to have increased anxiety behaviors studies have not detected additional behavioral abnormalities consistent with OCD behaviors such as excessive self-grooming.[87]

In other genetic mouse models of OCD and related disorders, the manipulated genes have not been studied and/or shown to contribute to risk in human OCD. Nevertheless, these too can provide additional tools to study the pathobiology of OCD. For example, mice with loss of function disruptions of the gene Hoxb8 show excess self-grooming leading to hair loss and skin lesions; unlike the Sapap3 and SLITRK5 knockout mice, these mice also excessively groom their normal cage mates. Although HOXB8 has not been shown to contribute to human OCD, the gene is highly expressed in brain regions thought to be involved in OCD, including the orbitofrontal cortex, anterior cingulate cortex, and striatum.[88] Thus, the model may have some construct validity, disrupting pathways similarly to other genetic causes of OCD even if the gene is not involved in human OCD, as well as face validity given the compulsive behaviors of the animals. Similarly, the 5HT2C receptor knockout mouse provides a promising model of compulsive behavior with face validity; compared with controls, the mice show more repetitive and organized behaviors, chewing more nonnutritive clay, producing a distinctly organized chewing pattern on plastic screens, and showing increased perseveration of a head dipping activity in a behavioral assay.[89] Finally, male aromatase knockout mice develop compulsive behaviors, such as excessive barbering, grooming, and wheel running. Interestingly, these mice have low catechol-O-methyltransferase (COMT) protein expression in the hypothalamus,[90] and in male humans, low COMT activity is associated with a higher risk of developing OCD.[91,92] Thus, this model again provides both face validity and possibly construct validity.

Thus, several animal models of OCD and related disorders exist valuable preclinical systems for exploring neurobiological mechanisms of these disorders as well as potential novel treatments. As knowledge of specific genetic factors that contribute to risk for human OCD expands, it will inform a richer understanding of the biological underpinnings of OCD and render preclinical models even more powerful tools.

## SUMMARY

Twin and family studies as well as newer population-based approaches and novel laboratory-based investigations have provided powerful insights into the substantial heritability in OCD and related disorders, supporting a significant genetic contribution to these disorders. GWAS and candidate gene studies have identified specific gene variants that may contribute a small portion of the total genetic risk to OCD and related disorders, allowing for the development of model systems in which to study the pathobiology and treatment of these disorders. Nevertheless, a substantial portion of the genetic risk lies in genes that remain unidentified. Ongoing and future work will continue to clarify the genetic architecture and risk profile in OCD and related disorders to allow improved assessment of individualized risk and the development of novel therapeutics.

## REFERENCES

1. Inouye E. Similar and dissimilar manifestations of obsessive-compulsive neuroses in monozygotic twins. Am J Psychiatry 1965;121:1171–5.
2. Clifford CA, Murray RM, Fulker DW. Genetic and environmental influences on obsessional traits and symptoms. Psychol Med 1984;14(4):791–800.
3. Jonnal AH, Gardner CO, Prescott CA, et al. Obsessive and compulsive symptoms in a general population sample of female twins. Am J Med Genet 2000; 96(6):791–6.
4. Eley TC, Bolton D, O'Connor TG, et al. A twin study of anxiety-related behaviors in pre-school children. J Child Psychol Psychiatry 2003;44(7):945–60.
5. Hudziak JJ, van Beijsterveldt CE, Althoff RR, et al. Genetic and environmental contributions to the child behavior checklist obsessive-compulsive scale. Arch Gen Psychiatry 2004;61:608–16.
6. Monzani B, Rijsdijk F, Cherkas L, et al. Prevalence and heritability of skin picking in an adult community sample: a twin study. Am J Med Genet B Neuropsychiatr Genet 2012;159B:605–10.
7. Mataix-Cols D, Boman M, Monzani B, et al. Population-based, multigenerational family clustering study of obsessive-compulsive disorder. JAMA Psychiatry 2013;70(7):709–17.
8. Monzani B, Rijsdijk F, Harris J, et al. The structure of genetic and environmental risk factors for dimensional representations of DSM-5 obsessive-compulsive spectrum disorders. JAMA Psychiatry 2014;71(2):182–9.
9. Iervolino AC, Rijsdijk FV, Cherkas L, et al. A multivariate twin study of obsessive-compulsive symptom dimensions. Arch Gen Psychiatry 2011;68(6):637–44.

10. van Grootheest DS, Cath DC, Beekman AT, et al. Twin studies on obsessive-compulsive disorder: a review. Twin Res Hum Genet 2005;8(5):450–8.

11. Novak CE, Keuthen NJ, Stewart SE, et al. A twin concordance study of trichotillomania. Am J Med Genet B Neuropsychiatr Genet 2009;150B:944–9.

12. Nordsletten AE, Monzani B, de la Cruz LF, et al. Overlap and specificity of genetic and environmental influences on excessive acquisition and difficulties discarding possessions: implications for hoarding disorder. Am J Med Genet B Neuropsychiatr Genet 2013;162B:380–7.

13. Ivanov VZ, Mataix-Cols D, Serlachius E, et al. Prevalence, comorbidity and heritability of hoarding symptoms in adolescence: a population based twin study in 15-year olds. PLoS One 2013;8(7):e69140.

14. Monzani B, Rijsdijk F, Iervolino AC, et al. Evidence for a genetic overlap between body dismorphic concerns and obsessive-compulsive symptoms in an adult female community sample. Am J Med Genet B Neuropsychiatr Genet 2012;159B: 376–82.

15. Leckman JF, Scholomskas D, Thompson WD, et al. Best estimate of lifetime psychiatric diagnosis: a methodological study. Arch Gen Psychiatry 1982;39(8): 879–83.

16. Pauls DL, Alsobrook JP 2nd, Goodman W, et al. A family study of obsessive-compulsive disorder. Am J Psychiatry 1995;152(1):76–84.

17. Nestadt G, Samuels J, Riddle M, et al. A family study of obsessive-compulsive disorder. Arch Gen Psychiatry 2000;57(4):358–63.

18. do Rosario-Campos MC, Leckman JF, Curi M, et al. A family study of early-onset obsessive-compulsive disorder. Am J Med Genet B Neuropsychiatr 2005; 136B(1):92–7.

19. Hanna G, Himle JA, Curtic GC, et al. A family study of obsessive–compulsive disorder with pediatric probands. Am J Med Genet 2005;134B:13–9.

20. Fyer AJ, Lipsitz JD, Mannuzza S, et al. A direct interview family study of obsessive-compulsive disorder. I. Psychol Med 2005;35(11):1611–21.

21. Grabe HJ, Ruhrmann S, Ettelt S, et al. Familiality of obsessive-compulsive disorder in nonclinical and clinical subjects. Am J Psychiatry 2006;163(11): 1986–92.

22. Bienvenu OJ, Samuels JF, Wuyek LA, et al. Is obsessive-compulsive disorder an anxiety disorder, and what, if any, are spectrum conditions? A family study perspective. Psychol Med 2012;42(1):1–13.

23. Fontenelle LF, Mendlowicz MV, Versiani M. The descriptive epidemiology of obsessive-compulsive disorder. Prog Neuropsychopharmacol Biol Psychiatry 2006;30(3):327–37.

24. Ruscio AM, Stein DJ, Chiu WT, et al. The epidemiology of obsessive-compulsive disorder in the National Comorbidity Survey Replication. Mol Psychiatry 2010; 15(1):53–63.

25. Black DW, Noyes R Jr, Goldstein RB, et al. A family study of obsessive-compulsive disorder. Arch Gen Psychiatry 1992;49(5):362–8.

26. Taylor S. Early versus late onset obsessive-compulsive disorder: evidence for distinct subtypes. Clin Psychol Rev 2011;31(7):1083–100.

27. Bienvenu OJ, Samuels JF, Riddle MA, et al. The relationship of obsessive-compulsive disorder to possible spectrum disorders: results from a family study. Biol Psychiatry 2000;48(4):287–93.

28. Brakoulias V, Starcevic V, Sammut P, et al. Obsessive-compulsive spectrum disorders: a comorbidity and family history perspective. Australas Psychiatry 2011; 19(2):151–5.

29. Lenane MC, Swedo SE, Rapoport JL, et al. Rates of obsessive compulsive disorder in first-degree relatives of patients with trichotillomania: a research note. J Child Psychol Psychiatry 1992;33(5):925–33.
30. Keuthen NJ, Altenburger EM, Pauls D. A family study of trichotillomania and chronic hair pulling. Am J Med Genet B Neuropsychiatr Genet 2014;165(2): 167–74.
31. Steinhausen HC, Bisgaard C, Munk-Jorgensen P, et al. Family aggregation and risk factors of obsessive-compulsive disorders in a nationwide three-generation study. Depress Anxiety 2013;30(12):1177–84.
32. Lee SH, Wray NR, Goddard ME, et al. Estimating missing heritability for disease from genome-wide association studies. Am J Hum Genet 2011;88:294–305.
33. Yang J, Manolio TA, Pasquale LR, et al. Genome partitioning of genetic variation for complex traits using common SNPs. Nat Genet 2011;43(6):519–25.
34. Yang J, Lee SH, Goddard ME, et al. GCTA: a tool for genomewide complex trait analysis. Am J Hum Genet 2011;88(1):76–82.
35. Davis LK, Yu D, Keenan CL, et al. Partitioning the heritability of Tourette syndrome and obsessive compulsive disorder reveals differences in genetic architecture. PLoS Genet 2013;9(10):e1003864.
36. Scharf JM, Yu D, Mathews CA, et al. Genomewide association study of Tourette's syndrome. Mol Psychiatry 2012;18(6):721–8.
37. Stewart SE, Yu D, Scharf JM, et al. Genomewide association study of obsessive-compulsive disorder. Mol Psychiatry 2013;18(7):788–98.
38. Mattheisen M, Samuels JF, Wang Y, et al. Genome-wide association study in obsessive-compulsive disorder: results from the OCGAS. Mol Psychiatry 2014. [Epub ahead of print]. http://dx.doi.org/10.1038/mp.2014.43.
39. Pe'er I, Yelensky R, Altshuler D, et al. Estimation of the multiple testing burden for genomewide association studies of nearly all common variants. Genet Epidemiol 2008;32(4):381–5.
40. Dudbridge F, Gusnanto A. Estimation of significance thresholds for genomewide association scans. Genet Epidemiol 2008;32(3):227–34.
41. Sullivan PF, Daly MJ, O'Donovan M. Genetic architectures of psychiatric disorders: the emerging picture and its implications. Nat Rev Genet 2012;13(8): 537–51.
42. Ferreira MA, O'Donovan MC, Meng YA, et al. Collaborative genome-wide association analysis supports a role for ANK3 and CACNA1C in bipolar disorder. Nat Genet 2008;40(9):1056–8.
43. Purcell SM, Wray NR, Stone JL, et al. Common polygenic variation contributes to risk of schizophrenia and bipolar disorder. Nature 2009;460(7256):748–52.
44. Stefansson H, Ophoff RA, Steinberg S, et al. Common variants conferring risk of schizophrenia. Nature 2009;460(7256):744–7.
45. Shi J, Levinson DF, Duan J, et al. Common variants on chromosome 6p22.1 are associated with schizophrenia. Nature 2009;460(7256):753–7.
46. Ripke S, O'Dushlaine C, Chambert K, et al. Genome-wide association analysis identifies 13 new risk loci for schizophrenia. Nat Genet 2013;45(10):1150–9.
47. Ripke S. Psychiatric Genomics Consortium Schizophrenia Working Group, World Congress of Psychiatric Genetics Annual Meeting. Boston, Massachusetts, October 17-21, 2013. p. 23. Available at: http://2013.ispg.net/wp-content/uploads/2013/10/2013-WCPG-Oral-Abstracts.pdf.
48. Pauls DL, Towbin KE, Leckman JF, et al. Gilles de la Tourette's syndrome and obsessive-compulsive disorder. Evidence supporting a genetic relationship. Arch Gen Psychiatry 1986;43(12):1180–2.

49. Grados MA, Riddle MA, Samuels JF, et al. The familial phenotype of obsessive-compulsive disorder in relation to tic disorders: the Hopkins OCD family study. Biol Psychiatry 2001;50(8):559–65.

50. Malhotra D, Sebat J. CNVs: harbingers of a rare variant revolution in psychiatric genetics. Cell 2012;148(6):1223–41.

51. Morrow EM. Genomic copy number variation in disorders of cognitive development. J Am Acad Child Adolesc Psychiatry 2010;49(11):1091–104.

52. Sanders SJ, Ercan-Sencicek AG, Hus V, et al. Multiple recurrent de novo CNVs, including duplications of the 7q11.23 Williams syndrome region, are strongly associated with autism. Neuron 2011;70(5):863–85.

53. Delorme R, Moreno-De-Luca D, Gennetier A, et al. Search for copy number variants in chromosomes 15q11-q13 and 22q11.2 in obsessive compulsive disorder. BMC Med Genet 2010;11:100.

54. Walitza S, Bove DS, Romanos M, et al. Pilot study on HTR2A promoter polymorphism, -1438G/A (rs6311) and a nearby copy number variation showed association with onset and severity in early onset obsessive-compulsive disorder. J Neural Transm 2012;119(4):507–15.

55. Sundaram SK, Huq AM, Wilson BJ, et al. Tourette syndrome is associated with recurrent exonic copy number variants. Neurology 2010;74(20):1583–90.

56. Fernandez TV, Sanders SJ, Yurkiewicz IR, et al. Rare copy number variants in Tourette syndrome disrupt genes in histaminergic pathways and overlap with autism. Biol Psychiatry 2012;71(5):392–402.

57. Nag A, Bochukova EG, Kremeyer B, et al. CNV analysis in Tourette syndrome implicates large genomic rearrangements in COL8A1 and NRXN1. PLoS One 2013;8(3):e59061.

58. McGrath LM, Yu D, Marshall C, et al. Copy number variation in obsessive-compulsive disorder and Tourette syndrome: a cross-disorder analysis. J Am Acad Child Adolesc Psychiatry, in press.

59. Robertson MM, Shelley BP, Dalwai S, et al. A patient with both Gilles de la Tourette's syndrome and chromosome 22q11 deletion syndrome: clue to the genetics of Gilles de la Tourette's syndrome? J Psychosom Res 2006;61(3): 365–8.

60. Clarke RA, Fang ZM, Diwan AD, et al. Tourette syndrome and klippel-feil anomaly in a child with chromosome 22q11 duplication. Case Rep Med 2009;2009: 361518.

61. Stewart SE, Mayerfeld C, Arnold PD, et al. Meta-analysis of association between obsessive-compulsive disorder and the 3' region of neuronal glutamate transporter gene SLC1A1. Am J Med Genet B Neuropsychiatr Genet 2013;162B(4): 367–79.

62. Taylor S. Molecular genetics of obsessive-compulsive disorder: a comprehensive meta-analysis of genetic association studies. Mol Psychiatry 2013;18(7): 799–805.

63. Abelson JF, Kwan KY, O'Roak BJ. Sequence variants in SLITRK1 are associated with Tourette's syndrome. Science 2005;310(5746):317–20.

64. Ercan-Sencicek AG, Stillman AA, Ghosh AK, et al. L-histidine decarboxylase and Tourette's syndrome. N Engl J Med 2010;362(20):1901–8.

65. Deng H, Le WD, Xie WJ, et al. Examination of the SLITRK1 gene in Caucasian patients with Tourette syndrome. Acta Neurol Scand 2006;114(6):400–2.

66. Keen-Kim D, Mathews CA, Reus VI, et al. Overrepresentation of rare variants in a specific ethnic group may confuse interpretation of association analyses. Hum Mol Genet 2006;15(22):3324–8.

67. Chou IC, Wan L, Liu SC, et al. Association of the Slit and Trk-like 1 gene in Taiwanese patients with Tourette syndrome. Pediatr Neurol 2007;37(6):404–6.
68. Scharf JM, Moorjani P, Fagerness J, et al. Lack of association between SLITRK1-var321 and Tourette syndrome in a large family-based sample. Neurology 2008; 70(16 Pt 2):1495–6.
69. Zimprich A, Hatala K, Riederer F, et al. Sequence analysis of the complete SLITRK1 gene in Austrian patients with Tourette's disorder. Psychiatr Genet 2008;18(6):308–9.
70. Miranda DM, Wigg K, Kabia EM, et al. Association of SLITRK1 to Gilles de la Tourette Syndrome. Am J Med Genet B Neuropsychiatr Genet 2009;150B(4):483–6.
71. Karagiannidis I, Rizzo R, Tarnok Z, et al. Replication of association between a SLITRK1 haplotype and Tourette Syndrome in a large sample of families. Mol Psychiatry 2012;17(7):665–8.
72. Wendland JR, Kruse MR, Murphy DL. Functional SLITRK1 var321, varCDfs and SLC6A4 G56A variants and susceptibility to obsessive-compulsive disorder. Mol Psychiatry 2006;11(9):802–4.
73. Zuchner S, Cuccaro ML, Tran-Viet KN, et al. SLITRK1 mutations in trichotillomania. Mol Psychiatry 2006;11(10):887–9.
74. Ozomaro U, Cai G, Kajiwara Y, et al. Characterization of SLITRK1 variation in obsessive-compulsive disorder. PLoS One 2013;8(8):e70376.
75. Tennessen JA, Bigham AW, O'Connor TD, et al. Evolution and functional impact of rare coding variation from deep sequencing of human exomes. Science 2012; 337(6090):64–9.
76. Karagiannidis I, Dehning S, Sandor P, et al. Support of the histaminergic hypothesis in Tourette syndrome: association of the histamine decarboxylase gene in a large sample of families. J Med Genet 2013;50(11):760–4.
77. Amat JA, Bronen RA, Saluja S, et al. Increased number of subcortical hyperintensities on MRI in children and adolescents with Tourette's syndrome, obsessive-compulsive disorder, and attention deficit hyperactivity disorder. Am J Psychiatry 2006;163(6):1106–8.
78. Graybiel AM. Habits, rituals, and the evaluative brain. Annu Rev Neurosci 2008; 31:359–87.
79. Lewis M, Kim SJ. The pathophysiology of restricted repetitive behavior. J Neurodev Disord 2009;1(2):114–32.
80. Muehlmann AM, Lewis MH. Abnormal repetitive behaviours: shared phenomenology and pathophysiology. J Intellect Disabil Res 2012;56(5):427–40.
81. Camilla d'Angelo LS, Eagle DM, Grant JE, et al. Animal models of obsessive-compulsive spectrum disorders. CNS Spectr 2014;19(1):28–49.
82. Welch JM, Lu J, Roriguiz RM, et al. Cortico-striatal synaptic defects and OCD-like behaviours in Sapap3-mutant mice. Nature 2007;448(7156):894–900.
83. Bienvenu OJ, Wang Y, Shugart YY, et al. Sapap3 and pathological grooming in humans: Results from the OCD collaborative genetics study. Am J Med Genet B Neuropsychiatr Genet 2009;150B(5):710–20.
84. Zuchner S, Wendland JR, Ashley-Koch AE, et al. Multiple rare SAPAP3 missense variants in trichotillomania and OCD. Mol Psychiatry 2009;14(1):6–9.
85. Crane J, Fagerness J, Osiecki L, et al. Family-based genetic association study of DLGAP3 in Tourette Syndrome. Am J Med Genet B Neuropsychiatr Genet 2011;156B(1):108–14.
86. Shmelkov SV, Hormigo A, Jing D. Slitrk5 deficiency impairs corticostriatal circuitry and leads to obsessive-compulsive-like behaviors in mice. Nat Med 2010;16(5):598–602.

87. Katayama K, Yamada K, Ornthanalai VG, et al. Slitrk1-deficient mice display elevated anxiety-like behavior and noradrenergic abnormalities. Mol Psychiatry 2010;15(2):177–84.
88. Greer JM, Capecchi MR. Hoxb8 is required for normal grooming behavior in mice. Neuron 2002;33(1):23–34.
89. Chou-Green JM, Holscher TD, Dallman MF, et al. Compulsive behavior in the 5-HT2C receptor knockout mouse. Physiol Behav 2003;78(4–5):641–9.
90. Hill RA, McInnes KJ, Gong EC, et al. Estrogen deficient male mice develop compulsive behavior. Biol Psychiatry 2007;61(3):359–66.
91. Karayiorgou M, Altemus M, Galke BL, et al. Genotype determining low catechol-O-methyltransferase activity as a risk factor for obsessive-compulsive disorder. Proc Natl Acad Sci U S A 1997;94(9):4572–5.
92. Pooley EC, Fineberg N, Harrison PJ. The met(158) allele of catechol-O-methyltransferase (COMT) is associated with obsessive-compulsive disorder in men: case-control study and meta-analysis. Mol Psychiatry 2007;12(6): 556–61.
93. Torgersen S. The oral, obsessive, and hysterical personality syndromes. A study of hereditary and environmental factors by means of the twin method. Arch Gen Psychiatry 1980;37:1272–7.
94. Carey G, Gottesman I. Twin and family studies of anxiety, phobic, and obsessive disorders. In: Klein DF, Rabkin JG, editors. Anxiety: new research and changing concepts. New York: Raven Press; 1981. p. 117–36.

# Cognitive Neuroscience of Obsessive-Compulsive Disorder

 CrossMark

Emily R. Stern, PhD[a,b,*], Stephan F. Taylor, MD[c]

## KEYWORDS

- Error monitoring • Conflict monitoring • Response inhibition • Switching
- Decision making • Reward • Default mode network • Perseverative cognition

## KEY POINTS

- Cognitive neuroscientific studies of obsessive-compulsive disorder (OCD) can be used to identify specific targets for treatment.
- The most consistent neuroimaging findings related to symptoms of OCD are hyperactivation in response to errors and hypoactivation during switching tasks, both occurring predominantly in the prefrontal cortex.
- This article proposes an additional model of OCD characterized by inflexible and inappropriate internally focused cognition, subserved by abnormal default mode network (DMN) activity.
- Given the complexity of the brain in general and OCD in particular, no single model is likely to fully explain the disorder.
- Together, the paradigms used in the cognitive neuroscientific study of OCD provide powerful probes that have already shed light on the underlying mechanisms of the disorder.

## INTRODUCTION

For the past several decades, neuroimaging techniques such as functional magnetic resonance imaging (fMRI) and positron emission tomography have been used to investigate neurocircuit functioning in obsessive-compulsive disorder (OCD). Although early

The authors have nothing to disclose.
[a] Department of Psychiatry, Icahn School of Medicine at Mount Sinai, One Gustave Levy Place, Box 1230, New York, NY 10029, USA; [b] Fishberg Department of Neuroscience, Friedman Brain Institute, Icahn School of Medicine at Mount Sinai, 1470 Madison Avenue, New York, NY 10029, USA; [c] Department of Psychiatry, University of Michigan, 4250 Plymouth Road, Ann Arbor, MI 48109, USA
* Corresponding author. Department of Psychiatry, Icahn School of Medicine at Mount Sinai, One Gustave Levy Place, Box 1230, New York, NY 10029.
E-mail address: emily.stern@mssm.edu

| Abbreviations | |
|---|---|
| dACC | Dorsal anterior cingulate cortex |
| DAN | Dorsal attention network |
| DLPFC | Dorsolateral prefrontal cortex |
| DMN | Default mode network |
| EF | Externally focused |
| fMRI | Functional magnetic resonance imaging |
| FPN | Frontal-parietal network |
| IF | Internally focused |
| IFG | Inferior frontal gyrus |
| MFC | Medial frontal cortical |
| MID | Monetary incentive delay |
| OCD | Obsessive-compulsive disorder |
| OFC | Orbitofrontal cortex |
| rACC | Rostral anterior cingulate cortex |
| SMA | Supplemental motor area |
| VMPFC | Ventromedial prefrontal cortex |

studies examining neural responses to symptom provocation in OCD are relevant for the disorder, they do not address whether basic cognitive-emotional mechanisms are impaired in the absence of direct symptom exacerbation. This article discusses findings from cognitive neuroscientific studies probing basic cognitive-emotional processes potentially at the core of OCD, focusing on those constructs for which there have been 3 or more studies comparing adults with OCD with a control group. It discusses results from studies examining conflict and error monitoring, response inhibition, task switching and reversal, decision making, reward processing, and emotional face processing in OCD. It concludes by proposing a model of OCD involving inflexibility of internally focused cognition, in which patients have difficulty disengaging from internally generated negative information. Several approaches not discussed here, such as correlations between neural activity and symptoms, effects of treatment, neurodevelopmental effects, and resting state functional connectivity, have substantially contributed to the understanding of OCD but are beyond the scope of this article.

A cognitive neuroscientific approach to the study of OCD has yielded critical insights into the neural mechanisms of the disorder, and these insights can be used to improve treatment. The most direct connection between cognitive neuroscientific studies of OCD and treatment development comes from the ability of neuroimaging studies to identify specific targets for treatment. Deep brain stimulation and transcranial magnetic stimulation have been used to correct abnormal neural functioning in psychiatric and neurologic disorders,[1] including OCD,[2-6] and investigation of cognitive-emotional processes in OCD has the potential to identify novel targets for these approaches. In addition, neurobiological targets can be modulated using real-time fMRI, which is a developing technology that trains individuals to modify activity in specific brain regions using neurofeedback of the fMRI blood oxygen level–dependent signal.[7] In addition, cognitive neuroscientific studies of OCD can help clarify the neurocircuit mechanisms underlying symptoms of the disorder in order to refine or develop pharmacologic and psychological interventions.

## CONFLICT AND ERROR MONITORING

Much research into the cognitive neuroscience of OCD has focused on conflict monitoring and error detection. This approach is based on the proposal that obsessions are caused by an overactive conflict or error signal continually telling the patient that something is wrong despite evidence to the contrary.[8] In this view, compulsions are behaviors that attempt to reduce this heightened conflict signal or to correct perceived errors. Cognitive conflict is typically studied in tasks in which there is a mismatch between what a subject would automatically do (ie, a prepotent response) and what is required in the task. The classic example of a conflict monitoring paradigm is the Stroop task, in which subjects must make a response according to the font color of a word that is the name of a color that is different from the font color (eg, the word blue written in red font). In this case, the prepotent response is to read the name of the word, but the task requires a response according to the color of the word, which creates conflict that significantly increases response times compared with trials in which the color and word name are the same.[9] Conflict monitoring in healthy controls usually implicates dorsal medial frontal cortical (MFC) regions including dorsal anterior cingulate cortex (dACC) and supplemental motor area (SMA) and pre-SMA,[10–13] but results from the many neuroimaging studies investigating this process in OCD do not present a coherent picture. Although some investigations have found hyperactivity of dorsal MFC during conflict in OCD,[14,15] other studies have identified reduced activity in this region[16,17] or no differences between patients and controls.[18,19] Many studies have reported differences between patients and controls during conflict monitoring in several other brain regions, including parietal cortex,[20,21] inferior frontal gyrus/insula,[22] ventral/rostral regions of MFC,[15,23,24] lateral[17,20] and medial[21] temporal cortex, and striatum including caudate nucleus and putamen.[16,17] However, these results are often contradictory, with some studies finding activations to be greater in OCD than in controls and other studies reporting the opposite effect. At present it is unknown whether these inconsistencies are caused by variability in task design and patient characteristics or whether brain mechanisms of conflict monitoring are not reliably altered in OCD.

Errors reflect a specific instance of conflict in which the intended or correct response does not match the response made by the subject. Similar to conflict monitoring, errors activate dorsal MFC regions including dACC and SMA. In addition, errors tend to elicit an emotional reaction related to frustration, disappointment, or fear of punishment and elicit activation of a broad range of brain regions including bilateral anterior insula, rostral ACC (rACC) and ventromedial prefrontal cortex (VMPFC), dorsolateral prefrontal cortex (DLPFC), and orbitofrontal cortex (OFC).[25] Anterior insula, rostral ACC/VMPFC, and OFC have been associated with valuation and emotion[26–29]; as such, activation of these brain regions to errors may reflect the neural processing of the emotional/motivational significance of mistakes. Support for this notion comes from a study by Taylor and colleagues[30] in which errors associated with a loss of money showed greater activation in rACC/VMPFC than errors involving no motivational consequences, with no effect of error consequence (loss of money vs no loss) on dorsal MFC regions processing conflict.

Patients with OCD show an increased neural response to errors in dACC,[14,31] rACC,[31] and lateral frontal cortex including OFC and DLPFC.[31] Fitzgerald and colleagues[16] found hyperactivity in VMPFC in a small group of patients with OCD, a finding that has been replicated in a larger study[18] that also identified hyperactivity in anterior insula. Despite some variation among the studies, overall these data suggest that patients with OCD respond more strongly to errors than healthy individuals, particularly in ventral frontal and insular regions involved in processing the value or emotional importance of the error. However, these studies examined OCD patients' responses to actual errors (and conflict), whereas the phenotype of the disorder is more consistent with the detection of errors (or conflict) where there are none (or at least where their presence is uncertain). Thus, although hyperactive error responses in OCD may reflect an important characteristic of the disorder related to sensitivity to mistakes, these studies do not directly probe the neural mechanisms associated with the feeling that something is wrong even in the absence of overt errors.

## RESPONSE INHIBITION/MOTOR OUTPUT SUPPRESSION

Unlike conflict or error monitoring models of OCD, in which compulsions are often viewed as secondary responses to the overactive conflict/error signals, studies of response inhibition examining the suppression of motor output in OCD are directly relevant for repetitive motor compulsions. Response inhibition is commonly studied using a go/no-go task (or variant thereof, such as the stop-signal task) in which subjects make button-press responses to frequent stimuli (go trials) and are required to inhibit responses to infrequently presented stimuli (no-go trials). Even though this task inevitably involves conflict monitoring between the frequent go and infrequent no-go trials, these paradigms additionally involve a specific motor suppression component not present in conflict studies. Although no-go trials are associated with activation of some of the same regions as for conflict monitoring, including dACC and SMA/pre-SMA,[32–35] they also elicit activation in subcortical structures including thalamus and basal ganglia, as well as predominantly right hemisphere lateral frontal and inferior parietal regions.[32–36] In a meta-analysis, right inferior frontal gyrus (IFG) has been most consistently associated with no-go trials,[33] which is supported by lesion and brain stimulation studies showing impaired response inhibition after inactivation of this region.[37,38]

It may be hypothesized that an OCD deficit in suppressing motor output would be associated with aberrant recruitment of the response suppression network, which would lead to more failed inhibitions on no-go trials. Although to our knowledge this analysis has not yet been performed, prior studies have compared patients with OCD with controls during successful inhibition in which motor output was appropriately suppressed on no-go trials. Reduced activity in SMA, ACC, right IFG, inferior parietal cortex, striatum, and thalamus has been found in patients with OCD during correct no-go trials,[20,39] which suggests reduced recruitment of the response suppression network even during inhibition success. However, OCD hyperactivity in caudate nucleus and thalamus,[31,39] as well as medial and lateral frontal regions, premotor cortex, middle temporal cortex, posterior cingulate cortex, and cerebellum,[20,31] has also been reported for successful inhibition, which has been interpreted as compensatory activation.[20] Given the variability of findings and the focus on neural differences during successful inhibitions (as opposed to inhibition failures, which would be most relevant for the disorder), further research is needed to determine whether dysfunction in a network for response inhibition is a core mechanism of OCD.

## TASK SWITCHING AND REVERSAL

Another approach to investigating basic mechanisms of OCD has focused on how patients switch attention between 2 or more different tasks, stimuli, or rewards. Rather than focusing on an overactive conflict/error signal or a failure to suppress motor output, these studies hypothesize that patients with OCD have an inflexibility that prevents them from shifting attention away from stimuli or features that are no longer relevant to the task at hand. Because switching deficits need not be limited to the motor domain, impaired switching in OCD may help to explain both obsessions and compulsions.

Many studies of switching have investigated neural activity associated with shifting attention between features or dimensions of stimuli (cognitive switching tasks). In a meta-analysis examining brain regions involved in cognitive switching and motor suppression, overlap between these processes were found in dACC/SMA, IFG, DLPFC, and inferior parietal cortex.[33] However, activations were more widespread and bilateral for cognitive switching than for motor suppression,[33,36] appearing to overlap with a frontal-parietal network (FPN) involved in executive function and task control.[40,41] Studies of brain activity in OCD during cognitive switching have found reduced activation in patients compared with controls in FPN as well as in OFC, caudate nucleus, temporal cortex, and medial parietal regions.[20,42,43] Two studies reported widespread reductions across the cortex and basal ganglia,[42,43] whereas 2 reported hypoactivations localized to only a few regions of frontal and parietal cortex.[20] In addition to hypoactivation of anterior prefrontal cortex extending into lateral OFC, a recent study also found increased dACC, putamen, and postcentral gyrus activity during task switching in OCD.[44]

Another type of switching that has been of interest in OCD involves reversing stimulus-reward contingencies (sometimes referred to as affective switching). In reversal tasks, the reward and punishment value of 2 stimuli switch unexpectedly so that the currently rewarded stimulus is punished and the previously punished stimulus is rewarded. There is some evidence to suggest that reversal of reward-punishment contingencies relies primarily on OFC rather than lateral prefrontal regions involved in cognitive switching.[36,45–47] Studies of reversal in OCD have examined neural activation on trials in which subjects made a reversal error that led to a successful switch compared with errors that did not lead to a successful switch, thereby isolating activity associated with the moment subjects learn that a switch is required.[48–50] For this comparison, patients with OCD show reduced activation in OFC, but, similar to results from cognitive switching studies, reductions were also found throughout FPN including DLPFC, bilateral insula, and lateral parietal cortex.[48–50] In one study, unaffected relatives of OCD also showed reduced activity in lateral OFC, DLPFC, and lateral parietal cortex during reversal,[48] suggesting that impaired frontal recruitment during reversal may be an endophenotype of the disorder.

Overall, these data support the notion that patients with OCD show hypoactivation in a variety of cortical regions during task switching and when reversing reward-punishment contingencies. Despite the dissociation of lateral and orbital frontal involvement in these processes, dysfunctional brain activity in OCD does not seem to be localized to one of these systems. Reduced recruitment of both DLPFC and OFC has been found when patients switch cognitive set as well as when they reverse reward contingencies. However, similar to the concerns discussed for the other approaches, interpretation of results from switching studies is complicated by the fact that neural differences between patients and controls being examined during successful switches (either at the time of the correct switch response or at the time of the error immediately before a correct switch) rather than for unsuccessful switches. Future work examining brain activity during switch failures might further elucidate the neural mechanisms of cognitive inflexibility in OCD.

## RISK AND UNCERTAINTY

OCD has been characterized as a disorder associated with impaired decision making.[51,52] OCD often manifests clinically as risk aversion and intolerance of uncertainty,[53,54] and, in experiments, patients with OCD show reduced risk taking[55] and excessive information gathering in the face of uncertainty.[56–59] In healthy individuals, risk and uncertainty are associated with activation of FPN,[60,61] with effects most consistently found in anterior insula and dorsal MFC.[61–66] In a recent study in which patients with OCD played an interactive game in which they could make risky or safe choices and anticipate outcomes of their choices, patients made fewer risky choices than controls and showed greater amygdala activation when anticipating outcomes of risky choices.[55] In a study focusing on uncertainty, Rotge and colleagues[67] found that patients with OCD showed reduced mid-OFC activity compared with controls for decisions that led to subsequent checking behavior. In another task investigating uncertainty, patients were required to make decisions based on evidence that was either uncertain (ie, the likelihoods for 2 different outcomes were similar) or certain (eg, the likelihood for one outcome was 100% and for the other was 0%).[68] For decisions based on certain evidence, patients with OCD reported more subjective uncertainty and showed increased activation of amygdala, parahippocampus and hippocampus, ventral anterior insula, lateral OFC, and VMPFC than controls, whereas for decisions based on uncertain evidence no group differences were found. In the above-described studies of Admon and colleagues[55] and Stern and colleagues,[68] hyperactivations in patients with OCD were found in brain regions not typically linked to risk and uncertainty in healthy populations, such as amygdala, parahippocampus and hippocampus, and VMPFC.[63] Recruitment of these additional limbic and paralimbic regions when processing risk and uncertainty may reflect greater emotion during decision making in OCD, or an excessive internal focus associated with default mode network (DMN) activity, as suggested later. However, differences between paradigms and the few studies investigating these behaviors in OCD suggest the need for additional study to better understand the scope of decision-making deficits in OCD.

## REWARD PROCESSING

A slightly different approach to understanding OCD proposes that patients have difficulty terminating inappropriate responses due to a reduced signal of goal attainment or satiety.[69] Within this framework, patients with OCD continue to engage in compulsive behaviors such as checking, washing, or repeating/ordering because the normal reward signal associated with successfully completing these tasks is not attained. In healthy individuals, rewards elicit activation in a network of brain regions including ventral striatum, thalamus, putamen, hippocampus, anterior insula, medial frontal cortex, and parietal cortex.[70] Prior studies in OCD have found altered activation in some of these regions during rewarding feedback, including reduced activity in VMPFC using a reversal paradigm.[49,50] However, using a version of the monetary incentive delay (MID) task,[71] Jung and colleagues[72] reported increased activity in cortical and subcortical regions including putamen and dorsal MFC to monetary reward feedback in patients with OCD, with no regions showing reduced activity compared with controls. In another study also using a version of the MID, patients with OCD showed reduced dorsal MFC activation compared with controls during reward feedback, as well as reduced activation in ventral striatum when anticipating an upcoming trial that could potentially provide reward.[73] This latter finding contrasts with 3 other studies showing no difference in striatal activation between patients with OCD and controls during anticipation of trials in which reward was possible.[72,74,75] Overall, it is not yet clear whether dysfunctional brain responses to reward contribute to OCD, although impaired recruitment of striatum during reward processing has not been consistently implicated in the disorder. Future neuroimaging work may benefit from examining reward processing from the standpoint of goal attainment or task completion, which may be particularly relevant for the symptoms of the disorder.

## EMOTIONAL FACE PROCESSING

Despite the importance of negative emotion in OCD, few studies have directly examined emotional processing in the disorder. It is possible that heightened neural activation to emotional stimuli in OCD could lead to the excessive fear and/or anxiety associated with obsessions. Experiments investigating the functional neuroanatomy of emotion often compare brain activity when viewing facial expressions of various emotions (including fear, disgust, happiness, sadness, and anger) with activity elicited by neutral faces or nonface control tasks.[76] Studies examining the neural correlates of emotional face processing in OCD have yielded conflicting results. A recent study found hyperactivation in OCD in visual cortex, DLPFC, posterior thalamus, and limbic regions including amygdala and parahippocampus when matching either happy or fearful facial expressions compared with matching nonface shapes.[77] There was also an effect of face valence, such that patients with OCD showed greater activation than controls in DLPFC and anterior insula for fearful compared with happy facial expressions. These data are consistent with a recent report of hyperactivation in OCD of visual cortex, anterior insula, OFC, and amygdala when matching fearful faces; amygdala was positively correlated with severity of aggressive and sexual/religious symptoms.[78] However, these more recent findings contrast with an earlier report of reduced amygdala activation in OCD when observing fearful, happy, and neutral faces compared with a fixation condition.[79] In addition, compared with neutral faces, facial expressions of disgust have been found to elicit greater activity in left OFC but reduced activity in thalamus in OCD, with no differences between patients and control subjects for fearful versus neutral faces.[80] These discrepancies may be caused by variability of task design and analyses, and further work is needed to determine whether patients with OCD have abnormalities in response to emotional stimuli other than faces.

## IMPAIRED FLEXIBILITY OF INTERNALLY FOCUSED COGNITION IN OCD
### New Approach to an Old Problem?

One of the most striking symptoms of patients with OCD is their propensity to get stuck in a thought, feeling, image, or behavior. As discussed earlier, previous studies investigating inflexibility in OCD have focused on how patients switch between attending to different pieces of external information,[20,42,44] such as sensory features of stimuli (eg, switching between color vs shape of stimuli). Although this basic level of task switching may be impaired in OCD, symptoms manifest clinically as difficulty switching attention away from internally generated and perpetuated fears of negative events (such as a person's home being broken into or contracting a disease) toward externally observable evidence indicating that the dreaded events will or did not happen (such as seeing that the door is locked or that the hands are clean). We propose here that a core dysfunction in OCD is an inflexibility of internally focused (IF) cognition.

The ability to flexibly switch attention between a perceptually decoupled IF state and a perceptually driven externally focused (EF) state is critical for efficient functioning. Estimates suggest that IF thought processes related to imagination and mental simulation, episodic memory, and introspection account for approximately 30% of all waking cognition.[81,82] At rest, individuals spontaneously switch between internal and external attentional states every 20 seconds, on average.[83] Although attentional state switching can occur outside of conscious awareness, such as when the brain unintentionally lapses into IF thought during mind wandering,[84] engaging with, or disengaging from, an IF state can be goal directed and even effortful. IF cognition can be adaptive and desirable when memory or imagination is used to regulate emotion (eg, remembering a safe plane flight when feeling afraid to fly) or solve a problem (eg, imagining how various scenarios will work out).[82,85–87] However, IF cognition becomes problematic when there is an inability to disengage from persistent thoughts about past or future events, sometimes referred to as perseverative cognition.[85–90] Perseverative cognition is associated with negative affect and is predictive of current and future mental disorder.[85–89,91] We suggest that abnormal IF cognition constitutes a key component of OCD.

Over the past decade, neuroimaging research has elucidated the neural mechanisms of IF and EF cognition. IF tasks activate the DMN, a large-scale system including VMPFC and anterior dorsomedial frontal cortex, medial parietal cortex including posterior cingulate and precuneus, lateral posterior inferior parietal cortex, lateral temporal cortex, parahippocampal gyrus, and hippocampus.[92–96] DMN activity decreases (or deactivates) during tasks requiring EF attention,[97,98] which may reflect the suspension of internal cognition when attention must be directed to information in the environment.[94,99,100] Activation in DMN (or a failure to deactivate) is associated with performance decrements during EF tasks of selective and sustained attention[96,101,102] but improved performance on IF tasks of episodic memory.[103–105]

In contrast with the role of DMN in IF cognition, EF tasks activate networks often referred to as task positive (in contrast with the deactivation seen in the DMN[41]). Several different formulations of these task-positive networks exist, but 2 dissociable networks consistently associated with the task-positive system are described here: the dorsal attention network (DAN) and the aforementioned FPN. The DAN is involved in visuospatial attention and motor planning and consists of precentral gyrus/frontal eye fields, superior parietal cortex, and posterior temporal and occipital cortex (including an area of motion-sensitive temporal cortex referred to as MT+).[95,106,107] The FPN is recruited by tasks tapping into higher-order cognitive functions involved in acting on or manipulating information, and consists of posterior regions of dorsal MFC (dACC and SMA/pre-SMA), DLPFC and IFG, anterior insula, inferior parietal cortex, and striatum.[33,90,95,106,107] The antagonist relationship between DMN and task-positive network activity during EF tasks is mirrored by negative correlations between these networks at rest,[108,109] which may be the basis for intrinsic competition between IF and EF attentional states.

Patients with OCD have repeatedly shown abnormality in various regions of DMN, which may be associated with impaired IF cognition. In a meta-analysis of fMRI data from several different task paradigms, Menzies and colleagues[110] found greater activation in OCD compared with controls within several regions including VMPFC, posterior cingulate cortex, and parahippocampus. Patients with OCD show reduced deactivation of VMPFC during EF tasks of error detection,[16,18] and greater activation of multiple DMN regions including VMPFC, parahippocampus and hippocampus, lateral temporal cortex, and posterior inferior parietal cortex during decision making,[68] suggesting impairment in suppressing neural substrates of IF cognition during certain EF tasks. Extending these findings to an IF cognition paradigm in which patients pondered moral dilemmas about causing harm to others, patients with OCD again showed greater activation of VMPFC and lateral temporal regions than controls.[111]

There is also some evidence that patients with OCD may not appropriately engage DMN-based IF cognition when it would be beneficial. In investigations of fear memory, a conditioned fear response is extinguished through repeated presentations of a conditioned stimulus, and extinction recall occurs when this extinction or safety information is remembered during later testing. Extinction recall has been characterized as a form of emotion regulation related to episodic memory[112] and involves both VMPFC and hippocampus.[113,114] In one recent study examining extinction recall in OCD, patients showed reduced VMPFC activity and greater electrodermal responses compared with controls,[115] suggesting an inability to implement memory-based emotion regulation in order to reduce fear. This finding is particularly intriguing because it raises the possibility that such a deficit may extend to other types of IF-based emotion regulation strategies (such as mental simulations and perspective-taking) as well as problem solving. Additional research is needed to test these hypotheses.

Overall, these data indicate that DMN functioning is abnormal in OCD, which may be the substrate for disruptions of IF cognition that characterize the disorder. Such altered DMN functioning may be caused by abnormal connectivity between DMN and FPN[116,117] as well as within DMN.[118–122] A lack of flexible IF cognition and DMN functioning could conceivably lead to multiple behavioral disturbances, including the excessive focus on internal thoughts and images that are the content of obsessions.

## SUMMARY

This article provides a selective review of neuroimaging correlates of psychological processes that could potentially underlie the complex symptom presentation of OCD. The most consistent findings were hyperactivation in response to errors and hypoactivation during switching tasks, with both effects occurring predominantly in prefrontal cortex. An additional model of the disorder is proposed, characterized by inflexible and inappropriate IF cognition, subserved by abnormal DMN activity. This conceptualization cannot explain all of the symptoms of this complex disorder, and it is likely that aberrant DMN functioning occurs in concert with dysfunction in other systems. For example, motor/habit functions involving frontostriatal circuits and interoceptive processes subserved by the insula may be important, particularly for compulsions. However, this novel conceptualization provides a jumping-off point for future work designed to improve understanding of mechanisms not only of OCD but also of comorbid internalizing disorders similarly characterized by perseverative cognition and DMN hyperactivity, such as depression.[123,124] Given the complexity of the brain in general and OCD in particular, no single model is likely to fully explain the disorder, and it is clear that the task chosen is critical for interpreting findings. Other approaches investigating habit formation,[125,126] loss expectancy,[72,127] image suppression,[128] performance feedback,[129] and working memory[130–133] have identified alterations in OCD that may also contribute to the phenomenology of the disorder. Taken together, the many paradigms used in the cognitive neuroscientific study of OCD provide powerful probes that have already shed light on the underlying mechanisms of the disorder. Future work would benefit from combining the strengths from these many approaches in order to explore neurocircuit functioning in OCD from a variety of perspectives.

## REFERENCES

1. Kopell BH, Greenberg B, Rezai AR. Deep brain stimulation for psychiatric disorders. J Clin Neurophysiol 2004;21(1):51–67.
2. Abelson JL, Curtis GC, Sagher O, et al. Deep brain stimulation for refractory obsessive-compulsive disorder. Biol Psychiatry 2005;57(5):510–6.
3. de Koning PP, Figee M, van den Munckhof P, et al. Current status of deep brain stimulation for obsessive-compulsive disorder: a clinical review of different targets. Curr Psychiatry Rep 2011;13(4):274–82.

4. Denys D, Mantione M, Figee M, et al. Deep brain stimulation of the nucleus accumbens for therapy-refractory obsessive-compulsive disorder. Eur Neuropsychopharmacol 2010;20:S235.

5. Goodman WK, Foote KD, Greenberg BD, et al. Deep brain stimulation for intractable obsessive compulsive disorder: pilot study using a blinded, staggered-onset design. Biol Psychiatry 2010;67(6):535–42.

6. Greenberg BD, Malone DA, Friehs GM, et al. Three-year outcomes in deep brain stimulation for highly resistant obsessive-compulsive disorder. Neuropsychopharmacology 2006;31(11):2384–93.

7. Sulzer J, Haller S, Scharnowski F, et al. Real-time fMRI neurofeedback: progress and challenges. Neuroimage 2013;76(1):386–99.

8. Pitman RK. A cybernetic model of obsessive-compulsive psychopathology. Compr Psychiatry 1987;28(4):334–43.

9. MacLeod CM. Half a century of research on the Stroop effect: an integrative review. Psychol Bull 1991;109(2):163–203.

10. Botvinick MM, Braver TS, Barch DM, et al. Conflict monitoring and cognitive control. Psychol Rev 2001;108(3):624–52.

11. Garavan H, Ross TJ, Kaufman J, et al. A midline dissociation between error-processing and response-conflict monitoring. Neuroimage 2003;20(2):1132–9.

12. Hester R, Fassbender C, Garavan H. Individual differences in error processing: a review and reanalysis of three event-related fMRI studies using the GO/NOGO task. Cereb Cortex 2004;14(9):986–94.

13. Ridderinkhof KR, Ullsperger M, Crone EA, et al. The role of the medial frontal cortex in cognitive control. Science 2004;306(5695):443–7.

14. Ursu S, Stenger VA, Shear MK, et al. Overactive action monitoring in obsessive-compulsive disorder: evidence from functional magnetic resonance imaging. Psychol Sci 2003;14(4):347–53.

15. Yucel M, Harrison BJ, Wood SJ, et al. Functional and biochemical alterations of the medial frontal cortex in obsessive-compulsive disorder. Arch Gen Psychiatry 2007;64(8):946–55.

16. Fitzgerald KD, Welsh RC, Gehring WJ, et al. Error-related hyperactivity of the anterior cingulate cortex in obsessive-compulsive disorder. Biol Psychiatry 2005;57(3):287–94.

17. Nakao T, Nakagawa A, Yoshiura T, et al. A functional MRI comparison of patients with obsessive-compulsive disorder and normal controls during a Chinese character Stroop task. Psychiatry Res 2005;139(2):101–14.

18. Stern ER, Welsh RC, Fitzgerald KD, et al. Hyperactive error responses and altered connectivity in ventromedial and frontoinsular cortices in obsessive-compulsive disorder. Biol Psychiatry 2011;69(6):583–91.

19. Viard A, Flament MF, Artiges E, et al. Cognitive control in childhood-onset obsessive-compulsive disorder: a functional MRI study. Psychol Med 2005;35(7):1007–17.

20. Page LA, Rubia K, Deeley Q, et al. A functional magnetic resonance imaging study of inhibitory control in obsessive-compulsive disorder. Psychiatry Res 2009;174(3):202–9.

21. van den Heuvel OA, Veltman DJ, Groenewegen HJ, et al. Disorder-specific neuroanatomical correlates of attentional bias in obsessive-compulsive disorder, panic disorder, and hypochondriasis. Arch Gen Psychiatry 2005;62(8):922–33.

22. Marsh R, Horga G, Parashar N, et al. Altered activation in fronto-striatal circuits during sequential processing of conflict in unmedicated adults with obsessive-compulsive disorder. Biol Psychiatry 2013;75(8):615–22.

23. Harrison BJ, Yucel M, Shaw M, et al. Evaluating brain activity in obsessive-compulsive disorder: preliminary insights from a multivariate analysis. Psychiatry Res 2006;147(2–3):227–31.
24. Nabeyama M, Nakagawa A, Yoshiura T, et al. Functional MRI study of brain activation alterations in patients with obsessive-compulsive disorder after symptom improvement. Psychiatry Res 2008;163(3):236–47.
25. Taylor SF, Stern ER, Gehring WJ. Neural systems for error monitoring: recent findings and theoretical perspectives. Neuroscientist 2007;13(2):160–72.
26. Harrison NA, Gray MA, Gianaros PJ, et al. The embodiment of emotional feelings in the brain. J Neurosci 2010;30(38):12878–84.
27. Kober H, Barrett LF, Joseph J, et al. Functional grouping and cortical-subcortical interactions in emotion: a meta-analysis of neuroimaging studies. Neuroimage 2008;42(2):998–1031.
28. Kringelbach ML, Rolls ET. The functional neuroanatomy of the human orbitofrontal cortex: evidence from neuroimaging and neuropsychology. Prog Neurobiol 2004;72(5):341–72.
29. Lebreton M, Jorge S, Michel V, et al. An automatic valuation system in the human brain: evidence from functional neuroimaging. Neuron 2009;64(3):431–9.
30. Taylor SF, Martis B, Fitzgerald KD, et al. Medial frontal cortex activity and loss-related responses to errors. J Neurosci 2006;26(15):4063–70.
31. Maltby N, Tolin DF, Worhunsky P, et al. Dysfunctional action monitoring hyperactivates frontal-striatal circuits in obsessive-compulsive disorder: an event-related fMRI study. Neuroimage 2005;24(2):495–503.
32. Aron AR, Poldrack RA. Cortical and subcortical contributions to stop signal response inhibition: role of the subthalamic nucleus. J Neurosci 2006;26(9):2424–33.
33. Buchsbaum BR, Greer S, Chang WL, et al. Meta-analysis of neuroimaging studies of the Wisconsin card-sorting task and component processes. Hum Brain Mapp 2005;25(1):35–45.
34. Garavan H, Hester R, Murphy K, et al. Individual differences in the functional neuroanatomy of inhibitory control. Brain Res 2006;1105:130–42.
35. Garavan H, Ross TJ, Stein EA. Right hemispheric dominance of inhibitory control: an event-related functional MRI study. Proc Natl Acad Sci U S A 1999;96(14):8301–6.
36. Robbins TW. Shifting and stopping: fronto-striatal substrates, neurochemical modulation and clinical implications. Philos Trans R Soc Lond B Biol Sci 2007;362(1481):917–32.
37. Aron AR, Fletcher PC, Bullmore ET, et al. Stop-signal inhibition disrupted by damage to right inferior frontal gyrus in humans. Nat Neurosci 2003;6(2):115–6.
38. Chambers CD, Bellgrove MA, Stokes MG, et al. Executive "brake failure" following deactivation of human frontal lobe. J Cogn Neurosci 2006;18(3):444–55.
39. Roth RM, Saykin AJ, Flashman LA, et al. Event-related functional magnetic resonance imaging of response inhibition in obsessive-compulsive disorder. Biol Psychiatry 2007;62(8):901–9.
40. Bressler SL, Menon V. Large-scale brain networks in cognition: emerging methods and principles. Trends Cogn Sci 2010;14(6):277–90.
41. Power JD, Cohen AL, Nelson SM, et al. Functional network organization of the human brain. Neuron 2011;72(4):665–78.
42. Gu BM, Park JY, Kang DH, et al. Neural correlates of cognitive inflexibility during task-switching in obsessive-compulsive disorder. Brain 2008;131:155–64.

43. Han JY, Kang DH, Gu BM, et al. Altered brain activation in ventral frontal-striatal regions following a 16-week pharmacotherapy in unmedicated obsessive-compulsive disorder. J Korean Med Sci 2011;26(5):665–74.
44. Remijnse PL, van den Heuvel OA, Nielen MM, et al. Cognitive inflexibility in obsessive-compulsive disorder and major depression is associated with distinct neural correlates. PLoS One 2013;8(4):e59600.
45. Dias R, Robbins TW, Roberts AC. Dissociation in prefrontal cortex of affective and attentional shifts. Nature 1996;380(6569):69–72.
46. Fellows LK, Farah MJ. Ventromedial frontal cortex mediates affective shifting in humans: evidence from a reversal learning paradigm. Brain 2003;126:1830–7.
47. Hampshire A, Owen AM. Fractionating attentional control using event-related fMRI. Cereb Cortex 2006;16(12):1679–89.
48. Chamberlain SR, Menzies L, Hampshire A, et al. Orbitofrontal dysfunction in patients with obsessive-compulsive disorder and their unaffected relatives. Science 2008;321(5887):421–2.
49. Remijnse PL, Nielen MM, van Balkom AJ, et al. Reduced orbitofrontal-striatal activity on a reversal learning task in obsessive-compulsive disorder. Arch Gen Psychiatry 2006;63(11):1225–36.
50. Remijnse PL, Nielen MM, van Balkom AJ, et al. Differential frontal-striatal and paralimbic activity during reversal learning in major depressive disorder and obsessive-compulsive disorder. Psychol Med 2009;39(9):1503–18.
51. Cavedini P, Gorini A, Bellodi L. Understanding obsessive-compulsive disorder: focus on decision making. Neuropsychol Rev 2006;16(1):3–15.
52. Sachdev PS, Malhi GS. Obsessive-compulsive behaviour: a disorder of decision-making. Aust N Z J Psychiatry 2005;39(9):757–63.
53. Steketee G, Frost RO. Measurement of risk-taking in obsessive compulsive disorder. Behav Cognit Psychother 1994;22:269–98.
54. Tolin DF, Abramowitz JS, Brigidi BD, et al. Intolerance of uncertainty in obsessive-compulsive disorder. J Anxiety Disord 2003;17(2):233–42.
55. Admon R, Bleich-Cohen M, Weizmant R, et al. Functional and structural neural indices of risk aversion in obsessive-compulsive disorder (OCD). Psychiatry Res 2012;203(2–3):207–13.
56. Fear CF, Healy D. Probabilistic reasoning in obsessive-compulsive and delusional disorders. Psychol Med 1997;27(1):199–208.
57. Foa EB, Mathews A, Abramowitz JS, et al. Do patients with obsessive-compulsive disorder have deficits in decision-making? Cognit Ther Res 2003; 27(4):431–45.
58. Milner AD, Beech HR, Walker VJ. Decision processes and obsessional behavior. Br J Soc Clin Psychol 1971;10(1):88–9.
59. Volans PJ. Styles of decision-making and probability appraisal in selected obsessional and phobic patients. Br J Soc Clin Psychol 1976;15(3):305–17.
60. Huettel SA. Behavioral, but not reward, risk modulates activation of prefrontal, parietal, and insular cortices. Cogn Affect Behav Neurosci 2006;6(2):141–51.
61. Krain AL, Wilson AM, Arbuckle R, et al. Distinct neural mechanisms of risk and ambiguity: a meta-analysis of decision-making. Neuroimage 2006;32(1):477–84.
62. Grinband J, Hirsch J, Ferrera VP. A neural representation of categorization uncertainty in the human brain. Neuron 2006;49(5):757–63.
63. Mohr PN, Biele G, Heekeren HR. Neural processing of risk. J Neurosci 2010; 30(19):6613–9.
64. Preuschoff K, Quartz SR, Bossaerts P. Human insula activation reflects risk prediction errors as well as risk. J Neurosci 2008;28(11):2745–52.

65. Stern ER, Gonzalez R, Welsh RC, et al. Medial frontal cortex and anterior insula are less sensitive to outcome predictability when monetary stakes are higher. Soc Cogn Affect Neurosci 2013. [Epub ahead of print].
66. Volz KG, Schubotz RI, von Cramon DY. Predicting events of varying probability: uncertainty investigated by fMRI. Neuroimage 2003;19(2 Pt 1):271–80.
67. Rotge JY, Langbour N, Dilharreguy B, et al. Contextual and behavioral influences on uncertainty in obsessive-compulsive disorder. Cortex 2012. http://dx.doi.org/10.1016/j.cortex.2012.12.010. pii:S0010-9452(12)00346-2. [Epub ahead of print].
68. Stern ER, Welsh RC, Gonzalez R, et al. Subjective uncertainty and limbic hyperactivation in obsessive-compulsive disorder. Hum Brain Mapp 2013;34(8):1956–70.
69. Szechtman H, Woody E. Obsessive-compulsive disorder as a disturbance of security motivation. Psychol Rev 2004;111(1):111–27.
70. Liu X, Hairston J, Schrier M, et al. Common and distinct networks underlying reward valence and processing stages: a meta-analysis of functional neuroimaging studies. Neurosci Biobehav Rev 2011;35(5):1219–36.
71. Knutson B, Fong GW, Bennett SM, et al. A region of mesial prefrontal cortex tracks monetarily rewarding outcomes: characterization with rapid event-related fMRI. Neuroimage 2003;18(2):263–72.
72. Jung WH, Kang DH, Han JY, et al. Aberrant ventral striatal responses during incentive processing in unmedicated patients with obsessive-compulsive disorder. Acta Psychiatr Scand 2011;123(5):376–86.
73. Figee M, Vink M, de Geus F, et al. Dysfunctional reward circuitry in obsessive-compulsive disorder. Biol Psychiatry 2011;69(9):867–74.
74. Choi JS, Shin YC, Jung WH, et al. Altered brain activity during reward anticipation in pathological gambling and obsessive-compulsive disorder. PLoS One 2012;7(9):e45938.
75. Kaufmann C, Beucke JC, Preusse F, et al. Medial prefrontal brain activation to anticipated reward and loss in obsessive-compulsive disorder. Neuroimage Clin 2013;2:212–20.
76. Phan KL, Wager T, Taylor SF, et al. Functional neuroanatomy of emotion: a meta-analysis of emotion activation studies in PET and fMRI. Neuroimage 2002;16(2):331–48.
77. Cardoner N, Harrison BJ, Pujol J, et al. Enhanced brain responsiveness during active emotional face processing in obsessive compulsive disorder. W J Biol Psychiatry 2011;12(5):349–63.
78. Via E, Cardoner N, Pujol J, et al. Amygdala activation and symptom dimensions in obsessive-compulsive disorder. Br J Psychiatry 2013;204(1):61–8.
79. Cannistraro PA, Wright CI, Wedig MM, et al. Amygdala responses to human faces in obsessive-compulsive disorder. Biol Psychiatry 2004;56(12):916–20.
80. Lawrence NS, An SK, Mataix-Cols D, et al. Neural responses to facial expressions of disgust but not fear are modulated by washing symptoms in OCD. Biol Psychiatry 2007;61(9):1072–80.
81. Kane MJ, Brown LH, McVay JC, et al. For whom the mind wanders, and when: an experience-sampling study of working memory and executive control in daily life. Psychol Sci 2007;18(7):614–21.
82. Smallwood J, Schooler JW. The restless mind. Psychol Bull 2006;132(6):946–58.
83. Vanhaudenhuyse A, Demertzi A, Schabus M, et al. Two distinct neuronal networks mediate the awareness of environment and of self. J Cogn Neurosci 2011;23(3):570–8.

84. Mason MF, Norton MI, Van Horn JD, et al. Wandering minds: the default network and stimulus-independent thought. Science 2007;315(5810):393–5.

85. Ottaviani C, Shapiro D, Couyoumdjian A. Flexibility as the key for somatic health: from mind wandering to perseverative cognition. Biol Psychol 2013;94(1):38–43.

86. Segerstrom SC, Stanton AL, Alden LE, et al. A multidimensional structure for repetitive thought: what's on your mind, and how, and how much? J Pers Soc Psychol 2003;85(5):909–21.

87. Watkins ER. Constructive and unconstructive repetitive thought. Psychol Bull 2008;134(2):163–206.

88. Brosschot JF, Gerin W, Thayer JF. The perseverative cognition hypothesis: a review of worry, prolonged stress-related physiological activation, and health. J Psychosom Res 2006;60(2):113–24.

89. Smith JM, Alloy LB. A roadmap to rumination: a review of the definition, assessment, and conceptualization of this multifaceted construct. Clin Psychol Rev 2009;29(2):116–28.

90. Smith SM, Fox PT, Miller KL, et al. Correspondence of the brain's functional architecture during activation and rest. Proc Natl Acad Sci U S A 2009; 106(31):13040–5.

91. Topper M, Emmelkamp PM, Ehring T. Improving prevention of depression and anxiety disorders: repetitive negative thinking as a promising target. Appl Prev Psychol 2010;14(1–4):57–71.

92. Addis DR, Wong AT, Schacter DL. Remembering the past and imagining the future: common and distinct neural substrates during event construction and elaboration. Neuropsychologia 2007;45(7):1363–77.

93. Andrews-Hanna JR. The brain's default network and its adaptive role in internal mentation. Neuroscientist 2012;18(3):251–70.

94. Buckner RL, Andrews-Hanna JR, Schacter DL. The brain's default network: anatomy, function, and relevance to disease. Ann N Y Acad Sci 2008;1124:1–38.

95. Spreng RN, Stevens WD, Chamberlain JP, et al. Default network activity, coupled with the frontoparietal control network, supports goal-directed cognition. Neuroimage 2010;53(1):303–17.

96. Stawarczyk D, Majerus S, Maquet P, et al. Neural correlates of ongoing conscious experience: both task-unrelatedness and stimulus-independence are related to default network activity. PLoS One 2011;6(2):e16997.

97. McKiernan KA, Kaufman JN, Kucera-Thompson J, et al. A parametric manipulation of factors affecting task-induced deactivation in functional neuroimaging. J Cogn Neurosci 2003;15(3):394–408.

98. Shulman GL, Fiez JA, Corbetta M, et al. Common blood flow changes across visual tasks: II. Decreases in cerebral cortex. J Cogn Neurosci 1997;9(5): 648–63.

99. Andrews-Hanna JR, Reidler JS, Sepulcre J, et al. Functional-anatomic fractionation of the brain's default network. Neuron 2010;65(4):550–62.

100. Gusnard DA, Akbudak E, Shulman GL, et al. Medial prefrontal cortex and self-referential mental activity: relation to a default mode of brain function. Proc Natl Acad Sci U S A 2001;98(7):4259–64.

101. Weissman DH, Roberts KC, Visscher KM, et al. The neural bases of momentary lapses in attention. Nat Neurosci 2006;9(7):971–8.

102. Wen X, Liu Y, Yao L, et al. Top-down regulation of default mode activity in spatial visual attention. J Neurosci 2013;33(15):6444–53.

103. Buckner RL, Wheeler ME. The cognitive neuroscience of remembering. Nat Rev Neurosci 2001;2(9):624–34.

104. Rugg MD, Vilberg KL. Brain networks underlying episodic memory retrieval. Curr Opin Neurobiol 2013;23(2):255–60.
105. Wagner AD, Shannon BJ, Kahn I, et al. Parietal lobe contributions to episodic memory retrieval. Trends Cogn Sci 2005;9(9):445–53.
106. Corbetta M, Shulman GL. Control of goal-directed and stimulus-driven attention in the brain. Nat Rev Neurosci 2002;3(3):201–15.
107. Vincent JL, Kahn I, Snyder AZ, et al. Evidence for a frontoparietal control system revealed by intrinsic functional connectivity. J Neurophysiol 2008;100(6): 3328–42.
108. Fox MD, Snyder AZ, Vincent JL, et al. The human brain is intrinsically organized into dynamic, anticorrelated functional networks. Proc Natl Acad Sci U S A 2005; 102(27):9673–8.
109. Fransson P. How default is the default mode of brain function? Further evidence from intrinsic BOLD signal fluctuations. Neuropsychologia 2006;44(14): 2836–45.
110. Menzies L, Chamberlain SR, Laird AR, et al. Integrating evidence from neuroimaging and neuropsychological studies of obsessive-compulsive disorder: the orbitofronto-striatal model revisited. Neurosci Biobehav Rev 2008;32(3): 525–49.
111. Harrison BJ, Pujol J, Soriano-Mas C, et al. Neural correlates of moral sensitivity in obsessive-compulsive disorder. Arch Gen Psychiatry 2012;69(7):741–9.
112. Quirk GJ, Beer JS. Prefrontal involvement in the regulation of emotion: convergence of rat and human studies. Curr Opin Neurobiol 2006;16(6):723–7.
113. Milad MR, Wright CI, Orr SP, et al. Recall of fear extinction in humans activates the ventromedial prefrontal cortex and hippocampus in concert. Biol Psychiatry 2007;62(5):446–54.
114. Quirk GJ, Garcia R, Gonzalez-Lima F. Prefrontal mechanisms in extinction of conditioned fear. Biol Psychiatry 2006;60(4):337–43.
115. Milad MR, Furtak SC, Greenberg JL, et al. Deficits in conditioned fear extinction in obsessive-compulsive disorder and neurobiological changes in the fear circuit. JAMA Psychiatry 2013;70(6):608–18 [quiz: 554].
116. Fitzgerald KD, Welsh RC, Stern ER, et al. Developmental alterations of frontal-striatal-thalamic connectivity in obsessive-compulsive disorder. J Am Acad Child Adolesc Psychiatry 2011;50(9):938–48.e3.
117. Stern ER, Fitzgerald KD, Welsh RC, et al. Resting-state functional connectivity between fronto-parietal and default mode networks in obsessive-compulsive disorder. PLoS One 2012;7(5):e36356.
118. Beucke JC, Sepulcre J, Talukdar T, et al. Abnormally high degree connectivity of the orbitofrontal cortex in obsessive-compulsive disorder. JAMA Psychiatry 2013;70(6):619–29.
119. Cocchi L, Harrison BJ, Pujol J, et al. Functional alterations of large-scale brain networks related to cognitive control in obsessive-compulsive disorder. Hum Brain Mapp 2012;33(5):1089–106.
120. Fontenelle LF, Harrison BJ, Pujol J, et al. Brain functional connectivity during induced sadness in patients with obsessive-compulsive disorder. J Psychiatry Neurosci 2012;37(4):231–40.
121. Jang JH, Kim JH, Jung WH, et al. Functional connectivity in fronto-subcortical circuitry during the resting state in obsessive-compulsive disorder. Neurosci Lett 2010;474(3):158–62.
122. Peng ZW, Xu T, He QH, et al. Default network connectivity as a vulnerability marker for obsessive compulsive disorder. Psychol Med 2014;44(7):1475–84.

123. Broyd SJ, Demanuele C, Debener S, et al. Default-mode brain dysfunction in mental disorders: a systematic review. Neurosci Biobehav Rev 2009;33(3): 279–96.

124. Hamilton JP, Furman DJ, Chang C, et al. Default-mode and task-positive network activity in major depressive disorder: implications for adaptive and maladaptive rumination. Biol Psychiatry 2011;70(4):327–33.

125. Rauch SL, Savage CR, Alpert NM, et al. Probing striatal function in obsessive-compulsive disorder: a PET study of implicit sequence learning. J Neuropsychiatry Clin Neurosci 1997;9(4):568–73.

126. Rauch SL, Wedig MM, Wright CI, et al. Functional magnetic resonance imaging study of regional brain activation during implicit sequence learning in obsessive-compulsive disorder. Biol Psychiatry 2007;61(3):330–6.

127. Ursu S, Carter CS. An initial investigation of the orbitofrontal cortex hyperactivity in obsessive-compulsive disorder: exaggerated representations of anticipated aversive events? Neuropsychologia 2009;47(10):2145–8.

128. Kocak OM, Ozpolat AY, Atbasoglu C, et al. Cognitive control of a simple mental image in patients with obsessive-compulsive disorder. Brain Cogn 2011;76(3): 390–9.

129. Becker MP, Nitsch AM, Schlosser R, et al. Altered emotional and BOLD responses to negative, positive and ambiguous performance feedback in OCD. Soc Cogn Affect Neurosci 2013. [Epub ahead of print].

130. Henseler I, Gruber O, Kraft S, et al. Compensatory hyperactivations as markers of latent working memory dysfunctions in patients with obsessive-compulsive disorder: an fMRI study. J Psychiatry Neurosci 2008;33(3):209–15.

131. Koch K, Wagner G, Schachtzabel C, et al. Aberrant anterior cingulate activation in obsessive-compulsive disorder is related to task complexity. Neuropsychologia 2012;50(5):958–64.

132. Nakao T, Nakagawa A, Nakatani E, et al. Working memory dysfunction in obsessive-compulsive disorder: a neuropsychological and functional MRI study. J Psychiatr Res 2009;43(8):784–91.

133. van der Wee NJ, Ramsey NF, Jansma JM, et al. Spatial working memory deficits in obsessive compulsive disorder are associated with excessive engagement of the medial frontal cortex. Neuroimage 2003;20(4):2271–80.

# Pediatric Acute-Onset Neuropsychiatric Syndrome

Tanya K. Murphy, MD, MS[a],*, Diana M. Gerardi, MA[a],
James F. Leckman, MD, PhD[b]

KEYWORDS

- PANDAS • Pediatric autoimmune neuropsychiatric disorder
- Streptococcal infections

KEY POINTS

- A subtype of obsessive-compulsive disorder (OCD) that consists of an abrupt and severe onset has been described.
- The clinical presentation of pediatric acute-onset neuropsychiatric syndrome (PANS) can be differentiated from classic pediatric OCD by its course and its more global neuropsychiatric dysfunction.
- The causal mechanism is unsettled, and it is possible that multiple triggers initiate a neuroimmune process that converges to a common pathway leading to the clinical presentation.
- Research is under way regarding potential treatments, but is currently limited.
- Empirical studies and case reports suggest that potential PANS treatments should consist mostly of therapies that target immune and infectious causes.

## OVERVIEW: NATURE OF PROBLEM

Pediatric autoimmune neuropsychiatric disorder associated with *Streptococcus* (PANDAS) is characterized by an abrupt (24–48 hours) onset of obsessive-compulsive disorder (OCD) and/or tics. Associated symptoms include emotional lability, separation anxiety, deterioration in handwriting, poor attention, and attention deficit/hyperactivity disorder (ADHD)-like impulsivity, deteriorating visual-spatial abilities, math and reading deficits, and enuresis (**Box 1**).[1] Neuropsychiatric symptoms tend to emerge 7 to 14 days after a group A streptococcal (GAS) infection. The course

Disclosures: See last page of article.
[a] Rothman Center for Pediatric Neuropsychiatry, USF Pediatrics, 880 6th Street South, Suite 460, Box 7523, St Petersburg, FL 33701, USA; [b] Child Study Center, Yale University School of Medicine, 230 S Frontage Road, New Haven, CT 06520, USA
* Corresponding author.
*E-mail address:* tmurphy@health.usf.edu

Psychiatr Clin N Am 37 (2014) 353–374
http://dx.doi.org/10.1016/j.psc.2014.06.001
0193-953X/14/$ – see front matter © 2014 Elsevier Inc. All rights reserved.

| Abbreviations | |
|---|---|
| ADHD | Attention deficit/hyperactivity disorder |
| ASO | Antistreptolysin |
| CaM kinase II | Calcium-calmodulin–dependent protein kinase II |
| CANS | Childhood acute neuropsychiatric symptoms |
| CBT | Cognitive-behavioral therapy |
| ELISA | Enzyme-linked immunosorbent assay |
| GAS | Group A streptococcal |
| IgG | Immunoglobulin G |
| IgM | Immunoglobulin M |
| IVIG | Intravenous immunoglobulin |
| MP | *Mycoplasma* pneumonia |
| NMDAR | *N*-methyl-ᴅ-aspartate receptor |
| NSAIDs | Nonsteroidal anti-inflammatory drugs |
| OCD | Obsessive-compulsive disorder |
| PANDAS | Pediatric autoimmune neuropsychiatric disorder associated with streptococcal infections |
| PANS | Pediatric acute-onset neuropsychiatric syndrome |
| PITANDS | Pediatric infection-triggered autoimmune neuropsychiatric disorders |
| RF | Rheumatic fever |
| SC | Sydenham chorea |
| TPE | Therapeutic plasma exchange |
| TS | Tourette syndrome |
| URI | Upper respiratory infection |

of the illness is classically or primarily relapsing/remitting, with symptom flares occurring months to years after the initial onset. Many PANDAS youth also display a sawtooth pattern characterized by dramatic flares followed by considerable improvement, but not fully remitting. A few will display a progressively deteriorative course with each relapse, and a few children will remain remitted after recovering from the initial episode.

Recently, a group of researchers and clinicians familiar with PANDAS met and established a reiteration of this subtype termed pediatric acute-onset neuropsychiatric syndrome (PANS).[2] PANS is characterized by a clinical presentation similar to that of PANDAS; however, the cause is not defined as being exclusively due to a GAS infection (**Box 2**). In addition, PANS does not account for patients presenting with tics without OCD.[2] In this iteration, food refusal and anorexia presentations are

---

**Box 1**
**Criteria for PANDAS**

1. Presence of obsessive-compulsive disorder (OCD) and/or a tic disorder

2. Prepubertal symptom onset

3. Episodic course characterized by acute, severe onset and dramatic symptom exacerbations

4. Neurological abnormalities (eg, choreiform movements) present during symptom exacerbations

5. Temporal relationship between Group A streptococcal (GAS) infections and symptom exacerbations

*Adapted from* Ahmad G, Duffy JM, Farquhar C, et al. Barrier agents for adhesion prevention after gynaecological surgery. Cochrane Database Syst Rev 2008;(2):CD000475.

---

**Box 2**
**Criteria for PANS**

1. Abrupt, dramatic overnight onset of OCD or severely restricted food intake

2. Concurrent presence of additional neuropsychiatric symptoms, with similarly severe and acute onset, from at least 2 of the following 7 categories:

   a. Anxiety

   b. Emotional lability and/or depression

   c. Irritability, aggression, and/or severe oppositional behaviors

   d. Behavioral (developmental) regression

   e. Deterioration in school performance

   f. Sensory or motor abnormalities, including heightened sensitivity to sensory stimuli, hallucinations, dysgraphia, complex motor and/or vocal tics

   g. Somatic signs and symptoms, including sleep disturbances, enuresis, or urinary frequency

3. Symptoms are not better explained by a known neurological or medical disorder, such as Sydenham chorea, systemic lupus erythematosus, Tourette disorder, or others

*From* Swedo S, Leckman J, Rose N. From research subgroup to clinical syndrome: modifying the PANDAS criteria to describe PANS. Pediatric Therapeutics 2012;2(113).

---

also included as a primary feature. Other iterations include pediatric infection-triggered autoimmune neuropsychiatric disorders (PITANDS) (**Box 3**) and childhood acute neuropsychiatric symptoms (CANS) (**Box 4**).

### *PANS OCD Versus Non-PANS OCD*

In many ways, the clinical presentation of OCD and tics is comparable in both PANS OCD and non-PANS OCD (**Table 1** presents a comparison of non-PANS with PANS OCD).[32] For example, both PANDAS and non-PANDAS youth have an increased

---

**Box 3**
**Criteria for PITANDS**

1. Pediatric onset (between age 3 years and beginning of puberty)

2. At some time, patient met criteria for OCD and/or a tic disorder

3. Sudden onset (with or without subclinical prodrome), and/or with a pattern of sudden, recurrent symptom exacerbations and remissions. Symptoms seem to have "exploded" in severity

4. Increased symptoms do not occur exclusively during stress or illness, are pervasive, and of severity to suggest need for treatment modifications. If untreated, last at least 4 weeks

5. During OCD and/or tic exacerbations, most patients will display abnormal neurological examination, frequently with adventitious movements (eg, mild chorea)

6. Evidence of an antecedent or concomitant infection (eg, positive throat culture, positive streptococcal serological findings, or history of illness)

7. Patients may or may not continue to have clinically significant symptoms between episodes of OCD and/or tic disorder

*Adapted from* Allen AJ, Leonard HL, Swedo SE. Case study: a new infection-triggered, autoimmune subtype of pediatric OCD and Tourette's syndrome. J Am Acad Child Adolesc Psychiatry 1995;34(3):310; with permission.

**Box 4**
**Criteria for CANS**

1. Appearance in childhood (age <18 years)

2. Acute onset

3. Infectious disorder, inflammatory disorder, or other association

4. Psychiatric signs, such as OCD, anxiety, psychosis, developmental regression, sensitivity to sensory stimuli, emotional lability

5. Motor signs, such as tics, dysgraphia, clumsiness, hyperactivity

6. Absence of abnormal magnetic resonance imaging

7. Can be monophasic or polyphasic

*Adapted from* Singer HS, Gilbert DL, Wolf DS, et al. Moving from PANDAS to CANS. J Pediatr 2012;160(5):729.

**Table 1**
**OCD versus PANS OCD**

| | OCD | PANS OCD |
|---|---|---|
| Age of onset | 10 y[3] | <7 y[2] |
| Gender relatedness | Age <15 y: males slightly higher than females. Female/male ratio increases post puberty[3] | Nearly 5:1 male-to-female ratio under age 8[2] |
| Course | Insidious onset; not episodic[3] | Dramatic and severe onset; episodic or saw-tooth course; long-term prognosis unknown[2] |
| Incidence | 2% of youth[3] | Unknown, estimate is 10%–20% of pediatric OCD (0.2%–0.4%) |
| Infectious trigger | No data available | Proposed association with infection but not required[2] |
| Motor signs | Increased findings of neurological soft signs, including choreiform movements[4] | "Choreiform" movements[2] |
| Neurocognitive findings | Oculomotor response inhibition deficits[5]; deficits in set shifting and inhibition[6–8]; deficits in cognitive flexibility and planning[9] | Poor attention and visual-spatial abilities; acute math and reading deficits, impulsivity; deficits in fine motor speed[1,10–12] |
| Involvement of basal ganglia | Strong support[13] | Good support[14–16] |
| Immune therapy response | No[12,17] | Some support for IVIG,[18] antibiotics[19–21] |
| Response to CBT | Yes[22–24] | Yes[25,26] |
| Response to serotonergic reuptake inhibitors | Yes[3,27] | Not studied, may be prone to activation[28] |
| Comorbidity (%) | Any tic disorder: 15–30<br>ADHD: 11–12<br>Separation anxiety: 30–52<br>Affective disorder: 25–62<br>Anxiety disorder: 26–75[27,29,30] | Any tic disorder: 55.3<br>ADHD: 44.6<br>Separation anxiety: 21<br>Affective disorder: 43<br>Anxiety disorder: 31[1,12,31] |

risk of OCD within the family.[33] However, key differences are observed in the onset, trajectory, and symptom attributes. As noted previously, PANDAS and PANS are characterized by a dramatic, almost overnight change in the child, whereas non-PANS OCD has an insidious onset. In addition, unlike non-PANS, PANS OCD often occurs concurrently with personality changes, new-onset ADHD, food refusal and weight loss, behavior regression, deterioration in handwriting and other fine motor skills, sleep disruption, psychosis, enuresis and pollakiuria (frequent urination), and mild to moderate cognitive dysfunction.[1,34]

### Brief History of PANDAS

Sydenham chorea (SC), a movement disorder that is a potential complication of rheumatic fever (RF), was described in 1848 as including acute-onset neuropsychiatric symptoms comprising irritability, emotionality, deterioration in handwriting and attention, and bizarre behaviors.[35] Osler noted that parents often described their choreic children as "completely changed," with some cases including acute-onset psychosis.[36] Since Sydenham and Osler, various associations between OCD, tics, and SC have been described in the medical literature, highlighting the struggle with diagnostic and causal clarity that past clinicians have encountered. Higher rates of SC have been documented in the medical history of patients with OCD,[37,38] and high rates of obsessive-compulsive symptoms are reported in youth with SC.[39–43] Because of this relationship, SC was proposed as a model for childhood autoimmune neuropsychiatric disorders, including OCD.[44]

Tic disorders triggered by infections are also another documented clinical presentation. In 1929, sinusitis was noted to lead to tics in 3 boys without significant premorbid psychiatric history, with sinus surgery correcting both the chronic sinusitis and tic flares.[45] It is notable that postoperative cultures contained, among other bacteria, *Streptococcus*. In 1965, a pediatric case of tics preceded by infection was described to be treated with neuroleptics and antibiotics.[46] In the late 1960s, haloperidol was advanced as a potential treatment for Tourette syndrome (TS),[47,48] eventually leading researchers to dedicate their efforts toward investigating neuroleptics, rather than antibiotics, as a treatment for tics.[49–51] Alternative treatments for tics, including the use of corticosteroids, have been reported.[52,53]

## GAS-ASSOCIATED TRIGGERS

With increased support of an association between acute-onset OCD/tic symptoms and GAS infection, the diagnostic criteria for PANDAS were formulated based on 50 cases, reported in 1998. Most of the subjects (77%) had some evidence of symptoms being preceded by GAS infection, including exacerbations associated with a positive throat culture or episode of scarlet fever, history of recent upper respiratory infection (URI) symptoms plus known GAS exposure, or sore throat or URI symptoms with fever in the absence of documented culture or titer.[1] Like the struggles of earlier clinicians with SC presentation,[35–38] the validity of PANDAS has been an ongoing debate within the medical community.[54–65] Although some studies[1,12,53,66,67] found support for a GAS association, others[59,68,69] have concluded that a significant temporal relationship did not exist between symptom exacerbation and GAS infection. This debate has been complicated in part by the fact that some of the cases identified originally as PANDAS in 2 prospective longitudinal studies may not have been true PANDAS cases.[59,68] Given the multitude of possible triggers (including various infections and life stress), as well as the heterogeneity, type of onset, and clinical severity of neuropsychiatric symptoms, it is not surprising that confusion and controversy exist over this clinical subtype.

Some youth with tics and/or OCD may have a unique susceptibility or reaction to GAS infections. TS and OCD youth are reported to have an average annual rate of new streptococcal infections of 0.42 infections per subject per year, in contrast to 0.28 infections per subject per year in healthy controls.[70] In a developmental pediatric practice, an increase in incidence of tics was noted to have occurred in temporal proximity to a GAS outbreak.[71] Children with tics or obsessive-compulsive symptoms have been shown to be more likely than healthy controls to have elevated antistreptolysin (ASO) titers.[72] In addition, patients with a tic disorder or OCD are more likely to have had a GAS infection within the 3 months before onset of symptoms.[53]

## INFECTIOUS TRIGGERS OTHER THAN GAS

Tic exacerbations following a cold have occurred in pediatric, but not adult, patients with tic disorders,[73] suggesting that other infectious triggers in addition to GAS should be considered in the etiology of PANS. Of interest, a temporal relationship between URI and the onset of tics in 2 adult patients was reported in a case study.[74] In addition, 3 adult patients reportedly developed dystonia, with sera containing anti–basal ganglia antibodies binding to antigens of molecular weight similar to those of SC, after a URI.[75]

In particular, *Mycoplasma* pneumonia (MP) has also been implicated in neurological sequelae,[76] and has been considered in the etiology of TS.[77] Müller and colleagues[78] noted a case in which 2 patients, who both experienced tic exacerbation after MP infection, were treated successfully with erythromycin for 4 weeks. In a study of 29 patients with TS, 59% of TS patients (compared with 3% of healthy controls) had positive or suspected positive antibody titers against MP.

Viruses, including influenza, have also been reported as a potential infectious trigger for acute-onset OCD and tics.[79] One subject, a 10-year-old boy, experienced acute-onset OCD, including contamination fears, and was successfully treated with plasmapheresis. Another subject, a 13-year-old boy, was treated with prednisone for acute-onset tics, and experienced symptom remittance for 2 weeks. Of note, this subject experienced a tic flare, potentially triggered by a viral respiratory infection and allergic reaction to an influenza immunization, weeks after prednisone treatment, and continued to suffer from tics despite a retrial of prednisone.

Lyme disease has been investigated as a potential infectious trigger in PANS, as OCD is often present in patients with Lyme disease.[80–82] Of note, the neuropsychiatric and cognitive symptoms of Lyme disease share some similarity with those of PANS, including distractibility, schoolwork deterioration, irritability/depression, insomnia, and sensitivity to light and/or sound.[83] Children with Lyme disease have also been reported to have oppositional behavior, anxiety disorders, and ADHD.[82] In addition, a case report described a child with Lyme disease who presented with acute-onset TS that resolved with antibiotic treatment.[84] However, no case reports have documented Lyme disease as a predecessor to acute-onset OCD symptoms.

## CLINICAL PRESENTATION OF PANDAS/PANS

Although co-occurring conditions are common in OCD (see **Table 1**), a key feature of PANDAS/PANS is the complexity and number of presenting symptoms. For example, ADHD is a common comorbidity in PANDAS youth. In a recent study by Murphy and colleagues,[12] PANDAS subjects (n = 41) were more likely to have comorbid ADHD (61%) than their non-PANDAS OCD peers (n = 68) (31%). In addition, psychosis (PANDAS = 12%, non-PANDAS = 9%) and separation anxiety (PANDAS = 29%, non-PANDAS = 22%) were more prevalent in the PANDAS group. ADHD exacerbations also seem to have a temporal relationship with GAS infections for PANDAS youth.[1] In a longitudinal study investigating possible associations between GAS infections and ADHD behaviors, schoolchildren with GAS infections were more likely to display ADHD symptoms than children who did not report GAS infections.[34] Elevated streptococcal titers have been associated with an ADHD diagnosis, even when controlling for the effects of chronic tic disorders and OCD comorbidity. Similarly, acute-onset behavioral problems, including ADHD symptoms, are more common during the winter months, the time during which the highest prevalence of GAS infections occurs.[85]

### Mood Symptoms

Mood symptoms of PANDAS are characterized by an abrupt onset concurrent with OCD onset. In the series of Swedo and colleagues[1] from 1998, the PANDAS group displayed emotional lability (66%), personality changes (54%), nighttime difficulties (50%), and separation anxiety (46%). PANDAS behaviors are often age-inappropriate, including behavioral regression, nighttime fears, change in school performance (eg, deterioration in math and reading), and oppositionality.[1,12,20,31]

### Sensory Issues

Sensory issues are often reported in PANS.[1,12,20,31] Sensitivity to light has been reported; for example, patients have abruptly begun refusing to go outside without sunglasses, or may not leave the house at all because of sensitivity to sunlight. This sensitivity extends to some PANS patients who insist on blinds being closed during the daytime. Anorexia and food refusal attributable to being "bothered" by the taste and texture of foods that the patients used to like is also common in PANS. Hallucinations have also been reported, such as smelling nonexistent fish. Tactile sensory issues have included refusal to wear clothes or shoes because they feel "too tight." In addition, sensitivity to sound has included requiring absolute quiet and use of noise-cancelling headphones when out of the house, in addition to inability to sit in the school lunchroom because of the noise. The abrupt onset of these symptoms is a defining characteristic of PANDAS/PANS, and is easily differentiated from sensory integration disorder and other disorders with insidious onset.

### Pollakiuria

Pollakiuria, a potential symptom of PANDAS/PANS, is the urge to urinate frequently without the physiological need. The etiology of pollakiuria is likely psychogenic.[86] Daytime urinary urgency and frequency in the absence of dysuria, fever, or incontinence has been reported in 41% to 58% of PANDAS youth.[12,20] By contrast, 25% of OCD and/or tic youth have been noted to experience pollakiuria.[12] Similarly, pollakiuria is a rare occurrence in TS.[87]

### Anorexia

Anorexia is another psychiatric illness that can be comorbid in PANDAS. Change in food intake has been a reported symptom in empirical studies of PANDAS youth.[31] As noted earlier, for many of these children the change in food intake has less to do with preoccupations with bodily appearance and more to do with restrictive eating because of sensory issues, for example, the "feel" or texture of the food and/or worries about choking.[2] However, case studies have reported acute-onset symptoms of classic anorexia nervosa after a GAS infection, with symptoms remitting with antibiotic therapy.[88–90] Similarly, anorexia is a common comorbidity in OCD,[91] with specific symptoms including contamination fears and hoarding or saving obsessions.[92]

### Clinical Symptom Timeline

In terms of symptom timeline, Bernstein and colleagues[31] noted that urinary urgency, hyperactivity, impulsivity, deterioration in handwriting, separation anxiety, and decline in school performance were common symptoms during the initial episode. In the sentinel episodes, inattention, mood swings, and oppositional behavior were common. Common obsessions included aggression and contamination, with compulsions including washing, cleaning, and checking. During exacerbations, mood lability, decline in school performance, change in personality, bedtime fears and rituals, and restlessness were noted.

Anecdotal reports of other abnormal movements (eg, dystonia, tremor, stereotypies, opsoclonus, myoclonus, paroxysmal choreoathetosis),[93] catatonia,[94] pervasive developmental disorders and schizophreniform symptoms,[95] body dysmorphia,[96] and conversion symptoms[97] occurring after a GAS infection also exist. However, empirical research has yet to validate these symptoms as occurring within the context of PANDAS/PANS.

## PATHOPHYSIOLOGY OF PANDAS/PANS

The current hypothesis regarding the pathophysiology of PANDAS is based on molecular mimicry, in that antibodies for GAS may target brain proteins, eventually leading to a clinical presentation of PANDAS. PANDAS children have been found to have significantly higher levels of antibodies that trigger calcium-calmodulin–dependent protein kinase II (CaM kinase II) production when compared with their OCD, ADHD, and TS peers in addition to healthy controls.[98,99] GAS antibodies may directly stimulate or block receptors of the basal ganglia, or affect immune complexes that lead to inflammation of the basal ganglia.[14,15] Cross-reactive antibodies may interfere with neuronal signals by increasing CaM kinase II production in the basal ganglia, eventually leading to dopamine dysregulation, and subsequently the clinical presentation characteristic of PANDAS. PANS pathophysiology is likely similar to postinfectious neurological sequelae such as that which occurs with MP and other infections.[2]

Anti–basal ganglia antibodies have been found using both enzyme-linked immunosorbent assay (ELISA) and Western blotting in the sera of tic-disorder youth who fulfilled the PANDAS criteria.[100] In a study using indirect tissue immunofluorescence, almost two-thirds of PANDAS youth, compared with less than 10% of children with active GAS infection without neuropsychiatric complications, displayed anti–basal ganglia antibodies.[101] However, another study found no significant differences in the anti–basal ganglia antibodies between PANDAS youth and healthy controls.[64] This discrepancy may be due to the use of a different tissue preparation. Another study using immunofluorescence found no association between the presence of autoantibodies and PANDAS or TS diagnosis.[72] However, this study used lower serum dilutions and confocal microscopy. In addition, another study found no differences between the autoantibodies in the serum of PANDAS and TS patients,[102] although this study has been criticized for multiple methodological issues.[103] Animal models have also provided compelling proof-of-onset evidence that these antibodies may play a role in the pathophysiology of PANDAS cases.[104–106]

## PANS ASSESSMENT

Acquiring a complete clinical history from the potential PANS child and his or her family is essential for identifying diagnostic features unique to PANS. For example, identifying drastic changes in symptom severity that correlate with illness will assist the physician in accurate diagnosis, and subsequent appropriate treatment. In addition to infectious triggers, course of illness and type of symptoms are the most important factors. Along with historical data, a comprehensive review of systems is necessary to rule out potential medical causes for the behavioral changes. Migratory pain in the large joints, fatigue, chest pain, or dyspnea suggests that RF needs to be ruled out. For example, in the possible connection between SC and PANDAS, a finding of chorea during physical examination should prompt more in-depth assessment, such as the consideration of ordering an echocardiogram to rule out rheumatoid carditis.

For children with severe and recent flare in neuropsychiatric symptoms, the presence of a GAS infection may be established with a rapid antigen test or throat culture. Checking family members whenever feasible may also be considered. Of note, GAS infections can be asymptomatic, and a child could be unknowingly exposed to streptococcal pharyngitis. Up to 20% of school-aged children may be asymptomatically infected with GAS, and 25% of asymptomatic family members of a child with GAS are actually infected.[107] Streptococcal pharyngitis can also go undiagnosed in preschool children, as their symptoms often include gastroenteritis with fewer tonsillar exudates and less cervical adenopathy than appear in school-age children.[108] Also noteworthy is that PANDAS symptom severity and chronicity has been correlated with the number of prior GAS infections.[20]

Because many healthy children have elevated levels of streptococcal antibodies, a single measurement will not prove or disprove PANDAS (**Table 2**). Ideally, streptococcal titers should be repeated within 3 to 8 weeks of baseline assessment of a

**Table 2**
**Diagnostic, results, and subsequent treatment**

| Potential Outcomes of Laboratory Tests | Considerations |
|---|---|
| Titers are not elevated | Younger patients may not have significant immune response even if infected[109]; 30% may not have titer elevation[110] |
| Elevated GAS titers | Titers may remain elevated 6–12 mo postinfection; elevated titers common in asymptomatic school-age children[111–113] |
| Positive rapid antigen or throat culture | Rapid antigen has sensitivity of 80%–90%. Culture has a sensitivity of 90%–95% for detection of GAS[114] |
| Acute and convalescent titers | 4-Fold increase in titer levels supports GAS as possible trigger[66] |
| IgG mycoplasma (MP) | The percentage of persons with acute infection that demonstrate a positive IgG response in the acute phase is <50%[115]; high presence of MP-specific IgG in healthy persons, which is likely due to prior MP infections[116] |
| IgM MP ELISA | 52% acute-phase sera-tested positive by various IgM assays, but 88% when convalescent sera were tested. IgM antibodies can sometimes persist for several weeks to months; single assay using the IgM ImmunoCard had a sensitivity of only 31.8% for detection of acute *M pneumoniae* infection in seropositive children with pneumonia, but this increased to 88.6% when paired sera were analyzed[115,117] |
| Positive MP polymerase chain reaction | Many individuals never progress to the severe lower respiratory phase of the infection, and up to 20% may be asymptomatic[118] |
| Positive rapid flu | Flu (most likely H1N1) may trigger some cases[2] |
| NMDAR antibody positive | NMDAR encephalitis[119]; slightly higher sensitivity with cerebrospinal fluid than sera[120,121] |

recent-onset illness or flare to assess for titer rises, which are more informative than an isolated ASO titer. Streptococcal antibody elevations with RF were discovered in 85% of patients after one serology test, and in more than 95% when multiple methods were used.[122,123] Owing to lags in symptom presentation (and likely symptoms attributable to other causes), 63% of SC patients had elevated ASO and anti-DNase B.[124] Similarly, PANDAS patients have high rates of streptococcal titer elevations when both ASO and anti-DNase B are used.[66] Antibody titers can remain elevated for months even without GAS, which underscores the importance of measuring both acute and convalescent titers.[66] In addition, as streptococcal titers often do not vary significantly over the course of 1 to 5 months,[66,111] reliance on clinical presentation is essential.

Assessment of the severity and characteristics of the symptoms is crucial, as gross motor neurological findings and/or cognitive/motor regression will signal that a neurological consultation and further testing is needed. Abnormalities typically will rule out PANDAS/PANS. In addition, altered sensorium, an abnormal electroencephalogram or magnetic resonance image, the presence of paraneoplastic antibodies, $N$-methyl-D-aspartate receptor (NMDAR) antibodies, or antithyroid peroxidase antibodies suggests other autoimmune encephalopathies rather than PANS. At present, no diagnostic measure will confirm PANS. **Box 5** summarizes the differential diagnosis.

### Identification of Risk Factors

Although specific risk factors for PANDAS have not been established, there are multiple risk factors that may play a role, such as recurrent GAS infections, subclinical GAS infections, misdiagnosed infections, infection exposures via close contacts, family history, and maternal auto immunity. Causes of recurrent GAS infections often include poor compliance or inadequate duration of antibiotic therapy, poor antibiotic penetration into tonsillar tissue, inactivation of the antibiotic resulting from β-lactamase–producing

---

**Box 5**
**Differential diagnosis of acute neuropsychiatric presentations**

Autoimmune or limbic encephalitis

- Postinfection
  - Acute disseminated encephalomyelitis[125]
  - Sydenham chorea[41]
  - PANS[2]
- Paraneoplastic/Idiopathic
  - NMDAR antibody encephalitis[125]
  - Voltage-gated antibody disorders[125]

Encephalitis, infectious[125]

Neuropsychiatric lupus[126]

Antiphospholipid antibody syndrome[126]

Trauma/stress

- Abuse, bereavement, bullying[127]

Metabolic/mitochondrial disorders

- Mitochondrial encephalomyopathy, lactic acidosis, and stroke-like episodes[125]
- Cerebral folate deficiency[128]

bacteria, lack of protective oral flora, or immunological defects.[125] Children with a history of recurrent streptococcal infections or a strong family history of RF, or both, may be especially susceptible. Among school-aged children, asking about sick contacts will help establish exposure to illness and particularly GAS. Although infection is likely the precipitating factor in PANDAS, genetics, similarly to OCD and TS, may be involved in susceptibility, disease onset and progression, symptomatology, and severity.[126] Maternal autoimmunity may be associated with an increased risk. In mothers of youth with tics and/or OCD, 16.8% had an autoimmune disease, in contrast to a rate of 5% in the community. In addition, 25% of mothers of youth with PANDAS had autoimmune disease, compared with only 13.4% of mothers of youth with OCD/tics.[127] Maternal antibodies to GAS or other inciting infections could hypothetically cross-react to fetal central nervous system tissue, and may cause subtle changes in brain development.[128,129] The presence or absence of maternal antibodies can possibly influence future immune defense against pathogens.[130] Research also suggests that although genetics are important when assessing for PANDAS, clinical presentations among identical siblings can vary from a typical PANDAS presentation to asymptomatic.[131]

---

**PANDAS Case**

*A 5-year-old boy with no significant premorbid psychiatric history began to have an overnight onset of severe food refusal because of fear of choking, vomiting, and stomachaches. His medical history was significant for frequent staphylococcal infections, and he was reportedly exposed to a GAS infection 3 months before symptom onset. One month after psychiatric symptom onset, the patient developed throat clearing and sniffing tics. He also began experiencing acute-onset severe irritability, mood lability, sleep disturbances, deterioration in school performance, and behavioral regression. He developed painful and frequent urination 2 months later, and had lost 4 lb (1.8 kg) because of his decreased appetite. Concurrent with the pollakiuria, the patient started having visual and sensory hallucinations, such as seeing "Curious George" and body parts on various objects, in addition to olfactory hallucinations. On evaluation in the emergency room, the patient's laboratory results showed elevated anti-DNAse B titer, other measures including NMDAR antibodies being normal. He continued to have "playful" hallucinations throughout the next month, triggered by visual or auditory stimuli. For example, he saw whales and dolphins in his room when his mother mentioned the beach, and once saw a penguin come up to him and say "Hi." Three months after initial symptom presentation, the patient started experiencing hyperactivity, mydriasis, and auditory hallucinations including hearing "sloppy" words and being woken up by imagined sirens. He was given intravenous immunoglobulin (IVIG) and was started on azithromycin therapy on the same day. One month after treatment began, the patient was 80% improved. He continued to have a few intrusive thoughts, but needed less reassurance. Two months later, the patient achieved remission of symptoms that have continued to date. He is being weaned off azithromycin (daily dose 3 mL) and continues to do "extremely well" according to his mother's reports during monthly follow-up phone calls.*

---

### Treatment Options

Although children clearly present with sudden and severe OCD, a definitive association between infection and OCD has yet to be established; however, research to establish protocols for diagnosis and treatment of PANS is under way nationally and internationally. Although multiple pharmacologic treatment options for PANDAS and PANS have been explored, there is currently no agent of choice.

### Pharmacotherapy

Penicillin, cephalosporin, and amoxicillin, which are all appropriate treatments for GAS infections,[132] have been correlated with OCD symptom remittance in PANDAS youth.[20,133] Azithromycin is another approved treatment for *Mycoplasma*, *Borrelia*, and GAS,[134] the most implicated triggers in PANS, and has been correlated with improvement in neuropsychiatric symptoms within 2 to 6 weeks of initiating treatment.[20,21] The mechanisms underlying these effects have not been systematically explored. Azithromycin has a longer duration of action, is believed to be less detrimental with respect to disruption of microflora in comparison with amoxicillin/clavulanate, and allows for once-daily dosing. The main drawback relates to reports of emergence of macrolide-resistant GAS[135] especially over longer courses of treatment.[136] A randomized placebo-controlled trial of azithromycin for PANS is in progress. In a small pilot study of cefdinir (N = 20) (14 mg/kg), children with recent-onset neuropsychiatric symptoms had improvements in OCD and tics.[137] Anecdotal testimony from parents and practitioners suggests that antibiotics can significantly reduce the severity of symptoms; however, research to support these claims is still needed. The response to antibiotics can occur as quickly as within 24 to 48 hours, but often the response is delayed until after 14 days of treatment. Some symptoms, such as tics and mood disturbance, may respond sooner than OCD or deficits in attention; however, this varies considerably among patients. Anecdotally, relapse can also occur within a few days of discontinuation. Prophylactic antibiotics have also been investigated as potential PANDAS treatment, with studies having shown possible benefit with penicillin and azithromycin.[19,21] Risks of long-term antibiotic therapy include increasing antibiotic-resistant organisms, allergic reactions, and gastrointestinal side effects. In addition, youth on long-term azithromycin should undergo electrocardiographic monitoring because of the risk of prolonged QTc interval.

*Therapeutic plasma exchange and intravenous immunoglobulin*
Other treatments for PANDAS such as therapeutic plasma exchange (TPE) and IVIG therapy have been examined in research and are not infrequently used in clinical practice. More research is needed regarding which patients are the best candidates for these therapies, and establishing when during the course of illness that these therapies should be introduced. IVIG is the infusion of immunoglobulins (antibodies) into the vein. This solution is composed of antibodies normally found in adult human blood that provide immunity against disease. IVIG products are derived from the plasma of a large number of individuals who have formed antibodies to a wide variety of bacteria, viruses, and other proteins. Plasma of all donors goes through several extensive screenings and testing for safety. The most common side effects include chills, low-grade fever, and headache. Rare serious side effects such as difficulty breathing, chest pain, seizures, and severe anaphylactic reactions have been reported. Similar to treatment of SC[138,139] IVIG was found to be superior in a randomized clinical trial for PANDAS.[18] A second IVIG study for PANS was recently completed, the results of which are pending. Of interest, IVIG was not effective in a double-blind, placebo-controlled study of adult patients with tics.[140]

TPE is another method that has been researched as a potential treatment,[18] and PANS/PANDAS has been included as an indication in the apheresis guidelines.[141] TPE is a process by which whole blood is removed from the patient, followed by the removal of plasma, and return of blood to the patient. TPE is thought to exert benefits by removing autoantibodies and antigen-antibody complexes. The treatment is often provided in an inpatient setting, and requires either a central or femoral catheter. Adverse effects are frequent and some can be serious.[142] One open-label trial[18] and a few cases have been reported in the scientific literature.[79,94] In one case, TPE resulted in improvement of OCD symptoms and a decrease in basal ganglia swelling, suggesting an immune-mediated process.[94] With minimal empirical support for its use in

PANS/PANDAS, this treatment option is generally reserved for those cases that remain severe and are resistant to other therapies. TPE has not been effective in non-PANS OCD.[17]

### Steroids and NSAIDs

Other less investigated treatments include steroids and NSAIDs. Two boys with TS reportedly experienced full tic remittance after treatment with prednisone augmented with corticotropin.[52] Case reports of NSAIDs for PANDAS youth are anecdotal and not well studied. However, a randomized, double-blind clinical trial found that fluoxetine with celecoxib was superior in OCD symptom reduction in adults when compared with fluoxetine with placebo.[143]

### Tonsillectomy

Many families query about the benefit of tonsillectomies for improving PANDAS/PANS symptoms. Recurrent GAS infections are certainly a common indication for surgery.[144–146] As histories of frequent GAS infections are not uncommon in patients with PANDAS, these surgical interventions have been explored as a potential PANDAS treatment.[147–150] However, until the efficacy of tonsillectomy has been prospectively explored, it is not recommended as a treatment for PANDAS without meeting already established guidelines,[144] such as tonsillar hypertrophy, obstructive sleep apnea, or recurrent throat infections. A recent study found that youth with PANS/PANDAS had high rates of tonsillectomies and adenoidectomies that predated the onset of OCD and tics.[151] No significant difference in streptococcal titer elevations was observed among participants who had previously had a surgical procedure and those without surgery.

### Multiple treatment methods

Many children, even after a mostly successful immune-based treatment, will have some residual symptoms that need to be addressed. As PANDAS is a condition that affects multiple domains, including the emotional, cognitive, and neurological, multiple treatment modalities used in conjunction are likely to produce optimal results. Therefore, these children should have the opportunity to receive the standard care for patients with OCD and TS, including medications (eg, guanfacine, aripiprazole, and fluoxetine in lower than typical starting doses) and therapies such as cognitive-behavioral therapy (CBT).[26] These evidence-based treatments may lessen the severity of a future flare. OCD symptoms are best treated with CBT unless they are too severe to engage in therapy.[25,26] CBT can help children remodel automatic responses to obsessions, teach skills that should prove helpful if symptoms do recur, and also help families with behavioral strategies to lessen the risk of disrupted functioning and accommodation. Children often report feeling empowered from coping, relaxation, and resiliency skills learned in CBT. Antidepressants approved for OCD[3] also help, but many of these children are prone to behavioral activation with a typical starting dose, but do well when started on a low dose (eg, sertraline at 6.25 mg) that is gradually increased as tolerated.[28] These medications may exert neuropsychiatric effects via immunomodulation and support of neurogenesis and repair mechanisms. Anti-inflammatory effects may result via suppression of interferon-$\gamma$, interleukin-1$\beta$, interleukin-2, tumor necrosis factor $\alpha$, natural killer cell cytotoxicity, and T-cell proliferation.[152] Patients with tics respond well to a variety of evidence-based pharmacological agents and behavioral treatments if they are needed to reduce symptom severity and impairment.[109] As PANDAS patients often demonstrate sensory issues in addition to acute-onset handwriting deterioration, occupational therapy can be a successful treatment option.[153]

## Management

For management of GAS infections, limiting exposure to sick contacts, in addition to adhering to scheduled vaccinations and complying with treatment, is always recommended. Good health practices that decrease the potential of a proinflammatory state, such as exercise, monitoring stress, and a healthy diet (eg, a diet low in refined sugars, omega-6 and omega-9 fatty acids) may improve general health and resilience.

Longitudinal studies measuring treatment outcomes for PANDAS subjects are limited in number. Factors predicting symptom trajectory, whether remission or chronic, have not yet been identified.[12]

## Future Perspective

Although it is evident that extensive research is needed in this area, the potential role of immune modulation as a therapeutic option for psychiatric disorders opens up a therapeutic avenue that may be a source of important therapeutic alternatives and increased mechanistic understanding of complex disorders with heterogeneous antecedents. The overlap between immune and central nervous system pathways and signaling molecules suggests that disruption of the immune system may have secondary effects that extend beyond its localized actions. Characteristic markers of immune activation, such as increased expression of proinflammatory cytokines, have been observed in psychiatric disorders and have been implicated in their pathology.

## DISCLOSURES

Dr T.K. Murphy has received research support from the following: NIH/NIMH: 1RO1MH093381-01A1, 5R34HD065274-02, 1R21MH087849-01A1, 5R01MH079489-04, Centers for Disease Control and Prevention: 5U01DD000509-02, NARSAD, International OCD Foundation, Otsuka Pharmaceuticals, AstraZeneca Pharmaceuticals, Sunovion, F. Hoffmann-LaRoche Ltd, Ortho-McNeil Janssen Pharmaceuticals, Shire Pharmaceuticals, Pfizer Inc, Transcept Pharmaceuticals, and Indevus Pharmaceuticals. She has received travel support from the Tourette Syndrome Association and honoraria from grand rounds lectures. She also receives book royalties from Lawrence Erlbaum, Inc and Taylor & Francis. Ms D.M. Gerardi has no potential conflicts of interest to report. Dr J.F. Leckman has received support from the following: National Institutes of Health (salary and research funding), Tourette Syndrome Association (research funding), Grifols, LLC (research funding), Klingenstein Third Generation Foundation (medical student fellowship program), John Wiley and Sons (book royalties), McGraw Hill (book royalties), Oxford University Press (book royalties).

## REFERENCES

1. Swedo SE, Leonard HL, Garvey M, et al. Pediatric autoimmune neuropsychiatric disorders associated with streptococcal infections: clinical description of the first 50 cases. Am J Psychiatry 1998;155(2):264–71.
2. Swedo S, Leckman J, Rose N. From research subgroup to clinical syndrome: modifying the PANDAS criteria to describe PANS. Pediatric Therapeutics 2012;2(113).
3. Geller DA, March J. Practice parameter for the assessment and treatment of children and adolescents with obsessive-compulsive disorder. Focus 2012; 10(3):360–73.
4. Wise SP, Rapoport JL. Obsessive-compulsive disorder: is it basal ganglia dysfunction. In: Rapoport JL, editor. Obsessive-compulsive disorder in children and adolescents. Washington, DC: American Psychiatric Press; 1989. p. 327–44.

5. Rosenberg DR, Averbach DH, O'Hearn KM, et al. Oculomotor response inhibition abnormalities in pediatric obsessive-compulsive disorder. Arch Gen Psychiatry 1997;54(9):831.

6. Bannon S, Gonsalvez CJ, Croft RJ, et al. Executive functions in obsessive–compulsive disorder: state or trait deficits? Aust N Z J Psychiatry 2006; 40(11–12):1031–8.

7. Chang SW, McCracken JT, Piacentini JC. Neurocognitive correlates of child obsessive compulsive disorder and Tourette syndrome. J Clin Exp Neuropsychol 2007;29(7):724–33.

8. Zandt F, Prior M, Kyrios M. Similarities and differences between children and adolescents with autism spectrum disorder and those with obsessive compulsive disorder: executive functioning and repetitive behaviour. Autism 2009;13(1):43–57.

9. Ornstein TJ, Arnold P, Manassis K, et al. Neuropsychological performance in childhood OCD: a preliminary study. Depress Anxiety 2010;27(4):372–80.

10. Hirschtritt ME, Hammond CJ, Luckenbaugh D, et al. Executive and attention functioning among children in the PANDAS subgroup. Child Neuropsychol 2009;15(2):179–94.

11. Lewin AB, Storch EA, Mutch PJ, et al. Neurocognitive functioning in youth with pediatric autoimmune neuropsychiatric disorders associated with streptococcus. J Neuropsychiatry Clin Neurosci 2011;23(4):391–8.

12. Murphy TK, Storch EA, Lewin AB, et al. Clinical factors associated with pediatric autoimmune neuropsychiatric disorders associated with streptococcal infections. J Pediatr 2012;160(2):314–9.

13. Rosenberg DR, Keshavan MS, O'Hearn KM, et al. Frontostriatal measurement in treatment-naive children with obsessive-compulsive disorder. Arch Gen Psychiatry 1997;54(9):824.

14. Giedd JN, Rapoport JL, Garvey MA, et al. MRI assessment of children with obsessive-compulsive disorder or tics associated with streptococcal infection. Am J Psychiatry 2000;157(2):281–3.

15. Giedd JN, Rapoport JL, Leonard HL, et al. Case study: acute basal ganglia enlargement and obsessive-compulsive symptoms in an adolescent boy. J Am Acad Child Adolesc Psychiatry 1996;35(7):913–5.

16. Kumar A, Williams MT, Chugani HT. Evaluation of basal ganglia and thalamic inflammation in children with pediatric autoimmune neuropsychiatric disorders associated with streptococcal infection and Tourette syndrome: a positron emission tomographic (PET) study using C-[R]-PK11195. J Child Neurol, in press.

17. Nicolson R, Swedo SE, Lenane M, et al. An open trial of plasma exchange in childhood-onset obsessive-compulsive disorder without poststreptococcal exacerbations. J Am Acad Child Adolesc Psychiatry 2000;39(10):1313–5.

18. Perlmutter SJ, Leitman SF, Garvey MA, et al. Therapeutic plasma exchange and intravenous immunoglobulin for obsessive-compulsive disorder and tic disorders in childhood. Lancet 1999;354(9185):1153–8.

19. Garvey MA, Perlmutter SJ, Allen AJ, et al. A pilot study of penicillin prophylaxis for neuropsychiatric exacerbations triggered by streptococcal infections. Biol Psychiatry 1999;45(12):1564–71.

20. Murphy ML, Pichichero ME. Prospective identification and treatment of children with pediatric autoimmune neuropsychiatric disorder associated with group A streptococcal infection (PANDAS). Arch Pediatr Adolesc Med 2002;156(4):356.

21. Snider LA, Lougee L, Slattery M, et al. Antibiotic prophylaxis with azithromycin or penicillin for childhood-onset neuropsychiatric disorders. Biol Psychiatry 2005; 57(7):788–92.

22. Storch EA, Björgvinsson T, Riemann B, et al. Factors associated with poor response in cognitive-behavioral therapy for pediatric obsessive-compulsive disorder. Bull Menninger Clin 2010;74(2):167–85.

23. Storch EA, Geffken GR, Merlo LJ, et al. Family-based cognitive-behavioral therapy for pediatric obsessive-compulsive disorder: comparison of intensive and weekly approaches. J Am Acad Child Adolesc Psychiatry 2007;46(4):469–78.

24. March JS, Foa E, Gammon P, et al. Cognitive-behavior therapy, sertraline, and their combination for children and adolescents with obsessive-compulsive disorder-The Pediatric OCD Treatment Study (POTS) randomized controlled trial. JAMA 2004;292(16):1969–76.

25. Storch EA, Gerdes AC, Adkins JW, et al. Behavioral treatment of a child with PANDAS. J Am Acad Child Adolesc Psychiatry 2004;43(5):510–1.

26. Storch EA, Murphy TK, Geffken GR, et al. Cognitive-behavioral therapy for PANDAS-related obsessive-compulsive disorder: findings from a preliminary waitlist controlled open trial. J Am Acad Child Adolesc Psychiatry 2006; 45(10):1171–8.

27. Geller DA, Wagner KD, Emslie G, et al. Paroxetine treatment in children and adolescents with obsessive-compulsive disorder: a randomized, multicenter, double-blind, placebo-controlled trial. J Am Acad Child Adolesc Psychiatry 2004;43(11):1387–96.

28. Murphy TK, Storch EA, Strawser MS. Selective serotonin reuptake inhibitor-induced behavioral activation in the PANDAS subtype. Prim Psychiatr 2006;13(8):87–9.

29. Langley AK, Lewin AB, Bergman RL, et al. Correlates of comorbid anxiety and externalizing disorders in childhood obsessive compulsive disorder. Eur Child Adolesc Psychiatry 2010;19(8):637–45.

30. Coskun M, Zoroglu S, Ozturk M. Phenomenology, psychiatric comorbidity and family history in referred preschool children with obsessive-compulsive disorder. Child Adolesc Psychiatry Ment Health 2012;6(1):36.

31. Bernstein GA, Victor AM, Pipal AJ, et al. Comparison of clinical characteristics of pediatric autoimmune neuropsychiatric disorders associated with streptococcal infections and childhood obsessive-compulsive disorder. J Child Adolesc Psychopharmacol 2010;20(4):333–40.

32. Murphy TK, Kurlan R, Leckman J. The immunobiology of Tourette's disorder, pediatric autoimmune neuropsychiatric disorders associated with Streptococcus, and related disorders: a way forward. J Child Adolesc Psychopharmacol 2010;20(4):317–31.

33. Lougee L, Perlmutter SJ, Nicolson R, et al. Psychiatric disorders in first-degree relatives of children with pediatric autoimmune neuropsychiatric disorders associated with streptococcal infections (PANDAS). J Am Acad Child Adolesc Psychiatry 2000;39(9):1120–6.

34. Murphy TK, Snider LA, Mutch PJ, et al. Relationship of movements and behaviors to Group A streptococcus infections in elementary school children. Biol Psychiatry 2007;61(3):279–84.

35. Sydenham T, Latham RG. The works of Thomas Sydenham, MD, vol. 2. London: Printed for the Sydenham Society; 1850.

36. Osler W. On Chorea and Choreiform Affections. London(UK): H.K. Lewis; 1894. p. 33–5.

37. Grimshaw L. Obsessional disorder and neurological illness. J Neurol Neurosurg Psychiatry 1964;27:229–31.

38. Keeler W, Bender L. A follow-up study of children with behavior disorder and Sydenham's chorea. Am J Psychiatry 1952;109(6):421–8.

39. Swedo SE, Rapoport JL, Cheslow D, et al. High prevalence of obsessive-compulsive symptoms in patients with Sydenham's chorea. Am J Psychiatry 1989;146(2):246–9.

40. Swedo SE, Leonard HL, Casey B, et al. Sydenham's chorea: physical and psychological symptoms of St Vitus dance. Pediatrics 1993;91(4):706–13.

41. Abbas S, Khanna S, Taly A. Obsessive-compulsive disorder and rheumatic chorea: is there a connection? Psychopathology 1996;29(3):193–7.

42. Asbahr FR, Negrão AB, Gentil V, et al. Obsessive-compulsive and related symptoms in children and adolescents with rheumatic fever with and without chorea: a prospective 6-month study. Am J Psychiatry 1998;155(8):1122–4.

43. Moore DP. Neuropsychiatric aspects of Sydenham's chorea: a comprehensive review. J Clin Psychiatry 1996;57(9):407–14.

44. Swedo SE. Sydenham's chorea: a model for childhood autoimmune neuropsychiatric disorders. JAMA 1994;272(22):1788–91.

45. Selling L. The role of infection in the etiology of tics. Arch Neurol Psychiatr 1929; 22(6):1163.

46. Langlois M, Force L. Nosologic and clinical revision of Gilles de la Tourette disease evoked by the action of certain neuroleptics on its course. Rev Neurol 1965;113(6):641.

47. Boris M. Gilles de la Tourette's syndrome: remission with haloperidol. JAMA 1968;205(9):648–9.

48. Shapiro AK, Shapiro E. Treatment of Gilles de la Tourette's syndrome with haloperidol. Br J Psychiatry 1968;114(508):345–50.

49. Goldstone S, Lhamon WT. The effects of haloperidol upon temporal information processing by patients with Tourette's syndrome. Psychopharmacology 1976; 50(1):7–10.

50. Messiha FS, Knopp W, Vanecko S, et al. Haloperidol therapy in Tourette's syndrome: neurophysiological, biochemical and behavioral correlates. Life Sci 1971;10(8):449–57.

51. Shapiro AK, Shapiro E, Wayne H. Treatment of Tourette's syndrome: with haloperidol, review of 34 cases. Arch Gen Psychiatry 1973;28(1):92.

52. Matarazzo EB. Tourette's syndrome treated with ACTH and prednisone: report of two cases. J Child Adolesc Psychopharmacol 1992;2(3):215–26.

53. Mell LK, Davis RL, Owens D. Association between streptococcal infection and obsessive-compulsive disorder, Tourette's syndrome, and tic disorder. Pediatrics 2005;116(1):56–60.

54. de Oliveira SK, Pelajo CF. Pediatric autoimmune neuropsychiatric disorders associated with streptococcal infection (PANDAS): a controversial diagnosis. Curr Infect Dis Rep 2010;12(2):103–9.

55. Gabbay V, Coffey B. Obsessive-compulsive disorder, Tourette's disorder, or pediatric autoimmune neuropsychiatric disorders associated with Streptococcus in an adolescent? Diagnostic and therapeutic challenges. J Child Adolesc Psychopharmacol 2003;13(3):209–12.

56. Gabbay V, Coffey BJ, Babb JS, et al. Pediatric autoimmune neuropsychiatric disorders associated with streptococcus: comparison of diagnosis and treatment in the community and at a specialty clinic. Pediatrics 2008;122(2): 273–8.

57. Giulino L, Gammon P, Sullivan K, et al. Is parental report of upper respiratory infection at the onset of obsessive-compulsive disorder suggestive of pediatric autoimmune neuropsychiatric disorder associated with streptococcal infection? J Child Adolesc Psychopharmacol 2002;12(2):157–64.

58. Kurlan R, Kaplan EL. The pediatric autoimmune neuropsychiatric disorders associated with streptococcal infection (PANDAS) etiology for tics and obsessive-compulsive symptoms: hypothesis or entity? Practical considerations for the clinician. Pediatrics 2004;113(4):883–6.

59. Kurlan R, Johnson D, Kaplan EL. Streptococcal infection and exacerbations of childhood tics and obsessive-compulsive symptoms: a prospective blinded cohort study. Pediatrics 2008;121(6):1188–97.

60. Larson M, Storch E, Murphy T. What are the diagnostic and treatment implications for PANDAS: pediatric autoimmune neuropsychiatric disorders associated with streptococcal infections. Curr Psychiatr 2005;4:33–48.

61. Macerollo A, Martino D. Pediatric autoimmune neuropsychiatric disorders associated with streptococcal infections (PANDAS): an evolving concept. Tremor Other Hyperkinet Mov (N Y) 2013;3. pii:tre-03-167-4158-7.

62. Murphy TK, Petitto JM, Voeller KKS, et al. Obsessive Compulsive Disorder: Is there an Association with Childhood Streptococcal Infections and Altered Immune Function? Seminars in Clinical Neuropsychiatry October 2001;6(4):266–76.

63. Perrin EM, Murphy ML, Casey JR, et al. Does group A beta-hemolytic streptococcal infection increase risk for behavioral and neuropsychiatric symptoms in children? Arch Pediatr Adolesc Med 2004;158(9):848–56.

64. Singer HS, Loiselle CR, Lee O, et al. Anti-basal ganglia antibodies in PANDAS. Mov Disord 2004;19(4):406–15.

65. Snider LA, Swedo SE. PANDAS: current status and directions for research. Mol Psychiatry 2004;9(10):900–7.

66. Murphy TK, Sajid M, Soto O, et al. Detecting pediatric autoimmune neuropsychiatric disorders associated with streptococcus in children with obsessive-compulsive disorder and tics. Biol Psychiatry 2004;55(1):61–8.

67. Leslie DL, Kozma L, Martin A, et al. Neuropsychiatric disorders associated with streptococcal infection: a case-control study among privately insured children. J Am Acad Child Adolesc Psychiatry 2008;47:1166–72.

68. Leckman JF, King RA, Gilbert DL, et al. Streptococcal upper respiratory tract infections and exacerbations of tic and obsessive-compulsive symptoms: a prospective longitudinal study. J Am Acad Child Adolesc Psychiatry 2011;50(2):108–18.e3.

69. Schrag A, Gilbert R, Giovannoni G, et al. Streptococcal infection, Tourette syndrome, and OCD. Is there a connection? Neurology 2009;73(16):1256–63.

70. Luo F, Leckman JF, Katsovich L, et al. Prospective longitudinal study of children with tic disorders and/or obsessive-compulsive disorder: relationship of symptom exacerbations to newly acquired streptococcal infections. Pediatrics 2004;113(6): e578–85.

71. Kiessling LS, Marcotte AC, Culpepper L. Antineuronal antibodies in movement disorders. Pediatrics 1993;92(1):39–43.

72. Morris CM, Pardo-Villamizar C, Gause CD, et al. Serum autoantibodies measured by immunofluorescence confirm a failure to differentiate PANDAS and Tourette syndrome from controls. J Neurol Sci 2009;276(1):45–8.

73. Hoekstra PJ, Manson WL, Steenhuis MP, et al. Association of common cold with exacerbations in pediatric but not adult patients with tic disorder: a prospective longitudinal study. J Child Adolesc Psychopharmacol 2005;15(2):285–92.

74. Edwards MJ, Dale RC, Church AJ, et al. Adult-onset tic disorder, motor stereotypies, and behavioural disturbance associated with antibasal ganglia antibodies. Mov Disord 2004;19(10):1190–6.

75. Edwards M, Dale R, Church A, et al. A dystonic syndrome associated with antibasal ganglia antibodies. J Neurol Neurosurg Psychiatry 2004;75(6):914–6.

76. Yiş U, Kurul SH, Çakmakçı H, et al. *Mycoplasma pneumoniae*: nervous system complications in childhood and review of the literature. Eur J Pediatr 2008; 167(9):973–8.
77. Müller N, Riedel M, Blendinger C, et al. Childhood Tourette's syndrome and infection with mycoplasma pneumoniae. Am J Psychiatry 2000;157:481–2.
78. Müller N, Abele-Horn M, Riedel M. Infection with *Mycoplasma pneumoniae* and Tourette's syndrome (TS): increased anti-mycoplasmal antibody titers in TS. Psychiatry Res 2004;129:119–25.
79. Allen AJ, Leonard HL, Swedo SE. Case study: a new infection-triggered, autoimmune subtype of pediatric OCD and Tourette's syndrome. J Am Acad Child Adolesc Psychiatry 1995;34(3):307–11.
80. Fallon B, Nields J, Parsons B, et al. Psychiatric manifestations of Lyme borreliosis. J Clin Psychiatry 1993;54(7):263–8.
81. Fallon BA, Nields JA. Lyme disease: a neuropsychiatric illness. Am J Psychiatry 1994;151(11):1571–83.
82. Fallon BA, Kochevar JM, Gaito A, et al. The underdiagnosis of neuropsychiatric Lyme disease in children and adults. Psychiatr Clin North Am 1998;21(3):693–703.
83. Tager FA, Fallon BA, Keilp J, et al. A controlled study of cognitive deficits in children with chronic Lyme disease. J Neuropsychiatry Clin Neurosci 2001;13(4):500–7.
84. Riedel M, Straube A, Schwarz MJ, et al. Lyme disease presenting as Tourette's syndrome. Lancet 1998;351(9100):418–9.
85. Snider LA, Seligman LD, Ketchen BR, et al. Tics and problem behaviors in schoolchildren: prevalence, characterization, and associations. Pediatrics 2002;110(2):331–6.
86. Asnes RS, Mones RL. Extraordinary urinary frequency. Pediatrics 1991;87(6):953.
87. Wang H, Chang H, Chang S. Pollakiuria in children with tic disorders. Chang Gung Med J 2005;28(11):773.
88. Calkin CV, Carandang CG. Certain eating disorders may be a neuropsychiatric manifestation of PANDAS: case report. J Can Acad Child Adolesc Psychiatry 2007;16(3):132.
89. Sokol MS, Gray NS. Case study: an infection-triggered, autoimmune subtype of anorexia nervosa. J Am Acad Child Adolesc Psychiatry 1997;36(8):1128–33.
90. Sokol MS. Infection-triggered anorexia nervosa in children: clinical description of four cases. J Child Adolesc Psychopharmacol 2000;10(2):133–45.
91. Rubenstein CS, Pigott TA, L'Heureux F, et al. A preliminary investigation of the lifetime prevalence of anorexia and bulimia nervosa in patients with obsessive compulsive disorder. J Clin Psychiatry 1992;53:309–14.
92. Hirani V, Serpell L, Willoughby K, et al. Typology of obsessive-compulsive symptoms in children and adolescents with anorexia nervosa. Eat Weight Disord 2010;15(1–2):e86–9.
93. Dale R, Heyman I, Surtees R, et al. Dyskinesias and associated psychiatric disorders following streptococcal infections. Arch Dis Child 2004;89(7):604–10.
94. Elia J, Dell ML, Friedman DF, et al. PANDAS with catatonia: a case report. Therapeutic response to lorazepam and plasmapheresis. J Am Acad Child Adolesc Psychiatry 2005;44(11):1145–50.
95. Kerbeshian J, Burd L, Tait A. Chain reaction or time bomb: a neuropsychiatric-developmental/neurodevelopmental formulation of tourettisms, pervasive developmental disorder, and schizophreniform symptomatology associated with PANDAS. World J Biol Psychiatry 2007;8(3):201–7.
96. Mathew SJ. PANDAS variant and body dysmorphic disorder. Am J Psychiatry 2001;158(6):963.

97. Kuluva J, Hirsch S, Coffey B. PANDAS and paroxysms: a case of conversion disorder? J Child Adolesc Psychopharmacol 2008;18(1):109–15.

98. Kirvan CA, Swedo SE, Heuser JS, et al. Mimicry and autoantibody-mediated neuronal cell signaling in Sydenham chorea. Nat Med 2003;9(7):914–20.

99. Kirvan CA, Swedo SE, Snider LA, et al. Antibody-mediated neuronal cell signaling in behavior and movement disorders. J Neuroimmunol 2006;179(1):173–9.

100. Church A, Dale R, Giovannoni G. Anti-basal ganglia antibodies: a possible diagnostic utility in idiopathic movement disorders? Arch Dis Child 2004;89(7):611–4.

101. Pavone P, Bianchini R, Parano E, et al. Anti-brain antibodies in PANDAS versus uncomplicated streptococcal infection. Pediatr Neurol 2004;30(2):107–10.

102. Singer HS, Hong JJ, Yoon DY, et al. Serum autoantibodies do not differentiate PANDAS and Tourette syndrome from controls. Neurology 2005;65(11):1701–7.

103. Dale R, Church A, Candler P, et al. Serum autoantibodies do not differentiate PANDAS and Tourette syndrome from controls. Neurology 2006;66(10):1612.

104. Brimberg L, Benhar I, Mascaro-Blanco A, et al. Behavioral, pharmacological, and immunological abnormalities after streptococcal exposure: a novel rat model of Sydenham chorea and related neuropsychiatric disorders. Neuropsychopharmacology 2012;37:2076–87.

105. Yaddanapudi K, Hornig M, Serge R, et al. Passive transfer of streptococcus-induced antibodies reproduces behavioral disturbances in a mouse model of pediatric autoimmune neuropsychiatric disorders associated with streptococcal infection. Mol Psychiatry 2009;15(7):712–26.

106. Cox CJ, Sharma M, Leckman JF, et al. Brain human monoclonal autoantibody from Sydenham chorea targets dopaminergic neurons in transgenic mice and signals dopamine D2 receptor: implications in human disease. J Immunol 2013;191(11):5524–41.

107. Schwartz RH, Wientzen RL, Pedreira F, et al. Penicillin V for group A streptococcal pharyngotonsillitis: a randomized trial of seven vs ten days' therapy. JAMA 1981;246(16):1790–5.

108. Schwartz RH, Hayden GF, Wientzen R. Children less than three-years-old with pharyngitis are group A streptococci really that uncommon? Clin Pediatr 1986;25(4):185–8.

109. Murphy TK, Toufexis MD. PANDAS: Immune Related OCD. In: McKay D, Storch E, editors. Handbook of Assessing Variants and Complications in Anxiety Disorders. New York: Springer; 2013. p. 193–9.

110. O'Connor SP, Darip D, Fraley K, et al. The human antibody response to streptococcal C5a peptidase. J Infect Dis 1991;163(1):109–16.

111. Johnson DR, Kurlan R, Leckman J, et al. The human immune response to streptococcal extracellular antigens: clinical, diagnostic, and potential pathogenetic implications. Clin Infect Dis 2010;50(4):481–90.

112. Kaplan EL, Rothermel CD, Johnson DR. Antistreptolysin O and anti-deoxyribonuclease B titers: normal values for children ages 2 to 12 in the United States. Pediatrics 1998;101(1):86–8.

113. Shet A, Kaplan EL. Clinical use and interpretation of group A streptococcal antibody tests: a practical approach for the pediatrician or primary care physician. Pediatr Infect Dis J 2002;21(5):420–6.

114. Gerber MA. Comparison of throat cultures and rapid strep tests for diagnosis of streptococcal pharyngitis. Pediatr Infect Dis J 1989;8(11):820–4.

115. Talkington DF, Shott S, Fallon MT, et al. Analysis of eight commercial enzyme immunoassay tests for detection of antibodies to Mycoplasma pneumoniae in human serum. Clin Diagn Lab Immunol 2004;11(5):862–7.

116. Waites KB. New concepts of *Mycoplasma pneumoniae* infections in children. Pediatr Pulmonol 2003;36(4):267–78.
117. Ozaki T, Nishimura N, Ahn J, et al. Utility of a rapid diagnosis kit for *Mycoplasma pneumoniae* pneumonia in children, and the antimicrobial susceptibility of the isolates. J Infect Chemother 2007;13(4):204–7.
118. Clyde WA. *Mycoplasma pneumoniae* respiratory disease symposium: summation and significance. Yale J Biol Med 1983;56(5–6):523.
119. Dalmau J, Lancaster E, Martinez-Hernandez E, et al. Clinical experience and laboratory investigations in patients with anti-NMDAR encephalitis. Lancet Neurol 2011;10(1):63–74.
120. Gresa-Arribas N, Titulaer MJ, Torrents A, et al. Antibody titres at diagnosis and during follow-up of anti-NMDA receptor encephalitis: a retrospective study. Lancet Neurol 2014;13:167–77.
121. Suh-Lailam BB, Haven TR, Copple SS, et al. Anti-NMDA-receptor antibody encephalitis: performance evaluation and laboratory experience with the anti-NMDA-receptor IgG assay. Clin Chim Acta 2013;421:1–6.
122. Ayoub EM, Wannamaker LW. Evaluation of the streptococcal desoxyribonuclease b and diphosphopyridine nucleotidase antibody tests in acute rheumatic fever and acute glomerulonephritis. Pediatrics 1962;29(4):527–38.
123. Stollerman GH, Lewis AJ, Schultz I, et al. Relationship of immune response to group A streptococci to the course of acute, chronic and recurrent rheumatic fever. Am J Med 1956;20(2):163–9.
124. Ayoub EM, Wannamaker LW. Streptococcal antibody titers in Sydenham's chorea. Pediatrics 1966;38(6):946–56.
125. Holm SE. Treatment of recurrent tonsillopharyngitis. J Antimicrob Chemother 2000;45(Suppl 1):31–5.
126. Murphy TK. Infections and Tic Disorders. In: Martino D, Leckman JF, editors. Tourette Syndrome. New York: Oxford University Press; 2013. p. 168–201.
127. Murphy T, Storch E, Turner A, et al. Maternal history of autoimmune disease in children presenting with tics and/or obsessive–compulsive disorder. J Neuroimmunol 2010;229(1):243–7.
128. Patterson PH. Maternal infection: window on neuroimmune interactions in fetal brain development and mental illness. Curr Opin Neurobiol 2002;12(1):115–8.
129. Vincent A, Deacon R, Dalton P, et al. Maternal antibody-mediated dyslexia? Evidence for a pathogenic serum factor in a mother of two dyslexic children shown by transfer to mice using behavioural studies and magnetic resonance spectroscopy. J Neuroimmunol 2002;130(1):243–7.
130. Mackay IR, Rosen FS, Zinkernagel RM. Maternal antibodies, childhood infections, and autoimmune diseases. N Engl J Med 2001;345(18):1331–5.
131. Lewin AB, Storch EA, Murphy TK. Pediatric autoimmune neuropsychiatric disorders associated with Streptococcus in identical siblings. J Child Adolesc Psychopharmacol 2011;21(2):177–82.
132. Shulman ST, Bisno AL, Clegg HW, et al. Clinical practice guideline for the diagnosis and management of group A streptococcal pharyngitis: 2012 update by the Infectious Diseases Society of America. Clin Infect Dis 2012;55(10):e86–102.
133. Falcini F, Lepri G, Rigante D, et al. PReS-FINAL-2252: descriptive analysis of pediatric autoimmune neuropsychiatric disorder associated with streptococcus infection (PANDAS) in a cohort of 65 Italian patients. Pediatr Rheumatol 2013; 11(Suppl 2):P242.
134. Ruuskanen O. Safety and tolerability of azithromycin in pediatric infectious diseases: 2003 update. Pediatr Infect Dis J 2004;23(2):S135–9.

135. Jacobs MR, Johnson CE. Macrolide resistance: an increasing concern for treatment failure in children. Pediatr Infect Dis J 2003;22(8):S131–8.
136. Strunk RC, Bacharier LB, Phillips BR, et al. Azithromycin or montelukast as inhaled corticosteroid-sparing agents in moderate-to-severe childhood asthma study. J Allergy Clin Immunol 2008;122(6):1138–44.e4.
137. Murphy TK, Parker-Athill EC, Lewin AB, et al. Cefdinir for New Onset Pediatric Neuropsychiatric Disorders: A Pilot Randomized Trial. Journal of Child & Adolescent Psychopharmacology, in press.
138. Walker K, Brink A, Lawrenson J, et al. Treatment of Sydenham chorea with intravenous immunoglobulin. J Child Neurol 2012;27:147–55.
139. Garvey MA, Snider LA, Leitman SF, et al. Treatment of Sydenham's chorea with intravenous immunoglobulin, plasma exchange, or prednisone. J Child Neurol 2005;20:424–9.
140. Hoekstra PJ, Minderaa RB, Kallenberg C. Lack of effect of intravenous immunoglobulins on tics: a double-blind placebo-controlled study. J Clin Psychiatry 2004;65(4):537–42.
141. Winters JL. Plasma exchange: concepts, mechanisms, and an overview of the American Society for Apheresis guidelines. Hematology Am Soc Hematol Educ Program 2012;2012(1):7–12.
142. Goldstein SL. Therapeutic apheresis in children: special considerations. Seminars in Dialysis 2012;25(2):165–70.
143. Sayyah M, Boostani H, Pakseresht S, et al. A preliminary randomized double-blind clinical trial on the efficacy of celecoxib as an adjunct in the treatment of obsessive–compulsive disorder. Psychiatry Res 2011;189(3):403–6.
144. Baugh RF, Archer SM, Mitchell RB, et al. Clinical practice guideline tonsillectomy in children. Otolaryngol Head Neck Surg 2011;144(Suppl 1):S1–30.
145. Frohna JG. Effectiveness of adenotonsillectomy in children with mild symptoms of throat infections or adenotonsillar hypertrophy: open, randomised controlled trial. J Pediatr 2005;146(3):435–6.
146. Blakley BW, Magit AE. The role of tonsillectomy in reducing recurrent pharyngitis: a systematic review. Otolaryngol Head Neck Surg 2009;140(3):291–7.
147. Alexander AA, Patel NJ, Southammakosane CA, et al. Pediatric autoimmune neuropsychiatric disorders associated with streptococcal infections (PANDAS): an indication for tonsillectomy. Int J Pediatr Otorhinolaryngol 2011;75(6):872–3.
148. Batuecas Caletrío Á, Sánchez González F, Santa Cruz Ruiz S, et al. PANDAS Syndrome: a new tonsillectomy indication? Acta Otorrinolaringol Esp 2008; 59(7):362–3 [in Spanish].
149. Heubi C, Shott SR. PANDAS: pediatric autoimmune neuropsychiatric disorders associated with streptococcal infections—an uncommon, but important indication for tonsillectomy. Int J Pediatr Otorhinolaryngol 2003;67(8):837–40.
150. Orvidas LJ, Slattery MJ. Pediatric autoimmune neuropsychiatric disorders and streptococcal infections: role of otolaryngologist. Laryngoscope 2001;111(9):1515–9.
151. Murphy TK, Lewin AB, Parker-Athill EC, et al. Tonsillectomies and adenoidectomies do not prevent the onset of pediatric autoimmune neuropsychiatric disorder associated with group A streptococcus. Pediatr Infect Dis J 2013;32:834–8.
152. Obregon D, Parker-Athill EC, Tan J, et al. Psychotropic effects of antimicrobials and immune modulation by psychotropics: implications for neuroimmune disorders. Neuropsychiatry (London) 2012;2(4):331–43.
153. Tona J. Pediatric autoimmune neuropsychiatric disorders. OT Practice 2011.

# Pharmacological Treatment of Obsessive-Compulsive Disorder

Christopher Pittenger, MD, PhD*, Michael H. Bloch, MD, MS

## KEYWORDS

- Obsessive-compulsive disorder • OCD • Pharmacotherapy • SSRI • Antidepressant
- Augmentation

## KEY POINTS

- About two thirds cases of obsessive-compulsive disorder will improve with appropriate pharmacotherapy.
- The mainstay of pharmacotherapy is the use of selective serotonin reuptake inhibitors.
- Second-line options include clomipramine and augmentation with neuroleptics.
- A substantial minority of patients remain refractory to aggressive pharmacotherapy.

| Abbreviations | |
|---|---|
| CBT | Cognitive behavioral therapy |
| MDD | Major depressive disorder |
| NMDA | N-methyl-d-aspartate |
| OCD | Obsessive compulsive disorder |
| SRI | Serotonin reuptake inhibitor |
| SSRI | Selective serotonin reuptake inhibitor |

## INTRODUCTION

Obsessive-compulsive disorder (OCD) can present a significant management challenge to the clinical psychiatrist. OCD affects approximately 1.3% of the population in any given year and up to 2.7% over the course of a lifetime.[1] Symptoms consist of obsessions and compulsions; although either alone suffices for a diagnosis, it is typical for a patient to have both.[2] Obsessions are repetitive, stereotyped thoughts

The authors have nothing to disclose.
Department of Psychiatry and Child Study Center, Yale University School of Medicine, 34 Park Street, New Haven, CT 06519, USA
* Corresponding author.
E-mail address: Christopher.pittenger@yale.edu

Psychiatr Clin N Am 37 (2014) 375–391
http://dx.doi.org/10.1016/j.psc.2014.05.006          psych.theclinics.com

that cause anxiety or distress. These obsessions are generally experienced as intrusive or egodystonic, and they are typically recognized as unrealistic or excessive; this distinguishes them from delusions, although the distinction can become unclear in some severe cases. Compulsions are ritualized actions that are undertaken to mitigate distress, often in response to obsessions. Typical obsessions and compulsions include preoccupations with contamination accompanied by repeated or ritualized washing; fear of harm to self or others accompanied by checking rituals; and a need for symmetry or order, accompanied by ordering or arranging compulsions.

OCD can be treated using pharmacotherapy, specialized psychotherapy, anatomically targeted treatments, or their combination.[3] First-line treatments include cognitive behavioral therapy (CBT) and pharmacotherapy with the selective serotonin reuptake inhibitors (SSRIs). In this article, the authors review evidence-based pharmacotherapies for OCD, as well as alternatives that may be considered in refractory patients. Other treatment modalities are reviewed in other articles in this issue.

Unfortunately, even with optimal treatment, many patients continue to experience significant symptoms. Remission of moderate or severe OCD is uncommon, and long-term management is often necessary. The development of new, more effective treatment interventions represents an urgent clinical need.

## SEROTONIN REUPTAKE INHIBITORS

The SSRIs are the mainstay of the pharmacologic treatment of OCD. The tricyclic antidepressant clomipramine was shown to be of benefit in the early 1980s,[4] but side effects limit its use as a first-line agent. Fluvoxamine was first shown to be beneficial in individuals with OCD by Goodman and colleagues[5] in 1989. Since then, more than 20 blinded, placebo-controlled studies have firmly established the efficacy of SSRI monotherapy in OCD.[6,7] Because of the combination of proven efficacy and a typically benign side-effect profile, SSRIs are the first-line pharmacological option for the treatment of OCD.[3]

Closer examination of these studies permits several generalizations with respect to the clinical use of SSRIs for OCD.

Although fluvoxamine was the first SSRI shown to be efficacious and is still often thought of (and marketed) as a preferred OCD drug, there is no evidence of differential benefit among the SSRIs[7]; the choice of agent is therefore best made from of side effects, drug interactions, patient preference, and similar considerations.

SSRIs are more efficacious in OCD when used at high doses, in excess of the typical dose range established by their suppliers (which are generally derived from studies of major depressive disorder [MDD]). For example, doses of up to 80 mg of fluoxetine, 40 mg of escitalopram, 300 mg of fluvoxamine, and 100 mg of paroxetine are often needed; sometimes even higher doses are used.[3] The benefit of these higher doses has been clearly shown by a meta-analysis of multiple studies.[8] Interestingly, this contrasts with the use of the same agents in the treatment of MDD, in which higher doses have been shown to carry a higher side-effect burden without increased benefit.[9] OCD symptoms typically also take longer to respond to SSRI monotherapy than do those of MDD; an adequate trial is 8 to 12 weeks.[3] The reasons for these differences between OCD and MDD response to SSRIs remain unclear.

Although these adages—higher dose and longer treatment—are widely accepted by OCD specialists, their relevance to clinical treatment of individual patients should not be overstated. The number needed to treat (NNT) for OCD patients treated with SSRI monotherapy at standard (antidepressant) doses is approximately 5, meaning that if 5 patients are treated with an SSRI, 1 can be expected to respond who would not have responded to placebo.[7,8] The NNT for a dose escalation from a medium dose to the higher doses noted earlier is 13 to 15.[8] Therefore, although there is clear, measurable benefit to escalating SSRI dosage, the probability that it will move an individual patient from being a 'nonresponder' to being a 'responder' is modest. There may, however, be smaller but still clinically meaningful improvements with dose escalation to which studies are insensitive because they typically use a categorical definition of treatment response.

With respect to the time to response, the picture is also more complicated than the simple statement that SSRIs take 8 to 12 weeks to work. Some patients experience subjective improvement much more rapidly. A recent meta-analysis examining the trajectory of symptom improvement, rather than the response rate at endpoint, suggests that benefit begins in the first weeks of treatment, although it may take many weeks to become clinically (and statistically) significant in many cases (Issari Y, Jakubovski E, Bartley CA, et al. Early onset of selective-serotonin reuptake inhibitors in obsessive-compulsive disorder, submitted for publication). Therefore, although the observation that SSRI response is typically slower in OCD than in MDD is correct, the suggestion that there is no response until after many weeks of treatment is an oversimplification.

Use of the SSRI citalopram merits particular mention. Although it is not approved by the Food and Drug Administration (FDA) for use in OCD, citalopram is as efficacious as the SSRIs that are approved[7] and has historically been frequently used because of its generally good tolerability. However, in 2011, the FDA issued a black-box warning against the use of citalopram doses in excess of 40 mg/d, due to a risk of electrocardiographic (ECG) abnormalities and a theoretical risk of arrhythmia.[10] Doses higher than 20 mg/d are not recommended in the elderly, and it is recommended that the drug be avoided altogether in individuals with a $QT_c$ of greater than 500 msec or with conditions that predispose to arrhythmia. (This effect appears to be smaller for escitalopram, which does not carry a similar FDA warning and is a reasonable alternative.[11]) The merit of this warning, which did not take into account the evidence for benefit from higher doses in OCD, has been questioned.[12] Nevertheless, its existence complicates the clinical use of citalopram at high doses for OCD, and many clinicians have switched to escitalopram or another SSRI as an alternative. Because all of the SSRIs have similar efficacy, there is little reason not to make such a switch. In individual patients who have clearly benefited from citalopram and do not wish to make a switch, ECG monitoring is advisable.

### Children and Adolescents

The use of SSRIs in children and adolescents differs in some ways from their use in adults. Although randomized, placebo-controlled trials clearly demonstrate benefits of SSRI in children with OCD, concerns regarding side effects are more substantial.[6] The added benefit from higher doses of SSRIs, which is clear in adults, has not been demonstrated in the pediatric population. Three of the SSRIs are approved by the FDA for use in children: fluoxetine (age 7 years and older), sertraline (age 6 years and older), and fluvoxamine (age 8 years and older). Clomipramine is also an FDA-approved drug for children aged 10 years and older.

### Clomipramine

The tricyclic antidepressant clomipramine was the first agent shown clearly to be beneficial in patients with OCD[4]; it was approved by the FDA for the treatment of OCD in 1989. Of the tricyclics, clomipramine is the most potent inhibitor of serotonin reuptake. It is sometimes described as an SRI, not an SSRI, because it also binds with high affinity to other receptors and reuptake sites. Meta-analysis suggests that clomipramine may be more efficacious than the SSRIs.[13] However, a variety of technical issues (such as drug dosing and the difficulty maintaining a blind in studies of clomipramine due to its side-effect profile) complicate this interpretation, and head-to-head trials comparing clomipramine with SSRIs have not shown it to be superior.[3] The fact that higher doses of SSRIs are more efficacious suggests that studies using standard SSRI doses may underestimate the benefit of these agents and therefore bias a comparison with clomipramine (for which dose elevation is not possible due to the risk of cardiac toxicity). On the other hand, the authors' recent meta-analysis suggests added benefit to clomipramine even when SSRI dosage is appropriately taken into account (Issari Y, et al, submitted for publication). It seems likely that clomipramine has a small added benefit, at least for some patients.

This modestly greater efficacy must be balanced against clomipramine's more problematic side effect and safety profile. In contrast to SSRIs, clomipramine has significant anticholinergic side effects (eg, dry mouth and constipation), antihistaminergic effects (eg, weight gain and sedation), and α-adrenergic blocking effects (eg, hypotension). It also has substantial arrhythmogenic potential; doses at or higher than the upper limit of the recommended dosing range, 250 mg, may require ECG monitoring, and cardiotoxicity in overdose is a concern. Clomipramine also carries a risk of seizure at doses higher than 250 mg. For all of these reasons, clomipramine is not generally considered a first-line agent. It remains an important alternative when SSRI monotherapy fails.[3]

One pharmacologic strategy that is sometimes used is the addition of clomipramine to an SSRI or the addition of an SSRI to clomipramine. The motivating logic is that this may capture the benefits of clomipramine without requiring doses that produce problematic side effects. However, controlled data on the use of these strategies are sparse[14] and do not provide clear guidance as to their efficacy. The combination of clomipramine with fluvoxamine can be problematic and is best avoided. Fluvoxamine is a potent inhibitor of the liver enzyme CYP2C19 and thus inhibits the metabolism of clomipramine to desmethylclomipramine, which can result in marked elevations of serum clomipramine when the 2 agents are coadministered, raising the risk of side effects such as seizure or arrhythmia.[15]

## Discontinuation of Treatment

Only a few studies have addressed the issue of how long to continue pharmacotherapy, once a clinical response has been achieved. This decision is of course a complex one in individual cases, with benefit being weighed in the context of side effects, patient attitudes, comorbidities, the potential for drug interactions, pregnancy and lactation, and other factors. OCD is often a chronic condition, and remission in moderate to severe cases is unfortunately uncommon. Treatment of an episode to remission followed by treatment discontinuation is, therefore, not a common clinical scenario.

This question can be addressed using a double-blind discontinuation study design, in which a group of stably treated patients are randomized to continue on their pharmacotherapy or be switched to a placebo. One recent study found much higher relapse rate in patients switched to placebo (52%) than those who continued on stable escitalopram (23%).[16] A meta-analysis of similar studies supports this conclusion, with relapse rates in individuals switched from stable active pharmacotherapy to placebo approximately double those in patients maintained on their SSRI pharmacotherapy.[17] In general, once symptom improvement on a stable medication regimen has been achieved, these results suggest that continuation of treatment is advisable, in the absence of intolerable side effects or other case-specific factors.

*Serotonin-norepinephrine Reuptake Inhibitors*

The efficacy of clomipramine led to the hypothesis that dual-acting serotonin-norepinephrine reuptake blockers (SNRIs) might be of greater benefit than SSRIs.[18] Indeed, an early open-label study of venlafaxine suggested that SNRIs are highly effective in the treatment of SSRI-refractory OCD, with response rates of 76% in 29 subjects.[19] However, although other uncontrolled case series have continued to suggest benefit, a subsequent double-blind crossover study suggested that venlafaxine may actually be less effective than paroxetine in the treatment of refractory OCD.[20] When 43 patients who failed to respond to 1 of these 2 agents were switched in a double-blind fashion to the alternative agent, the response rate to paroxetine (56%) was significantly higher than that to venlafaxine (19%).[20] Although there continues to be some theoretical rationale for the use of SNRIs, they cannot be recommended for OCD monotherapy by currently available data. Further research is needed.

## PHARMACOLOGICAL AUGMENTATION

Monotherapy with agents beyond the SRIs has not been shown to be of benefit in OCD. When SRI monotherapy fails, therefore, pharmacologic augmentation with other agents is a frequent recourse. Clear evidence exists for benefit from the addition of low-dose neuroleptics to stable SRIs. Numerous other agents have been investigated in this context, but the evidence for benefit is less clear. Nevertheless, because up to 30% of patients experience little benefit from the best evidence-based treatments, clinicians must in practice often turn to these less well-established strategies.

*Neuroleptic Augmentation*

Double-blind trials in the late 1990s demonstrated efficacy of augmentation of SSRI pharmacotherapy with low-dose typical and atypical antipsychotics in OCD. A recent meta-analysis of 9 double-blind, placebo controlled trials of augmentation with typical or atypical antipsychotics demonstrated their efficacy compared with placebo.[21,22] Approximately one-third of treatment-refractory OCD patients will respond to antipsychotic augmentation; the NNT is 4.6. OCD patients with comorbid tic disorders appear to respond particularly well to antipsychotic augmentation. There is no evidence that any particular antipsychotic commonly used as augmentation is better than any other, although the most convincing evidence for efficacy exists for haloperidol and risperidone. It should be noted that not all studies show positive results; one recent study found no benefit from the addition of risperidone to stable clomipramine treatment (whereas the addition of CBT was highly beneficial).[23] It is clear that not all patients benefit from neuroleptic augmentation; the patients included in this recent study had fewer tics and may have been less treatment-resistant than those in earlier studies, which may explain the discrepant results.

In general, antipsychotic augmentation should not be considered until 2 SRI trials of adequate dose and duration have been attempted, because of the more benign side-effect profile of the SRIs and the reasonable likelihood of response to extended treatment or a switch to a second agent. However, if significant symptoms persist after 2 such trials, augmentation with a low dose of an antipsychotic represents a realistic treatment option, especially in patients with a personal or family history of tics.

*Glutamatergic Agents: the N-Methyl-D-Aspartate Receptor*

Substantial recent interest has focused on the role of glutamate imbalance in OCD.[24] Polymorphisms in the gene for the major neuronal glutamate transporter have been associated with OCD, although the nature of any causative polymorphism remains unclear.[25] Several magnetic resonance spectroscopy studies have indicated abnormalities in glutamate and related molecules, although again the specific nature of the hypothesized disruption remains unclear.[26] Finally, a pair of studies examining cerebrospinal fluid in unmedicated adults with OCD has found elevated glutamate levels.[27,28] These findings have spurred interest in the use of glutamate modulators for pharmacological augmentation in SRI-refractory disease; several such agents are already approved for other indications. Because the data suggest an excess of extrasynaptic glutamate, antiglutamatergic modulators have been the most extensively investigated.

Agents targeting the N-methyl-d-aspartate (NMDA) class of glutamate receptor have received particular attention. The NMDA receptor has been targeted in several distinct ways, which may have distinct effects on neuronal function and circuit dynamics. Memantine, which is used for the treatment of Alzheimer disease, is a low-affinity noncompetitive NMDA blocker. A series of small uncontrolled studies have suggested benefit in both adults and children with OCD.[29–32] One of these studies suggested differential benefit in OCD compared with generalized anxiety disorder, indicating that there may be some diagnostic specificity to the effect.[30] More recently, a pair of blinded, placebo controlled studies from Iran examined memantine augmentation[33] or monotherapy[34] and found a surprisingly substantial benefit. The effects reported are substantially more robust than what is suggested by the previously reported open-label studies, reaching 100% response and 89% remission after 8 weeks of treatment. These studies are promising, but replication in other populations is needed to increase confidence in the generalizability of the results. On the other hand, as memantine is an FDA-approved medication with a rather benign side-effect profile at the doses used (typically 20 mg/d), empirical use in refractory patients may be reasonable even in the absence of definitive studies.

Several other studies have reported benefit from indirect modulators of the NMDA receptor. Glycine is a coagonist of the NMDA receptor and is required for its full activation. In a small study, blinded treatment with glycine (or placebo) appeared to improve symptoms, an effect that nearly reached significance in an analysis of completers.[35] Unfortunately, glycine was very poorly tolerated, and there were many dropouts. Another small, open-label study investigated the naturally occurring amino acid analogue sarcosine, which is an inhibitor of glycine reuptake and thus is predicted to indirectly increase synaptic glycine. There was a 20% reduction in OCD symptoms; this must be interpreted with caution in the absence of a placebo comparison group but is encouraging.[36]

A third set of studies have used the high-potency anesthetic NMDA blocker ketamine. These studies are motivated by the startling observation that a single challenge with ketamine can have rapid antidepressant effects lasting days or 1 to 2 weeks, even in treatment-refractory MDD.[37] Two fairly small studies of ketamine challenge in OCD have yielded conflicting results. In a placebo-controlled study of unmedicated patients, Rodriguez and colleagues[38] have shown a pattern of response very similar to what has been reported in MDD: a rapid improvement within hours of a ketamine infusion that lasts several days before symptoms return to baseline. In contrast, in a somewhat more ill group of patients, many of whom had comorbidities and many of whom were medicated, Bloch and colleagues[39] found no clinically significant benefit from ketamine. This second study did not have a placebo control group. However, many of the subjects were depressed, and many of these exhibited an improvement in their depressive symptoms. This provides an 'internal control' documenting the adequacy of the ketamine infusion. It remains unclear whether the discrepancy between these studies derives from methodological factors or from differences in the patient populations. Further research is needed. Regardless, ketamine is unlikely to become a major part of the pharmacologic armamentarium: as currently administered it requires intravenous infusion; the effects are transient; and both basic and clinical literature raise concerns about the neurotoxic potential of chronic ketamine exposure. As in depression, therefore, any benefit from ketamine challenge is likely to be more useful as a guide to the development of future therapeutics than as a new treatment option in its own right.

It is important to note that these 3 ways of modulating the NMDA receptor are fundamentally different from one another. Memantine chronically blocks NMDA receptor function; in both open-label and controlled studies, benefit has been seen after weeks. Glycine and sarcosine, in contrast, are positive modulators of NMDA function and may potentiate it. Finally, ketamine is a much more potent antagonist than memantine, but its use in studies to date is fundamentally different from that of memantine, consisting of an acute challenge rather than chronic treatment for weeks. These very different ways of targeting the receptor are likely to have fundamentally different effects on neuronal and circuit functioning. If ongoing research corroborates the benefit of more than one of these interventional strategies, an explanation for this fact will be called for.

### Other Glutamate-modulating Agents

A variety of other glutamate-modulating agents have been tried in OCD, chiefly in small, uncontrolled studies. A pair of open-label studies in profoundly refractory patients suggests benefit from the glutamate modulator riluzole, which is approved by the FDA for the treatment of amyotrophic lateral sclerosis[40,41]; however, controlled data have not yet been reported. Riluzole is generally well tolerated, and some patients have been on it continuously for years without problems.[41] Riluzole has several mechanisms of action; it remains unclear which may provide benefit in OCD.[42]

The antiepileptic topiramate is thought to modulate neuronal glutamate levels through its interaction with voltage-gated ion channels. Two controlled trials have suggested benefit from topiramate, at a variety of doses; there is some evidence of a greater effect on compulsions than on obsessions.[43,44] Cognitive, sedative, and weight-loss side effects may limit the use of topiramate in some cases.

Lamotrigine is an antiepileptic and mood stabilizer. It is thought to reduce neuronal glutamate outflow through its inhibition of certain voltage-gated sodium channels, a mechanism that overlaps with some of the effects of riluzole.[42] An initial investigation of lamotrigine in OCD provided no evidence of benefit.[45] However, a more recent randomized trial investigated lamotrigine augmentation of stable SSRI treatment and found marked benefit, with 50% responders in the lamotrigine group and none in the placebo group.[46] The reason for this discrepancy is unclear, and more work is needed.

The amino acid derivative N-acetylcysteine has both antioxidant and glutamate-modulating properties. It has been examined in a variety of conditions and is an attractive agent because it is available over-the-counter (OTC), is extremely affordable, and has few side effects. An early case report suggested benefit in OCD.[47] More recently, a placebo-controlled trial from Iran suggested marked benefit of the addition of N-acetylcysteine to stable SSRI treatment in adults with OCD.[48] More work is needed; but the many attractive characteristics of this agent may make it a viable option in some cases once better-proved strategies have been exhausted.

### Other pharmacologic augmentation strategies

A variety of other agents have been used to augment ineffective SSRI treatment; none are sufficiently well supported by the literature to have entered the standard of care, but small studies provide intriguing evidence of benefit in several cases.

### Mirtazapine

Mirtazapine is an α-2 adrenergic receptor antagonist and thus enhances norepinephrine release[49]; it also indirectly enhances serotonergic neurotransmission. A case series of 6 OCD patients suggested that mirtazapine is ineffective as an augmentation agent for treatment-refractory OCD.[19] However, in an unblinded trial of 49 treatment-naïve OCD patients, subjects receiving citalopram plus mirtazapine had an accelerated clinical response, with a significantly greater reduction in OCD severity at 4 weeks compared with citalopram plus placebo. Treatment response in the 2 groups equalized by 12 weeks[50]; this result suggests that mirtazapine may be helpful in accelerating the initial response to SRI pharmacotherapy but not in increasing the ultimate likelihood of response in those who fail initial SRI pharmacotherapy.

### Opioid augmentation

The endogenous opioid system has been postulated to be involved in OCD pathogenesis ever since it was noted that administration of the opioid antagonist naloxone exacerbated OCD symptoms.[51] A double-blind, placebo-controlled crossover trial of 23 treatment-refractory OCD patients demonstrated a significantly greater decrease in OCD symptoms in response to weekly oral morphine compared with placebo.[52] Two weeks of oral morphine produced a median decrease in Y-BOCS severity of 13%, with 7 of the 23 subjects (30%) being treatment responders.[52] Tramadol hydrochloride, an opioid agonist with lower abuse potential than morphine, has been studied as an augmentation agent for treatment-refractory OCD in an open-label trial. The 6 treatment-refractory OCD patients included in this study experienced an average decline of Y-BOCS scores of 26%.[53] Further double-blind studies are needed to establish the efficacy of tramadol as an augmentation agent in OCD.

### Ondansetron

Ondansetron is a 5-HT3 receptor agonist that is used as an antiemetic. Several small studies have suggested benefit from low doses of ondansetron and of the related agent granisetron in OCD.[54,55] The studies showing the clearest effects are again from Iran.[56,57] In December of 2012, Transcept Pharmaceuticals announced that a Phase 2 trial of ondansetron had not met its primary efficacy endpoint.[58] The role, if any, for 5-HT3 agonists as augmentation in refractory disease remains to be clarified.

### Caffeine

Caffeine was included as an active control in a pilot study of amphetamine augmentation in OCD. Both dextroamphetamine and caffeine led to significant improvements in refractory patients over 5 weeks.[59] The potential clinical use of these stimulants has not yet been followed-up in larger studies.

In sum, small studies of varying quality have led to several intriguing possibilities for augmentation strategies in OCD that is refractory to standard pharmacologic approaches. However, in none of these cases is such an approach supported by multiple high-quality studies. Further research is needed to address the unmet clinical needs of the substantial minority of OCD patients who do not respond to standard-of-care treatment.

## OVER-THE-COUNTER AGENTS

There has been significant interest in a variety of OTC agents for OCD.[60,61] These are often perceived as safer and more 'natural' than prescription pharmacotherapy, which makes them attractive to many patients. N-acetylcysteine, sarcosine, and glycine, which have been addressed earlier in the context of glutamate modulators, fall into this category. Unfortunately, variable quality control makes it difficult to use these less-regulated agents with confidence, and the research base guiding their use remains very thin. The authors have recently reviewed this literature and provide guidance for the use of OTC agents.[62] They do not extensively review the literature on these agents here but rather highlight those for which there is some substantive evidence of benefit. Most OTC agents are well tolerated, which is why they are lightly regulated; the typically low risk associated with their moderate use may make such a strategy reasonable, when preferred by individual patients, even when the evidence for benefit is less than robust.

### Myo-inositol

Myo-inositol has been examined in 2 small studies. The first found evidence of benefit from monotherapy.[63] A follow-up study from the same group found no benefit from the addition of myo-inositol to stable SSRI treatment.[64] The investigators suggest that this indicates an interaction, such that myo-inositol is only efficacious when used as mono-therapy. However, both of these studies, although well designed, were small. More work would be needed to substantiate the use of myo-inositol to the point that it could be recommended as part of the standard of care.

### Other Agents

Small studies have investigated several other agents, including kava, St.John's wort, borage, milk thistle, eicosapentaenoic acid, and tryptophan.[62] However, for none of these is there substantial evidence of benefit for OCD symptoms (although St. John's wort may be of benefit for comorbid depressive symptoms). Potential side effects are of concern in some cases, especially with chronic use of kava.

## COMBINATION TREATMENT

SSRI pharmacotherapy and behavioral and cognitive behavioral psychotherapy are considered first-line treatments for OCD. (Psychotherapies for OCD are reviewed elsewhere in this issue.) It is intuitive that their combination would be more efficacious than either alone. Surprisingly, careful studies suggest that this may not always be the case, at least in an idealized setting in adults.

In the pediatric population, the POTS trial (Pediatric OCD Treatment Study) compared CBT, sertraline, and their combination with placebo in 112 children with OCD.[65] All active treatments were superior to placebo and were well tolerated. Combination treatment was more effective than either CBT alone or sertraline alone, supporting synergistic benefit. A follow-up study found that the addition of CBT to stable pharmacotherapy can provide further improvement.[66] This pair of large, definitive studies establishes rather clearly that the combination of medication and psychotherapy is more effective than either one alone, in the pediatric population.

In adults, the benefits of combination therapy are less clear. A large study comparing expert CBT, clomipramine, and their combination to placebo found that the benefit of CBT exceeded that of clomipramine and that combination treatment provided no significant additional improvement.[67] A follow-up study from the same group looked at the addition of CBT to stable SRI treatment compared with risperidone augmentation. CBT was markedly superior.[23] These studies suggest that combination treatment may not provide benefit.

However, important caveats to this conclusion must be noted. The CBT provided in these studies was intensive (twice weekly) and was administered by particularly skilled experts at academic centers; it is likely to be more potent than CBT as practiced in the community, even by experienced practitioners. Medication in these studies was administered in a manualized, relatively inflexible way, which may not recapitulate typical pharmacological strategies. In clinical practice, most authorities continue to recommend combination therapy as having potential benefits above and beyond medication or therapy alone.[3] For example, some patients cannot tolerate the anxiety that is inherent to CBT until their symptoms are somewhat moderated by medication.

### Augmentation of Psychotherapy Through Enhancement of Plasticity

As our understanding of the brain processes underlying learning advances, an exciting prospect is that this knowledge can be harnessed to enhance the potency and specificity of psychotherapy. Although such synergistic strategies have not entered mainstream clinical practice, there are several promising initial steps in this direction, especially in the treatment of anxiety disorders.

The NMDA glutamate receptor, described earlier, has a key role in modulating the strength of connections between neurons, which is thought to be a key substrate for learning. In animals, enhancement of NMDA receptor function can enhance learning.[68] This observation has led to the idea that transient enhancement of NMDA function, in conjunction with focused psychotherapeutic interventions, might lead to improved efficacy.[69] An initial proof of concept of this approach was provided by Ressler, Davis, and colleagues in a seminal set of studies. In animals, they showed that D-cycloserine, a positive allosteric modulator of the NMDA receptor, enhanced extinction of learned fear in animals.[70] They then applied this strategy to the extinction-based treatment of acrophobia and found that D-cycloserine enhanced clinical response.[71]

Several studies have sought to apply this approach to the treatment of OCD. Results to date are mixed, with some studies showing enhanced efficacy or rate of responding in patients treated with D-cycloserine before CBT sessions.[72] Variables such as the dosage and the timing of D-cycloserine administration are likely to be key to any benefit. The effect of D-cycloserine appears to decrease over CBT sessions, which may indicate that the primary effect is on the rate of responding, rather than on the ultimate efficacy of the treatment.[72] D-cycloserine is reasonably well tolerated and is available at compounding pharmacies; this strategy is therefore available to clinicians, although it has not entered widespread use. These findings are valuable as a demonstration of the viability of plasticity-enhancing manipulations to optimize the response to CBT; further research in this area may lead to more dramatic interactive effects.

It is important to note that the targeting of the NMDA receptor using D-cycloserine is qualitatively different from the pharmacologic use of memantine, ketamine, or glycine, which has been discussed earlier. When D-cycloserine is used in conjunction with CBT, function of the NMDA receptor is acutely enhanced to potentiate plasticity. Glycine, and similar agents, seeks to chronically enhance NMDA receptor function. In contrast, ketamine transiently blocks the NMDA receptor, while memantine treatment has been used to chronically block it. Such disparate therapeutic strategies aimed at a single target, with some evidence of benefit for each, speaks to the centrality of this receptor in brain function and in psychopathology.

## PHARMACOGENETICS

There has been great excitement in recent years about pharmacogenetics: the possibility of using individual genetic data to predict drug response and/or side effects, and thus to meaningfully guide treatment choices. The appeal and theoretic potential of this approach cannot be denied. Because the response to medication treatment in OCD is highly heterogeneous and the disorder has a substantial genetic component, this may be a particularly appropriate context for a pharmacogenetic approach.

In MDD, significant work has been done in this area and has implicated polymorphisms in several genes as predictors of antidepressant response.[73,74] In contrast, progress in establishing genetic polymorphisms with predictive value in OCD has been relatively slow.[75] Over the past decade, our ability to gather genetic information has rapidly outstripped our knowledge of which polymorphisms are prognostically useful. Because several companies are now offering genotyping services to patients, it is increasingly critical for clinicians to be in a position to interpret such data.

Conceptually, there are 2 ways in which genetic polymorphisms may contribute to medication response. First, they could affect pharmacokinetics, by altering drug metabolism or transport; well-characterized polymorphisms in the liver's cytochrome P450 system or the blood brain barrier efflux pump are likely to fall into this category. Alternatively, polymorphisms in brain-expressed molecules related to hypothesized pathophysiologic mechanisms are more likely to alter a drug's pharmacodynamics, either by directly altering its interactions with its molecular targets or by changing the way interacting molecules or cellular processes respond to direct drug effects. Polymorphisms in components of the serotonergic and glutamatergic system are more likely to fall into this latter category, although it may not be possible (or necessary) to make this distinction with confidence *a priori*.

Examination of loci in pharmacogenetic studies can be done either in a targeted, hypothesis-driven fashion, by picking genes of potential interest with known polymorphisms and examining them in the target population, or in an exploratory fashion, in which the genome is queried more broadly to find loci associated with response (ie, pharmacogenomics). The latter approach requires many more subjects and has not yet been used in OCD.

The cytochrome P450 enzymes are highly polymorphic in the population and have a well-characterized role in drug metabolism, including in the metabolism of several drugs commonly used for the treatment of OCD. Given that polymorphisms in this system are well established to affect the rate at which different individuals metabolize specific drugs, and thus the concentration of active drug to enter the brain and the concentration of potentially active metabolites, this system represents a promising target for pharmacogenetic studies. A recent investigation examined P450 polymorphisms in 184 patients with OCD.[76] The strongest effect was an association of low-activity variants in the gene CYP2D6 with the number of past-failed treatment trials in these patients, which may be a surrogate marker for refractoriness. There was also a lower incidence of side effects from venlafaxine in individuals with normal ("extensive") CYP2D6 metabolic activity than those with lower metabolizing alleles perhaps due to the fact that venlafaxine is metabolized to an active metabolite, O-desmethylvenlafaxine, which is therefore reduced in low metabolizers. Trend-level effects suggested an influence of CYP2D6 metabolizer status on response to fluoxetine and of CYP2C19 status on response to sertraline. These findings require replication and do not yet provide clear guidance for the application of genetic data to treatment selection, but they represent a promising start to a potentially important new source of information to guide clinical decision making.

Other small studies in OCD have examined polymorphisms in genes more likely to be associated with pharmacodynamics, such as the serotonin receptor HTR2A, the serotonin transporter SLC6A4, the neurotransmitter brain-derived neurotrophic factor, and the monoamine metabolic enzyme catechol-O-methyltransferase. However, these studies have by and large been small and inconsistent.[75] More work is needed in this area.

## SUMMARY

Our treatments for OCD remain inadequate. Although most patients will respond to established pharmacotherapy and/or psychotherapeutic approaches, approximately a quarter do not. Furthermore, many of those who are classified as "responders" continue to have substantial symptoms and a chronic reduction in productivity and in quality of life.

The SSRIs are the mainstay of the pharmacologic treatment of OCD. Their combination of efficacy with relatively good tolerability is not matched by any other available agents. There is no known difference in the efficacy of different SSRIs, and thus the choice of agent is best guided by side effects, pharmacokinetic considerations, and patient preference. Higher doses and longer duration of treatment, relative to standard practice in the treatment of MDD, are often required. Clomipramine provides an alternative for monotherapy and may be marginally more effective, but its side-effect profile mitigates against its use as a first-line agent in most cases. When monotherapy fails, augmentation with low-dose neuroleptic (especially risperidone) or psychotherapy has good support in the literature. Other augmentation strategies are less well established but are often appropriate when first- and second-line approaches have been exhausted.

Perhaps the most important conclusion from this review of pharmacotherapeutic options is that there is a relative paucity of well-established treatment options in OCD, when SSRI treatment fails. This conclusion contrasts with MDD, schizophrenia, and many other major psychiatric conditions, in which numerous mechanistically distinct pharmacologic strategies are available and algorithms for stepped treatment are being developed. It is to be hoped that, as more research is done in the pathophysiology and treatment of OCD and related disorders, clinicians will have a broader array of treatment options in the future.

## REFERENCES

1. Kessler RC, Petukhova M, Sampson NA, et al. Twelve-month and lifetime prevalence and lifetime morbid risk of anxiety and mood disorders in the United States. Int J Methods Psychiatr Res 2012;21(3):169–84.
2. American Psychiatric Association, DSM-5 Task Force. Diagnostic and statistical manual of mental disorders: DSM-5. 5th edition. Washington, DC: American Psychiatric Association; 2013. p. 947 xliv.
3. Koran LM, Hanna GL, Hollander E, et al. Practice guideline for the treatment of patients with obsessive-compulsive disorder. Am J Psychiatry 2007;164(Suppl 7):5–53.
4. Insel TR, Murphy DL, Cohen RM, et al. Obsessive-compulsive disorder. A double-blind trial of clomipramine and clorgyline. Arch Gen Psychiatry 1983; 40(6):605–12.
5. Goodman WK, Price LH, Rasmussen SA, et al. Efficacy of fluvoxamine in obsessive-compulsive disorder. A double-blind comparison with placebo. Arch Gen Psychiatry 1989;46(1):36–44.

6. Soomro GM. Obsessive compulsive disorder. Clin Evid (Online) 2012;2012. pii: 1004.
7. Soomro GM, Altman D, Rajagopal S, et al. Selective serotonin re-uptake inhibitors (SSRIs) versus placebo for obsessive compulsive disorder (OCD). Cochrane Database Syst Rev 2008;(1):CD001765.
8. Bloch MH, McGuire J, Landeros-Weisenberger A, et al. Meta-analysis of the dose-response relationship of SSRI in obsessive-compulsive disorder. Mol Psychiatry 2010;15(8):850–5.
9. Bollini P, Pampallona S, Tibaldi G, et al. Effectiveness of antidepressants. Meta-analysis of dose-effect relationships in randomised clinical trials. Br J Psychiatry 1999;174:297–303.
10. FDA. FDA drug safety comunications: revised recommendations for celexa (citalopram hydrobromide) related to a potential risk of abnormal heart rhythms with high doses. 2012 [cited January 14, 2014].
11. Citalopram, escitalopram, and the QT interval. Med Lett Drugs Ther 2013; 55(1421):59.
12. Zivin K, Pfeiffer PN, Bohnert AS, et al. Safety of high-dosage citalopram. Am J Psychiatry 2014;171(1):20–2.
13. Ackerman DL, Greenland S. Multivariate meta-analysis of controlled drug studies for obsessive-compulsive disorder. J Clin Psychopharmacol 2002; 22(3):309–17.
14. Marazziti D, Golia F, Consoli G, et al. Effectiveness of long-term augmentation with citalopram to clomipramine in treatment-resistant OCD patients. CNS Spectr 2008;13(11):971–6.
15. Szegedi A, Wetzel H, Leal M, et al. Combination treatment with clomipramine and fluvoxamine: drug monitoring, safety, and tolerability data. J Clin Psychiatry 1996;57(6):257–64.
16. Fineberg NA, Tonnoir B, Lemming O, et al. Escitalopram prevents relapse of obsessive-compulsive disorder. Eur Neuropsychopharmacol 2007;17(6–7): 430–9.
17. Donovan MR, Glue P, Kolluri S, et al. Comparative efficacy of antidepressants in preventing relapse in anxiety disorders - a meta-analysis. J Affect Disord 2010; 123(1–3):9–16.
18. Dell'Osso B, Nestadt G, Allen A, et al. Serotonin-norepinephrine reuptake inhibitors in the treatment of obsessive-compulsive disorder: a critical review. J Clin Psychiatry 2006;67(4):600–10.
19. Hollander E, Friedberg J, Wasserman S, et al. Venlafaxine in treatment-resistant obsessive-compulsive disorder. J Clin Psychiatry 2003;64(5):546–50.
20. Denys D, van Megen HJ, van der Wee N, et al. A double-blind switch study of paroxetine and venlafaxine in obsessive-compulsive disorder. J Clin Psychiatry 2004;65(1):37–43.
21. Bloch MH, Landeros-Weisenberger A, Kelmendi B, et al. A systematic review: antipsychotic augmentation with treatment refractory obsessive-compulsive disorder. Mol Psychiatry 2006;11(7):622–32.
22. Dold M, Aigner M, Lanzenberger R, et al. Antipsychotic augmentation of serotonin reuptake inhibitors in treatment-resistant obsessive-compulsive disorder: a meta-analysis of double-blind, randomized, placebo-controlled trials. Int J Neuropsychopharmacol 2013;16(3):557–74.
23. Simpson HB, Foa EB, Liebowitz MR, et al. Cognitive-behavioral therapy vs risperidone for augmenting serotonin reuptake inhibitors in obsessive-compulsive disorder: a randomized clinical trial. JAMA Psychiatry 2013;70(11):1190–9.

24. Pittenger C, Bloch MH, Williams K. Glutamate abnormalities in obsessive compulsive disorder: neurobiology, pathophysiology, and treatment. Pharmacol Ther 2011;132(3):314–32.

25. Stewart SE, Mayerfeld C, Arnold PD, et al. Meta-analysis of association between obsessive-compulsive disorder and the 3' region of neuronal glutamate transporter gene SLC1A1. Am J Med Genet B Neuropsychiatr Genet 2013; 162B(4):367–79.

26. Brennan BP, Rauch SL, Jensen JE, et al. A critical review of magnetic resonance spectroscopy studies of obsessive-compulsive disorder. Biol Psychiatry 2013; 73(1):24–31.

27. Bhattacharyya S, Khanna S, Chakrabarty K, et al. Anti-brain autoantibodies and altered excitatory neurotransmitters in obsessive-compulsive disorder. Neuropsychopharmacology 2009;34(12):2489–96.

28. Chakrabarty K, Bhattacharyya S, Christopher R, et al. Glutamatergic dysfunction in OCD. Neuropsychopharmacology 2005;30(9):1735–40.

29. Pasquini M, Biondi M. Memantine augmentation for refractory obsessive-compulsive disorder. Prog Neuropsychopharmacol Biol Psychiatry 2006;30(6): 1173–5.

30. Poyurovsky M, Weizman R, Weizman A, et al. Memantine for treatment-resistant OCD. Am J Psychiatry 2005;162(11):2191–2.

31. Stewart SE, Jenike EA, Hezel DM, et al. A single-blinded case-control study of memantine in severe obsessive-compulsive disorder. J Clin Psychopharmacol 2010;30(1):34–9.

32. Feusner JD, Kerwin L, Saxena S, et al. Differential efficacy of memantine for obsessive-compulsive disorder vs. generalized anxiety disorder: an open-label trial. Psychopharmacol Bull 2009;42(1):81–93.

33. Ghaleiha A, Entezari N, Modabbernia A, et al. Memantine add-on in moderate to severe obsessive-compulsive disorder: randomized double-blind placebo-controlled study. J Psychiatr Res 2013;47(2):175–80.

34. Haghighi M, Jahangard L, Mohammad-Beigi H, et al. In a double-blind, randomized and placebo-controlled trial, adjuvant memantine improved symptoms in inpatients suffering from refractory obsessive-compulsive disorders (OCD). Psychopharmacology (Berl) 2013;228(4):633–40.

35. Greenberg WM, Benedict MM, Doerfer J, et al. Adjunctive glycine in the treatment of obsessive-compulsive disorder in adults. J Psychiatr Res 2009;43(6): 664–70.

36. Wu PL, Tang HS, Lane HY, et al. Sarcosine therapy for obsessive compulsive disorder: a prospective, open-label study. J Clin Psychopharmacol 2011; 31(3):369–74.

37. Krystal JH, Sanacora G, Duman RS. Rapid-acting glutamatergic antidepressants: the path to ketamine and beyond. Biol Psychiatry 2013;73(12): 1133–41.

38. Rodriguez CI, Kegeles LS, Levinson A, et al. Randomized controlled crossover trial of ketamine in obsessive-compulsive disorder: proof-of-concept. Neuropsychopharmacology 2013;38(12):2475–83.

39. Bloch MH, Wasylink S, Landeros-Weisenberger A, et al. Effects of ketamine in treatment-refractory obsessive-compulsive disorder. Biol Psychiatry 2012; 72(11):964–70.

40. Coric V, Taskiran S, Pittenger C, et al. Riluzole augmentation in treatment-resistant obsessive-compulsive disorder: an open-label trial. Biol Psychiatry 2005;58(5):424–8.

41. Pittenger C, Kelmendi B, Wasylink S, et al. Riluzole augmentation in treatment-refractory obsessive-compulsive disorder: a series of 13 cases, with long-term follow-up. J Clin Psychopharmacol 2008;28(3):363–7.
42. Pittenger C, Coric V, Banasr M, et al. Riluzole in the treatment of mood and anxiety disorders. CNS Drugs 2008;22(9):761–86.
43. Berlin HA, Koran LM, Jenike MA, et al. Double-blind, placebo-controlled trial of topiramate augmentation in treatment-resistant obsessive-compulsive disorder. J Clin Psychiatry 2011;72(5):716–21.
44. Mowla A, Khajeian AM, Sahraian A, et al. Topiramate augmentation in resistant OCD: a double-blind placebo-controlled clinical trial. CNS Spectr 2010;15(11): 613–7.
45. Kumar TC, Khanna S. Lamotrigine augmentation of serotonin re-uptake inhibitors in obsessive-compulsive disorder. Aust N Z J Psychiatry 2000;34(3): 527–8.
46. Bruno A, Mico U, Pandolfo G, et al. Lamotrigine augmentation of serotonin reuptake inhibitors in treatment-resistant obsessive-compulsive disorder: a double-blind, placebo-controlled study. J Psychopharmacol 2012;26(11):1456–62.
47. Lafleur DL, Pittenger C, Kelmendi B, et al. N-acetylcysteine augmentation in serotonin reuptake inhibitor refractory obsessive-compulsive disorder. Psychopharmacology (Berl) 2006;184(2):254–6.
48. Afshar H, Roohafza H, Mohammad-Beigi H, et al. N-acetylcysteine add-on treatment in refractory obsessive-compulsive disorder: a randomized, double-blind, placebo-controlled trial. J Clin Psychopharmacol 2012;32(6):797–803.
49. de Boer T. The pharmacologic profile of mirtazapine. J Clin Psychiatry 1996; 57(Suppl 4):19–25.
50. Pallanti S, Quercioli L, Koran LM. Citalopram intravenous infusion in resistant obsessive-compulsive disorder: an open trial. J Clin Psychiatry 2002;63(9): 796–801.
51. Insel TR, Pickar D. Naloxone administration in obsessive-compulsive disorder: report of two cases. Am J Psychiatry 1983;140(9):1219–20.
52. Koran LM, Aboujaoude E, Bullock KD, et al. Double-blind treatment with oral morphine in treatment-resistant obsessive-compulsive disorder. J Clin Psychiatry 2005;66(3):353–9.
53. Shapira NA, Keck PE Jr, Goldsmith TD, et al. Open-label pilot study of tramadol hydrochloride in treatment-refractory obsessive-compulsive disorder. Depress Anxiety 1997;6(4):170–3.
54. Pallanti S, Bernardi S, Antonini S, et al. Ondansetron augmentation in treatment-resistant obsessive-compulsive disorder: a preliminary, single-blind, prospective study. CNS Drugs 2009;23(12):1047–55.
55. Pallanti S, Bernardi S, Antonini S, et al. Ondansetron augmentation in patients with obsessive-compulsive disorder who are inadequate responders to serotonin reuptake inhibitors: improvement with treatment and worsening following discontinuation. Eur Neuropsychopharmacol 2014;24(3):375–80.
56. Askari N, Moin M, Sanati M, et al. Granisetron adjunct to fluvoxamine for moderate to severe obsessive-compulsive disorder: a randomized, double-blind, placebo-controlled trial. CNS Drugs 2012;26(10):883–92.
57. Soltani F, Sayyah M, Feizy F, et al. A double-blind, placebo-controlled pilot study of ondansetron for patients with obsessive-compulsive disorder. Hum Psychopharmacol 2010;25(6):509–13.
58. Transcept Pharmaceuticals, I. Transcept Pharmaceuticals announces that a Phase 2 clinical trial of TO = 2061 as adjunctive therapy for obsessive-compulsive

disorder did not meet primary endpoint. 2012. Available at: http://ir.transcept.com/releasedetail.cfm?ReleaseID=728327. Accessed February 17, 2014.

59. Koran LM, Aboujaoude E, Gamel NN. Double-blind study of dextroamphetamine versus caffeine augmentation for treatment-resistant obsessive-compulsive disorder. J Clin Psychiatry 2009;70(11):1530–5.

60. Sarris J, Camfield D, Berk M. Complementary medicine, self-help, and lifestyle interventions for obsessive compulsive disorder (OCD) and the OCD spectrum: a systematic review. J Affect Disord 2012;138(3):213–21.

61. Camfield DA, Sarris J, Berk M. Nutraceuticals in the treatment of obsessive compulsive disorder (OCD): a review of mechanistic and clinical evidence. Prog Neuropsychopharmacol Biol Psychiatry 2011;35(4):887–95.

62. Kichuk SA, Carlton RM, Pittenger C. Over-the-counter supplements in the treatment of obsessive compulsive disorder: practical considerations and evidence. Newsletter of the International OCD Foundation 2013;Summer 2013:17–20.

63. Fux M, Levine J, Aviv A, et al. Inositol treatment of obsessive-compulsive disorder. Am J Psychiatry 1996;153(9):1219–21.

64. Fux M, Benjamin J, Belmaker RH. Inositol versus placebo augmentation of serotonin reuptake inhibitors in the treatment of obsessive-compulsive disorder: a double-blind cross-over study. Int J Neuropsychopharmacol 1999;2(3):193–5.

65. Pediatric OCD Treatment Study (POTS) Team. Cognitive-behavior therapy, sertraline, and their combination for children and adolescents with obsessive-compulsive disorder: the Pediatric OCD Treatment Study (POTS) randomized controlled trial. JAMA 2004;292(16):1969–76.

66. Franklin ME, Sapyta J, Freeman JB, et al. Cognitive behavior therapy augmentation of pharmacotherapy in pediatric obsessive-compulsive disorder: the Pediatric OCD Treatment Study II (POTS II) randomized controlled trial. JAMA 2011;306(11):1224–32.

67. Foa EB, Liebowitz MR, Kozak MJ, et al. Randomized, placebo-controlled trial of exposure and ritual prevention, clomipramine, and their combination in the treatment of obsessive-compulsive disorder. Am J Psychiatry 2005;162(1):151–61.

68. Myers KM, Carlezon WA Jr, Davis M. Glutamate receptors in extinction and extinction-based therapies for psychiatric illness. Neuropsychopharmacology 2011;36(1):274–93.

69. Krystal JH, Tolin DF, Sanacora G, et al. Neuroplasticity as a target for the pharmacotherapy of anxiety disorders, mood disorders, and schizophrenia. Drug Discov Today 2009;14(13–14):690–7.

70. Walker DL, Ressler KJ, Lu KT, et al. Facilitation of conditioned fear extinction by systemic administration or intra-amygdala infusions of D-cycloserine as assessed with fear-potentiated startle in rats. J Neurosci 2002;22(6):2343–51.

71. Ressler KJ, Rothbaum BO, Tannenbaum L, et al. Cognitive enhancers as adjuncts to psychotherapy: use of D-cycloserine in phobic individuals to facilitate extinction of fear. Arch Gen Psychiatry 2004;61(11):1136–44.

72. Norberg MM, Krystal JH, Tolin DF. A meta-analysis of D-cycloserine and the facilitation of fear extinction and exposure therapy. Biol Psychiatry 2008;63(12):1118–26.

73. Gvozdic K, Brandl EJ, Taylor DL, et al. Genetics and personalized medicine in antidepressant treatment. Curr Pharm Des 2012;18(36):5853–78.

74. Kato M, Serretti A. Review and meta-analysis of antidepressant pharmacogenetic findings in major depressive disorder. Mol Psychiatry 2010;15(5):473–500.

75. Brandl EJ, Muller DJ, Richter MA. Pharmacogenetics of obsessive-compulsive disorders. Pharmacogenomics 2012;13(1):71–81.
76. Brandl EJ, Tiwari K, Zhou X, et al. Influence of CYP2D6 and CYP2C19 gene variants on antidepressant response in obsessive-compulsive disorder. Pharmacogenomics J 2014;14(2):176–81.

# Neuromodulation in Obsessive-Compulsive Disorder

Melisse Bais, MD[a], Martijn Figee, MD, PhD[a],
Damiaan Denys, MD, PhD[a,b,*]

## KEYWORDS

- Neuromodulation • Obsessive-compulsive disorder (OCD)
- Electroconvulsive therapy (ECT) • Transcranial direct current stimulation (tDCS)
- Transcranial magnetic stimulation (TMS) • Deep brain stimulation (DBS) • Efficacy
- Review

## KEY POINTS

- Neuromodulation techniques in obsessive-compulsive disorder (OCD) involve electroconvulsive therapy (ECT), transcranial direct current stimulation (tDCS), transcranial magnetic stimulation (TMS), and deep brain stimulation (DBS).
- ECT has no place in the treatment of OCD, except for the treatment of comorbid depression or psychosis.
- One case report on tDCS of the dorsolateral prefrontal cortex (DLPFC) found no effects in OCD.
- Low-frequency TMS applied to the premotor or orbitofrontal cortex investigated in 90 patients with refractory OCD revealed good tolerability and significant improvement of obsessive-compulsive and affective symptoms. Beneficial effects disappeared, however, after discontinuation of TMS, and in most sham-controlled studies, TMS was not better than sham stimulation.
- DBS shows a response rate of 60% in open and sham-controlled studies in more than 100 patients with refractory OCD.
- All DBS targets for OCD are located subcortically within the frontostriatal network.
- In OCD, it can be concluded that DBS, although more invasive, is the most efficacious technique.

---

Disclosure statement: No potential conflict of interest.
[a] Department of Psychiatry, Academic Medical Center, Meibergdreef 5, Amsterdam 1105 AZ, The Netherlands; [b] Neuromodulation & Behavior group, Netherlands Institute for Neuroscience, Royal Netherlands Academy of Arts and Sciences, Meibergdreef 47, Amsterdam 1105 BA, The Netherlands
* Corresponding author. Department of Psychiatry, Academic Medical Center, University of Amsterdam, Postbox 75867, Amsterdam 1070 AW, The Netherlands.
E-mail address: ddenys@gmail.com

Psychiatr Clin N Am 37 (2014) 393–413
http://dx.doi.org/10.1016/j.psc.2014.06.003
0193-953X/14/$ – see front matter © 2014 Elsevier Inc. All rights reserved.

psych.theclinics.com

| Abbreviations | |
|---|---|
| ALIC | Anterior limb of internal capsule |
| CBT | Cognitive behavioral therapy |
| CSTC | Orbitofronto-striato-thalamo-cortical |
| DBS | Deep brain stimulation |
| DLPFC | Dorsolateral prefrontal cortex |
| ECT | Electroconvulsive therapy |
| fMRI | Functional magnetic resonance imaging |
| GPi | Globus pallidus interna |
| ITP | Inferior thalamic peduncle |
| NAcc | Nucleus accumbens |
| OCD | Obsessive-compulsive disorder |
| OFC | Orbitofrontal cortex |
| rTMS | Repetitive TMS |
| SMA | Supplementary motor area |
| STN | Subthalamic nucleus |
| tDCS | Transcranial direct current stimulation |
| TMS | Transcranial magnetic stimulation |
| VC | Ventral capsule |
| VC/VS | Ventral capsule, ventral striatum |
| VS | Ventral striatum |
| Y-BOCS | Yale Brown Obsessive-Compulsive Scale |

## INTRODUCTION

OCD is considered one of the most disabling psychiatric disorders, causing serious impairment in patients' daily functioning and affecting professional, social, and personal lives.[1] Thanks to a wide range of available pharmacologic treatments and cognitive behavioral therapy (CBT), most patients can be treated to a satisfactory level. However, 10% of patients experience inadequate response and remain severely ill.[2] Therefore, new treatment strategies are required. In the last decades, neuromodulating techniques have emerged as promising alternatives for the treatment of OCD. Different from the rather aspecific pharmacologic modulation of drug therapy, neuromodulation techniques enable modulation of distinct neuronal circuits by targeting specific brain structures. OCD may be particularly suitable for these interventions because of its strong link to discrete neuroanatomic networks. Neuroimaging studies have consistently related OCD to aberrant activity within the orbitofronto-striato-thalamo-cortical (CSTC) network.[3–5] A major advantage of neuromodulation is its potential of adjustable and reversible brain network manipulation. Neuromodulating techniques that have been investigated in OCD during the past decades include ECT, tDCS, TMS, and DBS. This article reviews the literature on the efficacy and applicability of these devices for the treatment of OCD.

## ELECTROCONVULSIVE THERAPY

ECT was widely used for the treatment of OCD until the 1980s.[6] However, a 1985 review of the literature concluded that ECT was ineffective in the treatment of OCD.[7] As of yet, ECT has no place in OCD treatment guidelines.[8,9] The literature on ECT for OCD is sparse, controlled trials are lacking, and most studies report limited effect. For an overview of recent studies on ECT in OCD, see **Table 1**. Although a 4-week trial of 10 open ECT sessions in 9 treatment-resistant patients with OCD yielded a mean

**Table 1**
**Studies of electroconvulsive therapy in the treatment of obsessive-compulsive disorder**

| Study, Year | N | Diagnosis | Intervention | Follow-up | Outcome |
|---|---|---|---|---|---|
| Khanna et al,[10] 1988 | 9 | OCD | 10 sessions (2–3 sessions weekly) 4 patients unilateral | 6 mo | LOI symptoms: 9 points (30%) decrease direct after ECT sessions, 6 mo: pretreatment level |
| Casey & Davis,[13] 1994 | 1 | OCD/MDD | 6 sessions bilateral | 1 y: maintenance ECT 24 sessions in total | No scale: good to moderate response after 1 y |
| Maletzky et al,[12] 1994 | 32 | OCD/MDD | MMECT: mean 3.5 sessions, mean 11.3 seizures | 1 y: maintenance MMECT NS (5 subjects) | MOCI: 7.7 points decrease (35%) after 1 y |
| Thomas & Kellner,[14] 2003 | 1 | OCD/MDD | 1 session unilateral | 24 wk | No scale: remission of symptoms after 24 wk |
| Strassnig et al,[15] 2004 | 1 | TS/OCD | 9 sessions (3 sessions weekly) unilateral | 1 y: maintenance ECT 1 session monthly | No scale: minimal symptoms |
| Chaves et al,[16] 2005 | 1 | SZ/OCD | 6 sessions (2 sessions weekly) bilateral | 6 mo | Y-BOCS: 34 points (68%) decrease after 6 mo |
| Hanisch et al,[17] 2009 | 1 | SAD/OCD | 6 sessions (3 sessions weekly) unilateral | 42 wk: maintenance ECT 1 session every 2 wk | Y-BOCS: 24 points (85%) decrease after 42 wk |
| Loi & Bonwick,[18] 2010 | 1 | OCD | 6 sessions (3 sessions weekly) unilateral | Follow-up NS: maintenance ECT 1 session every 3 wk | No scale: remission of symptoms |
| Makhinson et al,[19] 2012 | 1 | AN/OCD/Catatonia | 6 sessions bilateral | 1 mo | No scale: mild return of OCD symptoms |
| Raveendra-nathan et al,[20] 2012 | 1 | OCD | 14 sessions (3 weekly) bilateral | 6 mo: maintenance ECT 2 times 3 sessions after that 1 session weekly | Y-BOCS: 30 points (75%) decrease directly after last ECT session, 6 mo: 15 points (37.5%) decrease |
| D'urso et al,[21] 2012 | 1 | Catatonia/OCD | 8 sessions (2–3 weekly) bilateral | 6 mo | Y-BOCS: 16 points (42%) decrease after 6 mo |
| Bülbül et al,[22] 2013 | 1 | Bipolar/OCD | 13 sessions (3 sessions weekly) bilateral | 2 y: maintenance ECT 45 sessions in total | Y-BOCS: 27 points (82%) decrease after 2 y |

*Abbreviations:* AN, anorexia nervosa; LOI, Leyton Obsessional Inventory; MDD, major depressive disorder; MMECT, multiple monitored electroconvulsive therapy; MOCI, Maudsley Obsessive Compulsive Inventory; N, number of patients; NS, not specified; SAD, schizoaffective disorder; SZ, schizophrenia; TS, Tourette syndrome; Y-BOCS, Yale-Brown Obsessive Compulsive Scale.

30% reduction in obsessive-compulsive symptoms directly after the ECT administration period, symptoms returned to pretreatment level at 6 months follow-up.[10] No differences were noted between unilateral ECT in 4 patients and bilateral ECT in the other 5 patients. The authors report that patients with obsessive-compulsive personality traits responded worse to ECT. This result corresponds to observations in DBS for OCD, whereby subjects with perfectionism and more egosyntonic symptoms benefit less from DBS than patients without these symptoms.[11] Maletzky and colleagues[12] reported long-term efficacy of ECT in 32 patients with refractory OCD using multiple monitored ECT in which several seizures are induced within a single treatment session. An average of 4 bilateral ECT sessions totaling 11 seizures resulted in a mean 35% improvement of obsessive-compulsive symptoms at 1-year follow-up. Obsessive-compulsive symptoms improved independently from depressive symptoms. All patients received continuous drug therapy after discontinuation of ECT, and 5 patients received maintenance ECT. More recent case reports have also suggested favorable results of ECT for OCD.[13–22] However, in most of these cases, OCD was present as a comorbid condition with a primary unipolar or bipolar depression, psychotic disorders, catatonia, or anorexia nervosa. Moreover, in most patients, the effects were short term only, in which case weekly to monthly sessions of maintenance ECT were required for a reported period of 6 to 24 months to retain favorable effects.[13,15,17,18,22]

In conclusion, the available literature on ECT is limited to case reports and open uncontrolled studies. Except for one positive open study in 32 patients and 3 case reports, all other studies indicate that ECT may only be beneficial for OCD on the short term and require maintenance treatment for at least 6 months. Considering the need for general anesthesia, this would make ECT a risky treatment option for OCD. Furthermore, ECT was predominantly efficacious for OCD with comorbid mood or psychotic disorders. Therefore, the authors suggest that to date ECT should be used in OCD only to treat these comorbid disorders.

## TRANSCRANIAL DIRECT CURRENT STIMULATION

tDCS is a cheap and noninvasive technique consisting of a battery-powered device and 2 electrodes that can be placed on the head for electrical cortical stimulation through the skull. An electrical current is sent from the positively charged anodal electrode through the skull and brain toward the negatively charged cathode, or vice versa. Anodal stimulation assumedly induces depolarization and thus increased cortical excitability, whereas cathodal stimulation induces hyperpolarization and reduced cortical excitability.[23]

For a long time, tDCS was not implemented as a regular treatment option because the results varied widely. However, improved knowledge of the neurocircuitry underlying neuropsychiatric disease has reignited interest for tDCS treatment in disorders such as Parkinson disease, depression, schizophrenia, addiction, and posttraumatic stress disorder.[24–26] As OCD is related to hyperactivity of the orbitofrontal-subcortical circuit, tDCS could potentially normalize this by modulating excitability of the orbitofrontal or dorsolateral prefrontal cortices. To date, only 1 case report investigated the efficacy of tDCS in OCD.[27] After 10 daily sessions of cathodal stimulation (2 mA for 20 minutes) over the DLPFC, no changes were observed in obsessive-compulsive symptoms with real or sham stimulation, although active stimulation decreased anxiety and depressive symptoms. Neither did the authors find that tDCS in this patient reduced prefrontal hyperactivity with resting-state functional magnetic resonance imaging (fMRI). Based on this single case report, cathodal tDCS over the DLPFC seems to alter anxiety and depression symptoms rather than obsessive-compulsive symptoms. However, anodal tDCS of the DLPFC should still be explored, as this may alleviate OCD symptoms by increasing DLPFC excitability. Moreover, cathodal inhibitory tDCS aimed at the orbitofrontal cortex (OFC) may reduce its hyperactivity in OCD.

## REPETITIVE TRANSCRANIAL MAGNETIC STIMULATION

TMS is a noninvasive technique for modulation of local excitability by sending short-pulsed electricity through a coil placed over the head, which induces a rapidly changing magnetic field leading to depolarization or hyperpolarization of superficial cortical neurons.[28] Various studies have demonstrated an increase in neural excitability after high-frequency (5–20 Hz) stimulation[29] and inhibition of neural excitability after low-frequency (0–5 Hz) stimulation.[30,31] Hence, TMS could be effective for OCD by modulating cortical excitability, thereby normalizing hyperactivity of the connected corticostriatal network. As TMS alters neural excitability only transiently, repetitive TMS (rTMS) is required when used for treating OCD. In 1997, Greenberg and colleagues[32] were the first to investigate rTMS of the DLPFC in patients with OCD. Thereafter, various groups have investigated rTMS for OCD in the DLPFC, OFC, and the supplementary motor area (SMA).

### Efficacy

Since 1997, numerous studies have investigated the efficacy of rTMS in patients with OCD at the 3 different cortical targets (DLPFC, OFC, and SMA). Eleven randomized controlled studies totaling 307 subjects with OCD were published. In addition, 3 case studies were performed in an open design. For an overview, see **Table 2**. In 2013, Berlim and colleagues[33] published a meta-analysis on randomized and sham-controlled trials of rTMS for OCD.

### Dorsolateral prefrontal cortex

Assuming that OCD pathophysiology is characterized by hyperactivity of the orbitofrontal-subcortical circuit, high-frequency (excitatory) rTMS to the DLPFC could possibly normalize OFC hyperactivity via activation of the inhibitory indirect pathway or via direct connections between the DLPFC and OFC. High-frequency TMS to the left DLPFC in healthy subjects was shown to modulate dopamine release in the ipsilateral OFC and dorsal caudate nucleus,[34,35] whereas low-frequency (inhibitory) DLPFC TMS reduced regional blood flow in the OFC.[36] Greenberg and colleagues[32] were the first to administer high-frequency rTMS (20 Hz) for 20 minutes to the left and right DLPFC in 12 patients with OCD, which was compared with rTMS to the mid-occipital cortex as a control condition. Although compulsions and depressive symptoms significantly decreased after right and left DLPFC stimulation and not after stimulation in the control condition, these beneficial effects did not last longer than 8 hours. In a second study, ten 2.5-minute sessions of high-frequency (10 Hz) rTMS were administered to the right ($n = 6$) or left ($n = 6$) DLPFC in 12 patients with refractory OCD.[37] After 1 month, a significant decrease of 10.25 points (24%) was shown on the Yale Brown Obsessive-Compulsive Scale (Y-BOCS).[38,39] This result became nonsignificant after correction for depression scores. Five subsequent randomized controlled trials (RCTs) confirmed that rTMS to the DLPFC is not efficacious for OCD. There was no significant improvement in OCD symptoms when sham TMS was compared with 18 sessions of low-frequency (1 Hz) TMS to the right DLPFC in 18 patients with OCD,[40] 10 sessions of high-frequency (10 Hz) TMS to the right DLPFC in 21 patients with OCD,[30] or 30 sessions of high-frequency (10 Hz) TMS to the right DLPFC in 27 patients with OCD,[41] although depression scores did improve

**Table 2**
Studies of repetitive transcranial magnetic stimulation in the treatment of obsessive-compulsive disorder

| Study, Year | Target | N | Parameters | Time | Mean Y-BOCS Decrease, Points (%) |
|---|---|---|---|---|---|
| Greenberg et al,[32] 1997 | Intervention: right LPFC or left LPFC | 12 | 20 Hz, 80% MT | 1 session of 20 min; measurement after 8 h | Compulsions decreased (not quantified) |
| | Control: midoccipital | 12[a] | 20 Hz, 80% MT | 1 session of 20 min; measurement after 8 h | Compulsions decreased |
| Sachdev et al,[37] 2001 | Intervention: right PFC | 6 | 10 Hz, 110% MT | 10 sessions of 2.5 min in 2 wk; measurement 4 wk after last session | 15.2 (56) |
| | Control: left PFC | 6 | 10 Hz, 110% MT | 10 sessions of 2.5 min in 2 wk; measurement 4 wk after last session | 6 (27) |
| Alonso et al,[40] 2001 | Intervention: right DLPFC | 10 | 1 Hz, 110% MT | 18 sessions of 20 min in 6 wk; measurement after 10 wk | 3.4 (14) |
| | Control: right DLPFC | 8 | Sham condition (perpendicular placed coil over the same area, 1 Hz, 20% MT) | 18 sessions of 20 min in 6 wk; measurement after 10 wk | 0.3 (1) |
| Prasko et al,[42] 2006 | Intervention: left DLPFC | 15 | 1 Hz, 110% MT | 10 sessions of 30 min in 2 wk; measurement 2 wk after last session | 8.4 (28) |
| | Control: left DLPFC | 15 | Sham condition | 10 sessions of 30 min in 2 wk; measurement 2 wk after last session | 6.5 (28) |
| Sachdev et al,[43] 2007 | Intervention: left DLPFC | 10 | 10 Hz, 110% MT | 10 sessions of 2.5 min in 2 wk; measurement directly after last session | 5.8 (22) |
| | Control: left DLPFC | 8 | Sham condition (inactive coil and active coil 1 m away with same parameters) | 10 sessions of 2.5 min in 2 wk; measurement directly after last session | 4.9 (21) |
| Bishnoi et al,[81] 2010 | Intervention: DLPFC | 1 | 10 Hz, 110% MT | 30 sessions in 6 wk followed by 30 sessions once a week; measurements 3 mo after last session | 27 (84) |

| Study | Group | N | Parameters | Sessions | Y-BOCS mean (SD) |
|---|---|---|---|---|---|
| Sarkhel et al,[30] 2010 | Intervention: right DLPFC | 21 | 10 Hz, 110% MT | 10 sessions in 2 wk; measurements 2 wk after last session | 5 (19) |
| | Control: right DLPFC | 21[a] | Sham condition (45° angle to the head, 10 Hz, 110% MT) | 10 sessions in 2 wk; measurements 2 wk after last session | 4.19 (17) |
| Mansur et al,[41] 2011 | Intervention: right DLPFC | 13 | 10 Hz, 110% MT | 30 sessions in 6 wk; measurements 6 wk after last session | 5 (17) |
| | Control: right DLPFC | 14 | Sham condition (deactivated coil same position) | 30 sessions in 6 wk; measurements 6 wk after last session | 2.9 (10) |
| Ruffini et al,[44] 2009 | Intervention: left OFC | 16 | 1 Hz, 80% MT | 15 sessions of 10 min in 3 wk; measurements 12 wk after last session | 4.8 (15) |
| | Control: left OFC | 7 | Sham condition (coil perpendicular to the scalp) | 15 sessions of 10 min in 3 wk; measurements 12 wk after last session | 1.8 (6) |
| Mantovani et al,[46] 2006 | Intervention: SMA | 7 | 1 Hz, 100% MT | 10 sessions of 20 min in 2 wk; measurements 2 wk after last session | 10.4 (29) |
| Mantovani et al,[47] 2010 | Intervention: SMA | 9 | 1 Hz, 100% MT | 20 sessions of 20 min in 4 wk; measurement direct after last session | 6.6 (25) |
| | Control: SMA | 9 | Sham condition (Magstim sham coil) | 20 sessions of 20 min in 4 wk; measurement direct after last session | 3.2 (12) |
| Gomes et al,[49] 2012 | Intervention: SMA | 12 | 1 Hz, 100% MT | 10 sessions of 20 min in 2 wk; measurements after 12 wk | 12.7 (35) |
| | Control: SMA | 10 | Sham condition (Neurosoft sham coil) | 10 sessions of 20 min in 2 wk; measurements after 12 wk | 2.4 (6) |
| Kang et al,[48] 2009 | Intervention: right DLPC/SMA | 10 | Right DLPC: 1 Hz, 100% MT, SMA: 1 Hz 100% MT | 10 sessions of 10 min in 2 wk; measurements 2 wk after last session | 2.9 (11) |
| | Control: right DLPC/SMA | 10 | Sham condition (coil 45° angle from the scalp) | 10 sessions of 10 min in 2 wk; measurements 2 wk after last session | 3.4 (13) |
| Mantovani et al,[50] 2010 | Intervention: fMRI-guided pre-SMA | 2 | 1 Hz, 100% MT | 10 sessions of 30 min in 2 wk; measurement direct after last session | 11.5 (41) |

*Abbreviations:* LPFC, lateral prefrontal cortex; MT, motor threshold; N, number of patients; PFC, prefrontal cortex; Y-BOCS, Yale-Brown Obsessive Compulsive Scale.

[a] The same patients as in the intervention group.

significantly in the last 2 studies. Similarly, 10 sessions of low-frequency TMS (1 Hz, 30 patients with OCD)[42] or high-frequency TMS (10 Hz, 18 patients with OCD)[43] applied to the left DLPFC were not significantly better than sham TMS. In conclusion, there is no convincing evidence for the efficacy of high- or low-frequency rTMS to either the left or right DLPFC in OCD.

### Orbitofrontal cortex

Low-frequency rTMS to the OFC may reduce obsessive-compulsive symptoms by inhibiting OFC hyperactivity. Only 1 RCT studied the effects of rTMS to the OFC in OCD.[44] Low-frequency (1 Hz) rTMS to the left OFC was administered for 15 sessions to 16 therapy-resistant patients with OCD, whereas 7 patients with OCD received the same amount of sham sessions. All patients were blinded and received concurrent pharmacologic treatment with no modification throughout the study. A significant and specific Y-BOCS decrease of 19.7% was shown with active TMS compared with sham TMS (6.7% decrease) until week 10 after the end of the treatment, without significant improvement of depressive or anxiety symptoms. However, after 10 weeks, the significant difference between real and sham TMS was lost. Therefore, based on this single study, it seems that low-frequency left OFC TMS has a moderately positive effect specifically on obsessive-compulsive symptoms but only in the short term.

### Supplementary motor area

Pathologic excitability of motor cortical regions may underlie reduced inhibition of compulsions in OCD. TMS has been used first to evoke measures of motor inhibition, confirming defective inhibition and associated excessive motor cortical excitability in OCD.[45] Next, rTMS to the supplementary motor area (SMA) was tried as a treatment method. The first open-label pilot study of Mantovani and colleagues[46] included 7 patients with OCD (2 with comorbid Tourette syndrome). Subjects were treated with low-frequency (1 Hz) rTMS to the bilateral SMA for 10 sessions, which was added to ongoing pharmacotherapy. At the second week of treatment, statistically significant clinical improvement was shown with a Y-BOCS reduction of 10.4 points (29%) and an improvement on depressive scores of 9.9 points (48%), which remained stable after 3 months. Improvement of obsessions and compulsions was significantly correlated with improved measures of motor excitability and motor inhibition. The same group tried to replicate these results in 2010 in a sham-controlled double-blind design.[47] Eighteen patients with OCD were assigned to 20 sessions of sham or active low-frequency (1 Hz) rTMS to the bilateral SMA. Although mean Y-BOCS scores decreased significantly in the active group with 6.6 points (25.4%) versus a decrease of 3.2 points (12.0%) in the sham group, this difference was not statistically significant. At the end of the 20 sessions, 6 of 11 patients (54%) in the active rTMS group versus 2 of 10 patients (20%) in the sham group were considered as responders with a Y-BOCS reduction of greater than 30%, but again this difference was not statistically significant. Kang and colleagues[48] tried to combine 2 TMS regimes for OCD, stimulating the DLPFC and the SMA together. However, 10 open sham or active sessions of low-frequency (1 Hz) rTMS to the right DLPFC and bilateral SMA in 20 patients with OCD resulted in similar improvements of obsessive-compulsive and depressive symptoms between sham and real TMS.

The only sham-controlled study that did find significant benefits of SMA rTMS versus sham was by Gomes and colleagues[49] Ten sessions (2 weeks) of low-frequency (1 Hz) rTMS to the bilateral SMA in 12 patients with OCD led to a mean Y-BOCS reduction of 35% with 7 of 12 responders at 14 weeks follow-up, which was significantly better than sham TMS in 10 patients with OCD, where a mean

Y-BOCS reduction of 6% was observed with only 1 of 10 responders. Mantovani and colleagues[50] reported promising results after 10 open sessions of rTMS in 2 patients with refractory OCD (27% and 54% Y-BOCS reductions) when the coil was individually navigated to the SMA based on functional magnetic resonance activity during a motor finger tapping task.

### Side Effects

Overall, the side effects of rTMS are mild and transient, and the treatment is well tolerated. The most severe adverse event that can be induced by high-frequency rTMS is an epileptic seizure. However, this side effect was never observed in the studies previously discussed. Side effects that have been reported most often were headache and scalp discomfort, which were always transient.[30,49] Other effects like tearfulness, facial muscle twitching, hearing changes, and dizziness were described sporadically. Side effects are more often reported with high-frequency rTMS than with low-frequency rTMS.[47,51] No cognitive side effects have been mentioned in the various treatment studies of rTMS in OCD.

### Summary

The efficacy of low- and high-frequency rTMS to the left or right DLPFC, the OFC, or the SMA has been investigated in more than 300 obsessive-compulsive patients since 1997. It is hard to draw conclusions, as most study samples were likely underpowered and studies differed greatly from each other with respect to target, stimulation parameters, sham condition, number of sessions, and patient characteristics. Although open and double-blind sham-controlled studies demonstrate significant improvement of obsessive-compulsive symptoms with low-frequency rTMS to the SMA and OFC during or between sessions, these effects seem to disappear after discontinuation of TMS or follow-up results longer than 3 months are lacking. All but one sham-controlled rTMS studies failed to show statistically significant advantage of active over sham stimulation. Nevertheless, a recent meta-analysis of 10 RCTs totaling 282 patients with OCD suggested a significant and medium-sized difference in obsessive-compulsive symptoms, favoring active over sham rTMS.[33] Moreover, pooled outcomes in these largely treatment-refractory patients suggested that rTMS augmentation has comparable efficacy as other augmentation strategies. In addition, the noninvasive character and mild side effects make rTMS an attractive augmentation strategy. Finally, low-frequency rTMS seems to temporarily reduce obsessive-compulsive symptoms by inhibiting excessive excitability of hyperactive cortical regions such as the OFC and SMA, thereby improving patients' ability to inhibit and control obsessive-compulsive responding. Therefore, TMS could be a promising technique to enhance the effects of exposure-based therapies when given before each exposure session.

### DEEP BRAIN STIMULATION

Contrary to the transient and superficial neural modulation of tDCS and TMS, DBS allows for a more enduring modulation of subcortical structures. About 1 or 2 electrodes of just more than a millimeter thick are surgically placed into subcortical structures for electrical modulation via a battery-operated pulse generator implanted just below the clavicle. DBS targets for OCD were originally adopted from experience with stereotactic ablation, which was until then an accepted last-resort strategy for refractory OCD. Based on the efficacy of anterior capsulotomy for OCD,[52] high-frequency DBS of the same target was expected to improve OCD by producing a functional and reversible lesion. Subsequently, other targets within the CSTC network were explored. After the first positive results of DBS in the original anterior limb of internal capsule (ALIC) target in 1999,[53] targeting shifted more toward the ventral capsule, ventral striatum (VC/VS) and nucleus accumbens (NAcc). The subthalamic nucleus (STN) was tried after positive results on obsessive-compulsive symptoms from STN DBS in patients with Parkinson disease and comorbid OCD. Finally, case studies report on DBS in other nodes of the CSTC network, that is, the inferior thalamic peduncle (ITP) or globus pallidus interna (GPi).

### Efficacy

During the past 15 years, the efficacy of DBS has been reported in 8 double-blind controlled studies and 10 case studies. For an overview, see **Table 3**. More than 150 patients with OCD have been treated with DBS in the internal capsule or its connected network structures. In the following sections, efficacy studies of DBS in OCD are discussed separately per target. When evaluating the studies mentioned later, it should be noted that patient samples and DBS targets from different studies often overlap. Owing to the more invasive character of DBS relative to TMS, inclusion and response criteria in DBS studies have been more stringent and uniform: patients are all fully refractory to regular pharmacotherapy and behavioral therapy and have an illness duration of at least 5 years and Y-BOCS scores of at least 25 to 30. Response was generally defined as 35% or more improvement on the Y-BOCS. Depressive symptoms, global functioning, and anxiety symptoms were usually included as secondary outcome measures.

### Anterior limb of internal capsule

DBS of the ALIC in patients suffering from refractory OCD was initiated in 1998 at the Karolinska Institute in Stockholm, where 2 patients received bilateral implantation, but these results were never published (S. Andreewitch, personal communication, 2010). In 1999, the Leuven group published the first results of bilateral ALIC DBS in 4 patients with OCD.[53] In 3 of 4 patients, beneficial effects were observed but not objectified by Y-BOCS scores. These 4 patients and 2 others were followed up for a period of at least 21 months, at which time 3 patients were responders with a 35% or more decrease in symptoms.[54] Moreover, the actual DBS effects seemed to outweigh placebo effects, as an average symptom change of 12.5 points (40%) was observed between double-blinded on and off stimulation. A subsequent case-report of ALIC DBS in 1 patient described a 79% Y-BOCS reduction at 3-month follow-up and complete remission at 10-month follow-up.[55] The setting was on a much lower voltage (2 V) than that Nuttin used in his study (4–10.5 V). These initial positive effects of ALIC DBS could not be fully replicated in a double-blind controlled study performed by the Michigan Group.[56] Of the 4 patients, only 1 patient had a decrease of more than 35% in the double-blind phase. Nevertheless, this patient further improved with 73% at 8 months follow-up, and another patient improved with 44% when intensive behavioral therapy was added. Only in these 2 responding patients, decreased OFC activity was found on positron emission tomographic scans, suggesting that ALIC DBS can improve OCD when it is able to restore the inhibitory function of the ventral CSTC pathway.

Based on these first studies in small OCD samples, ALIC DBS seemed to have only modestly positive effects, which warranted exploration of other targets. As high voltages were often needed to achieve positive effects with ALIC DBS, and because the most distal parts of the ALIC electrodes were located in the ventral striatum (VS) and NAcc, these ventral targets were subsequently explored for treatment of OCD.

*Ventral capsule/ventral striatum*

In 2006, Greenberg and colleagues[57] were the first to target the more ventral part of the internal capsule (VC) and the VS. This target was chosen based on positive experiences of Gamma Knife lesions and DBS in more ventral regions of the ALIC, impinging inferiorly on the VS.[57,58] Moreover, a case report suggested positive results of ventral striatal (caudate nucleus) DBS in a patient with combined OCD and depression.[59] In the study by Greenberg and colleagues,[57] 10 patients received 3 years of bilateral VC/VS DBS in an open-label manner, which resulted in a mean decline in Y-BOCS of 12.3 points (36%) and 4 of 8 responders. These first positive results with VC/VS DBS were replicated in a randomized double-blind controlled study in 2010.[60] Six patients with OCD were implanted with bilateral VC/VS electrodes, after which 3 patients received active stimulation, whereas the other 3 patients received 1 month of sham stimulation and 1 month of true stimulation. Although Y-BOCS reductions did not significantly differ after 1 month of sham versus active stimulation, improvement was observed in either group only when the device was activated. At 1-year follow-up, there was an average Y-BOCS decrease of 15.7 points (47%) and 4 of the 6 patients responded to DBS. In all 6 patients, 1 year DBS significantly improved comorbid depressive symptoms. In the same year, Greenberg and colleagues[61] combined data of 4 centers, including patients implanted in the ALIC[54] and VC/VS,[57,60] with the most distal contacts often being placed in the NAcc. In a total of 26 patients, a mean Y-BOCS decrease of 13.1 points (38%) was shown after 3 to 36 months of DBS. The percentage of patients meeting the full response criterion was 61.5% (16 of 26) at 23 to 36 months follow-up. Finally, 2 open studies reported efficacy of VC/VS DBS for OCD, with a mean Y-BOCS decrease of 22.2 points (60%) after 24 months in 4 patients[62] and a decrease of 12.2 points (33%) after 15 months in another 4 patients.[63] Again, in both patient groups, a significant decrease in depressive symptoms was also observed.

Overall, beneficial effects on OCD and depressive symptoms were observed in uncontrolled DBS studies when stimulating the VC/VS, but patient samples have been small and the only controlled study did not show significant benefits of active over sham stimulation at 2 months postsurgery. Although ALIC and VC/VS DBS efficacy seems to be comparable, lower voltages are generally needed to achieve efficacy when stimulating VC/VS, suggesting that the VS is decisive for efficacy of DBS in OCD.

*Nucleus accumbens*

In 2003, Sturm and colleagues[64] implanted the electrodes in a way that the anterior and ventral capsule (VC) and the shell of the NAcc could be stimulated selectively. The rationale behind this targeting was based on the aforementioned studies that used internal capsule electrodes ending in the NAcc. Moreover, the NAcc has a central role in mediating neural activity between the amygdaloid complex, basal ganglia, mediodorsal thalamus, and prefrontal cortex, all crucially involved in the pathophysiology of OCD.[3] Four patients were implanted in the study of Sturm. The first patient improved with bipolar stimulation over the 2 distal electrode leads and not with stimulation of the internal capsule, which suggests that effective stimulation occurred in the NAcc itself. Moreover, bilateral stimulation did not improve the effects of right-sided unilateral stimulation. Therefore, the other 3 patients were implanted only unilaterally in the right NAcc. In a 24- to 30-weeks follow-up period, nearly total recovery from both anxiety and OCD symptoms in 3 of 4 patients was reported. However, no scale was used to register the improvement. The only patient without response seemed to have the electrode placed outside the NAcc. The same group failed to replicate efficacy of unilateral right NAcc DBS using a double-blind controlled design in 10

**Table 3**
Studies of deep brain stimulation in the treatment of obsessive-compulsive disorder

| Target | Study, Year | N | Parameters | Follow-up | Mean Y-BOCS Decrease, Points (%) | Responders,[a] n (%) | Y-BOCS On vs Off, Points |
|---|---|---|---|---|---|---|---|
| ALIC | Nuttin et al,[53] 1999 | 4 | 100 Hz, 210 μs, 4.7–5.0 V | NM | NA | 3 (75)[b] | NA |
| ALIC | Anderson et al,[55] 2003 | 1 | 100 Hz, 210 μs, 2.0 V | 3 mo | 27 (79) | 1 (100) | NA |
| STN | Chabardès et al,[70] 2013 | 4 | 130 Hz, 60 μs, 1.2–4.0 V | 6 mo | 21.2 (65) | 3 (75) | NA |
| ALIC | Nuttin et al,[54] 2003 | 6 | 100 Hz, 210/450 μs, 4.0–10.5 V | 31 mo; crossover phase: 3 mo on 5–10 wk off | NM | 3 (50) | 19.8 vs 32.3 |
| ALIC | Abelson et al,[56] 2005 | 4 | 130/150 Hz, 60/210 μs, 5.0–10.5 V | 4–23 mo; crossover phase: 4 blinded on-off periods | 9.8 (30) | 2 (50) | 26.5 vs 29.3 |
| VC/VS | Greenberg et al,[57] 2006 | 10 | 100–130 Hz, 90–210 μs, 8–17 V | 36 mo | 12.3 (36) | 4 (40) | NA |
| VC/VS | Goodman et al,[60] 2010 | 6 | 135 Hz, 90–210 μs, 3.3–8.5 V | 12 mo; staggered onset: 30 or 60 d stimulation following surgery | 15.7 (47) | 4 (67) | NM reduction: 5.33 vs 0.67 |
| ALIC - VC/VS | Greenberg et al,[61] 2010c | 26 | 100–130 Hz, 90–450 μs, 2–10.5 V | 3–36 mo | 13.1 (38) | 16 (62) | NA |
| VC/VS | Roh et al,[62] 2012 | 4 | 90–130 Hz, 90–270 μs, 2–5 V | 24 mo | 22.2 (60) | 4 (100) | NA |
| VC/VS | Tsai et al,[63] 2012 | 4 | 130 Hz, 210 μs, 2–8 V | 15 mo | 12.2 (33) | 2 (50) | NA |
| Right NAcc | Sturm et al,[64] 2003 | 4 | 130 Hz, 90 μs, 2–6, 5 V | 24–30 mo | NA | 3 (75)[b] | NA |

| | | N | | | | | |
|---|---|---|---|---|---|---|---|
| NAcc-VC/VS | Aouizerate et al,[59,82] 2004, 2005 | 1 | 130 Hz, 120 μs, 4 V | 27 mo | 13 (52) | 1 (100) | NA |
| NAcc | Denys et al,[11] 2010 | 16 | 130 Hz, 90 μs, 3.5–5.0 V | 21 mo; crossover phase: 2 wk on 2 wk off | 17.5 (52) | 9 (56) | NM difference: 8.3 |
| NAcc | Franzini et al,[83] 2010 | 2 | 130 Hz, 90 μs, 5/5.5 V | 24–27 mo | 13 (38) | 1 (50) | NA |
| Right NAcc | Huff et al,[65] 2010 | 10 | 145 Hz, 90–140 μs, 3.5–6.5 V | 12 mo; crossover phase: 3 mo on 3 mo off | 6.8 (21) | 1 (10) | 27.9 vs 31.1 |
| STN | Mallet et al,[68] 2002 | 2 | 185+130 Hz, 60+90 μs, 3.1+3.2 V | 6 mo | 20 (81) | 2 (100) | NA |
| STN | Fontaine et al,[67] 2004 | 1 | 185 Hz, 60 μs, Right = 3.5 V; left = 1.3 V | 12 mo | 31 (97) | 1 (100) | NA |
| STN | Mallet et al,[69] 2008 | 16 | 130 Hz, 3 60 μs, 2.0 ± 0.9 V | No follow-up; crossover: 3 mo on 3 mo off | 13.3 (41) | NA | 19 vs 28 |
| Left STN–left NAcc | Barcia et al,[71] 2014 | 2 | 130 Hz, 90 μs, 3.5–4.0 V | 15–36 mo | 12.5 (38) | 2 (100) | NA |
| ITP | Jiménez et al,[72] 2013 | 6 | 130 Hz, 450 μs, 5.0 V | 12 mo | 18.3 (51) | 6 (100)[d] | NA |
| GPi | Nair et al,[73] 2014 | 4 | 120–160 Hz, 90 μs, 2.3–4.4 mA | 3–26 mo | NA | 4 (100)[e] | NA |

*Abbreviations:* N, number of patients; NA, not applicable; NM, not mentioned.

a Responders defined as ≥35% reduction on the Y-BOCS.
b No scale: mentioned that effect was found.
c Combined study, including Nuttin (2003), Greenberg (2006), Goodman (2010).
d Six patients responded after 12 months; 3 patients were lost to follow-up after 36 months.
e Obsessive Compulsive Inventory scale >85% reduction in 4 patients.

patients with OCD.[65] After 12 months DBS, the mean Y-BOCS reduction was 6.8 points (21%) and only 1 of 10 patients had a Y-BOCS reduction of more than 35%. The blinded phase did not show a significant difference in Y-BOCS between on and off stimulation. A second double-blind controlled study performed by the authors' group[11] used the NAcc core instead of the shell as a target, and stimulation was performed bilaterally instead of unilaterally. In 16 patients with OCD, a significant Y-BOCS difference of 8.3 points (25%) was shown comparing active and sham DBS. In the open phase, there was a mean decline of 15.7 (46%) on the Y-BOCS score, in which 9 of 16 patients were responders with a remarkable symptom reduction of 72%. In addition, a significant reduction in anxiety and depressive symptoms was found. Different from previous studies, CBT was systematically added to the treatment after a first Y-BOCS reduction of 6 points. Anxiety and depression improved mainly during the initial phase of DBS treatment, whereas obsessive-compulsive symptoms continued to improve during subsequent CBT, which seemed to be particularly effective in decreasing compulsive behaviors and avoidance. Improvement in this study was observed only using the dorsal electrode in the area of the NAcc core around the border of the internal capsule, rather than in the NAcc shell that was targeted by Sturm and colleagues Thus, stimulation of both the NAcc and the VC seems essential for efficacy in OCD. Potentially, stimulation of this crossroad enables modulation of the NAcc as well as the adjacent limbic and prefrontal regions involved in OCD pathophysiology. In agreement, a recent study showed that DBS of this region in 16 patients with OCD modulated fMRI reward responses in the NAcc and found that OCD symptom improvement correlated with normalized functional connectivity between the NAcc and prefrontal cortex.[66]

### Subthalamic nucleus

The STN is a long-known DBS target for Parkinson disease and became an interesting option for OCD when positive effects of STN DBS were reported in patients with combined Parkinson disease and OCD.[67,68] Efficacy of STN DBS was confirmed in a double-blind controlled multicenter study in 16 patients with OCD.[69] Obsessive-compulsive symptoms were significantly lower after active STN stimulation compared with sham stimulation, with a Y-BOCS difference of 9 points (32%). Active stimulation resulted in a mean Y-BOCS decrease of 8.9 points (31%). After the first 3 months of open DBS treatment, 75% of the patients were responders, although response was defined as at least 25% Y-BOCS decrease instead of the usual 35%. Contrary to studies using internal capsule and VS targets, no significant effects on depression and anxiety symptoms were found with STN DBS. This result was replicated in a subsequent case series that included 2 patients of the previous study and 2 additional ones. In these 4 patients with OCD, 6 months of STN DBS resulted in a mean Y-BOCS decline of 21.2 points (65%), without effects on depressive or anxiety symptoms.[70]

In conclusion, case series and 1 controlled study demonstrate efficacy of bilateral STN DBS for OCD. However, unlike DBS at the VC and VS, STN stimulation does not affect anxiety or mood. In one study, 2 patients with OCD were implanted with electrodes in both the STN and the NAcc.[71] Combined stimulation improved both obsessive-compulsive and affective symptoms, and double-blind testing of all possible combinations showed that unilateral stimulation of the left NAcc combined with the left STN was most beneficial.

### Inferior thalamic penduncle

The ITP consists of white matter fibers connecting the thalamus and OFC and may thus be another target for modulation of aberrant activity in the CSTC circuit. One open study investigated DBS at the ITP in 6 patients with OCD.[72] One year of bilateral bipolar ITP stimulation resulted in a mean Y-BOCS decrease of 18.3 points (51%). ITP DBS did not affect comorbid drug abuse that was present in 3 patients.

### Anteromedial globus pallidus internus

The anteromedial GPi is a common target for DBS in the treatment of Gilles de la Tourette and movement disorders such as dystonia and Parkinson disease. However, its position within the corticostriatal network would make the GPi also an interesting DBS target for OCD. Nair and colleagues[73] reported an impressive improvement of obsessive-compulsive symptoms with GPi DBS in 4 patients with Gilles de la Tourette and prominent OCD symptoms. About 3 to 26 months of GPi DBS resulted in complete OCD resolution in 2 patients, with the other 2 experiencing a greater than 85% reduction in scores on the obsessive-compulsive inventory scale.

### Complications and Side Effects of DBS

Different from tDCS and rTMS, DBS is invasive and has to be applied in the long term. Therefore, appropriate attention should be paid to complications and side effects.

Surgery-related intracerebral hemorrhage or infection rates of 1% to 2% are generally reported in DBS studies for movement disorders.[74] Although the average age of implanted patients with OCD is low, high numbers of surgery-related hemorrhage were noted in DBS studies for OCD, that is, 1 of 17 patients with OCD receiving STN DBS[69] and 2 of 26 patients receiving VC/VS DBS.[61] Similarly, surgical wound infection was mentioned in 1 of 16 patients with NAcc DBS,[11] 1 of 26 patients with VC/VS DBS,[61] and 2 of 17 patients with STN DBS.[69] With regard to device-related problems, electrode breakage was reported in 1 of 4 patients[56] and in 1 of 26 patients,[61] and various studies noted that patient disturbingly felt the material within their body.[11,54] Stimulation-related side effects consist predominantly of mood changes, in particular transient hypomanic symptoms during acute stimulation at various targets, although more often with acute VC/VC and NAcc stimulation.[75] Other transient side effects consist of olfactory or gustatory symptoms, nausea, fear, panic, and impulsivity, often related to higher voltages and to more ventral electrode positions.[76,77] Mild and transient concentration problems, forgetfulness, word-finding problems, and confusion are sometimes reported.[11,72] Based on the available studies that investigated long-term cognitive functioning after DBS, no substantial cognitive decline was found in a total of 56 implanted patients with OCD. On the contrary, most studies reported cognitive improvement after DBS.[78]

### Summary

Although DBS is more invasive than the other devices, it enables long-term efficacy with fewer side effects. In case series, open and controlled studies, DBS of various targets improves obsessive-compulsive symptoms, with 21% to 75%, and on average 60% responders, and significant benefits of active over sham stimulation in the anterior and ventral capsule, VS, or STN. All effective DBS targets for OCD are part of the CSTC circuit and have comparable efficacy. However, stimulation centered around the ventral regions of the internal capsule and striatum improves depression and anxiety, whereas this does not occur with STN stimulation. DBS is well tolerated, as surgery-related hemorrhage and infections are rare and most side effects are mild and transient. Efficacy of DBS depends on bilateral stimulation, although combined unilateral stimulation of the NAcc and STN was shown to be a promising option.

Two studies have suggested that the efficacy of DBS may be improved if patients are followed up with behavioral therapy to overcome remaining compulsive and avoidant behaviors.[11,56] Finally, efficacy of DBS varies substantially between individual patients, which might be improved when stimulation parameters could be adjusted based on clinical response predictors. Based on the available DBS studies, however, it is difficult to distinguish reliable predictors, although studies report acute mood changes preceding further response at the ventral striatal targets. Moreover, normalization of excessive frontostriatal connectivity in OCD, as measured with resting-state fMRI, correlates with obsessive-compulsive symptom improvement in response to NAcc DBS.[66] As frontostriatal connectivity is simple to measure with robust outcomes in OCD,[66,79,80] this may be a promising prediction marker. It might even be used for the future development of closed-loop DBS systems that are able to recognize pathologic network activity for automatic adjustment of stimulation parameters.

## SUMMARY

Neuromodulation research in OCD suggests that stimulation techniques have great therapeutic potential for severely ill patients who failed to respond to pharmacologic or behavioral therapy. In contrast to conventional strategies, neuromodulation allows direct and adjustable manipulation of aberrant brain networks underlying OCD.

ECT is only indicated in patients with OCD with primary depressive or psychotic disorders, whereas tDCS for OCD needs more investigation. Low-frequency rTMS is a more recent noninvasive method for decreasing cortical excitability, which has proved to be an effective augmentation strategy in OCD when applied over the orbitofrontal or premotor cortices. Although efficacy and tolerability of TMS may be comparable with pharmacologic augmentation, TMS has to be applied on a daily basis and has no proven long-term efficacy. Although DBS is invasive, it is the most promising device-based intervention for refractory OCD, with long-term responder rates of more than 60% and good tolerability. Efficacy and tolerability of the various subcortical DBS targets within the corticostriatal network are comparable. Striatal DBS enhances the effects of subsequent behavioral therapy potentially by reducing anxiety, and it should be explored if cortical TMS could do the same by improving cortical regulation of anxiety. Finally, TMS and DBS trials provide important insights into networks that can be effectively modulated for treatment of a variety of symptoms. Not only obsessions and compulsions but also anxiety and depression are reduced with electrical modulation of the orbitofrontal and premotor cortex, internal capsule, and NAcc. Frontostriatal network changes may be critically involved in DBS-induced improvement of obsessive-compulsive symptoms, and this knowledge could be used to develop prediction markers, optimize stimulation settings, and design treatment devices that can identify and adjust pathologic brain network patterns in OCD.

## REFERENCES

1. Blomstedt P, Sjöberg RL, Hansson M, et al. Deep brain stimulation in the treatment of obsessive-compulsive disorder. World Neurosurg 2013;80(6):e245–53.
2. Denys D. Pharmacotherapy of obsessive-compulsive disorder and obsessive compulsive spectrum disorders. Psychiatr Clin North Am 2006;29(2):553–84.
3. Saxena S, Rauch S. Functional neuroimaging and the neuroanatomy of obsessive-compulsive disorder. Psychiatr Clin North Am 2000;23(3):563–86.
4. Rauch SL, Dougherty DD, Malone D, et al. A functional neuroimaging investigation of deep brain stimulation in patients with obsessive-compulsive disorder. J Neurosurg 2006;104(4):558–65.

5. Menzies L, Chamberlain SR, Laird AR, et al. Integrating evidence from neuroimaging and neuropsychological studies of obsessive-compulsive disorder: the orbitofronto-striatal model revisited. Neurosci Biobehav Rev 2008;32(3):525–49.
6. Jenike MA, Baer L, Minichiello WE. Somatic treatments for obsessive-compulsive disorders. Compr Psychiatry 1987;28(3):250–63.
7. Ottosson JO. Use and misuse of electroconvulsive treatment. Biol Psychiatry 1985;20(9):933–46.
8. National Institute for Health and Care Excellence. Obsessive-compulsive disorder: core interventions in the treatment of obsessive-compulsive disorder and body dysmorphic disorder. London: National Institute for Health and Care Excellence; 2005. Available at: http://www.nice.org.uk/guidance/CG31.
9. American Psychiatric Association. Practice guideline for the treatment of patients with obsessive-compulsive disorder. Arlington (VA): American Psychiatric Association; 2007. Available at: http://psychiatryonline.org/guidelines.aspx.
10. Khanna S, Gangadhar B, Sinha VK, et al. Electroconvulsive therapy in obsessive-compulsive disorder. Convuls Ther 1988;4(4):314–20.
11. Denys D, Mantione M, Figee M, et al. Deep brain stimulation of the nucleus accumbens for treatment-refractory obsessive-compulsive disorder. Arch Gen Psychiatry 2010;67(10):1061–8.
12. Maletzky B, McFarland B, Burt A. Refractory Obsessive Compulsive Disorder and ECT. Convuls Ther 1994;10(1):34–42.
13. Casey D, Davis M. Obsessive-compulsive disorder responsive to electroconvulsive therapy in an elderly woman. South Med J 1994;87(8):862–4.
14. Thomas SG, Kellner CH. Remission of major depression and obsessive-compulsive disorder after a single unilateral ECT. J ECT 2003;19(1):50–1.
15. Strassnig M, Hugo R, Muller N. Electroconvulsive therapy in a patient with Tourette's syndrome and co-morbid obsessive compulsive disorder. World J Biol Psychiatry 2004;5:164–6.
16. Chaves M, Crippa J, Morais SL, et al. Electroconvulsive therapy for coexistent schizophrenia and obsessive-compulsive disorder. J Clin Psychiatry 2005; 66(4):540–4.
17. Hanisch F, Friedemann J, Piro J, et al. Maintenance electroconvulsive therapy for comorbid pharmacotherapy-refractory obsessive-compulsive and schizoaffective disorder. Eur J Med Res 2009;14:367–8.
18. Loi S, Bonwick R. Electroconvulsive therapy for treatment of late-onset obsessive compulsive disorder. Int Psychogeriatr 2010;22(5):830–1.
19. Makhinson M, Furst BA, Shuff MK, et al. Successful treatment of co-occurring catatonia and obsessive-compulsive disorder with concurrent electroconvulsive therapy and benzodiazepine administration. J ECT 2012; 28(3):e35–6.
20. Raveendranathan D, Srinivasaraju R, Ratheesh A, et al. Treatment-refractory OCD responding to maintenance electroconvulsive therapy. J Neuropsychiatry Clin Neurosci 2012;24(2):E16–7.
21. D'Urso G, Mantovani A, Barbarulo AM, et al. Brain-behavior relationship in a case of successful ECT for drug refractory catatonic OCD. J ECT 2012;28(3): 190–3.
22. Bülbül F, Copoglu US, Alpak G, et al. Maintenance therapy with electroconvulsive therapy in a patient with a codiagnosis of bipolar disorder and obsessive-compulsive disorder. J ECT 2013;29(2):e21–2.
23. Paulus W. Transcranial electrical stimulation (tES - tDCS; tRNS, tACS) methods. Neuropsychol Rehabil 2011;21(5):602–17.

24. Kuo MF, Paulus W, Nitsche MA. Therapeutic effects of non-invasive brain stimulation with direct currents (tDCS) in neuropsychiatric diseases. Neuroimage 2014;85:948–60.

25. Jansen JM, Daams JG, Koeter MW, et al. Effects of non-invasive neurostimulation on craving: a meta-analysis. Neurosci Biobehav Rev 2013;37(10 Pt 2): 2472–80.

26. Marin MF, Camprodon JA, Dougherty DD, et al. Device-based brain stimulation to augment fear extinction: implications for PTSD treatment and beyond. Depress Anxiety 2014;10:1–10.

27. Volpato C, Piccione F, Cavinato M, et al. Modulation of affective symptoms and resting state activity by brain stimulation in a treatment-resistant case of obsessive-compulsive disorder. Neurocase 2013;19(4):360–70.

28. Barker A, Jalinous R, Freeston I. Non-invasive magnetic stimulation of human motor cortex. Lancet 1985;1:1106–7.

29. Fitzgerald PB, Fountain S, Daskalakis ZJ. A comprehensive review of the effects of rTMS on motor cortical excitability and inhibition. Clin Neurophysiol 2006; 117(12):2584–96.

30. Sarkhel S, Sinha VK, Praharaj SK. Adjunctive high-frequency right prefrontal repetitive transcranial magnetic stimulation (rTMS) was not effective in obsessive-compulsive disorder but improved secondary depression. J Anxiety Disord 2010;24(5):535–9.

31. Speer AM, Kimbrell TA, Wassermann EM, et al. Opposite effects of high and low frequency rTMS on regional brain activity in depressed patients. Biol Psychiatry 2000;48(12):1133–41.

32. Greenberg BD, George MS, Martin JD, et al. Effect of prefrontal repetitive transcranial magnetic stimulation in obsessive-compulsive disorder: a preliminary study. Am J Psychiatry 1997;154(6):867–9.

33. Berlim MT, Neufeld NH, Van den Eynde F. Repetitive transcranial magnetic stimulation (rTMS) for obsessive-compulsive disorder (OCD): an exploratory meta-analysis of randomized and sham-controlled trials. J Psychiatr Res 2013; 47(8):999–1006.

34. Cho SS, Strafella AP. rTMS of the left dorsolateral prefrontal cortex modulates dopamine release in the ipsilateral anterior cingulate cortex and orbitofrontal cortex. PLoS One 2009;4(8):e6725.

35. Strafella AP, Paus T, Barrett J, et al. Repetitive transcranial magnetic stimulation of the human prefrontal cortex induces dopamine release in the caudate nucleus. J Neurosci 2001;21(15):RC157.

36. Knoch D, Treyer V, Regard M, et al. Lateralized and frequency-dependent effects of prefrontal rTMS on regional cerebral blood flow. Neuroimage 2006; 31(2):641–8.

37. Sachdev P, McBride R, Mitchell PB, et al. Right versus left prefrontal transcranial magnetic stimulation for obsessive-compulsive disorder: a preliminary investigation. J Clin Psychiatry 2001;62(12):981–4.

38. Goodman W, Price L, Rasmussen S, et al. The Yale-Brown Obsessive Compulsive Scale. I. Development, use, and reliability. Arch Gen Psychiatry 1989; 46(11):1006–11.

39. Goodman W, Price L, Rasmussen S, et al. The Yale-Brown Obsessive Compulsive Scale. II. Validity. Arch Gen Psychiatry 1989;46(11):1012–6.

40. Alonso P, Pujol J, Cardoner N, et al. Right prefrontal repetitive transcranial magnetic stimulation in obsessive-compulsive disorder: a double-blind, placebo-controlled study. Am J Psychiatry 2001;158(7):1143–5.

41. Mansur CG, Myczkowki ML, de Barros Cabral S, et al. Placebo effect after prefrontal magnetic stimulation in the treatment of resistant obsessive-compulsive disorder: a randomized controlled trial. Int J Neuropsychopharmacol 2011; 14(10):1389-97.

42. Prasko J, Pasková B, Záleský R, et al. The effect of repetitive transcranial magnetic stimulation (rTMS) on symptoms in obsessive compulsive disorder. A randomized, double blind, sham controlled study. Neuroendocrinol Lett 2006;27(3): 327-32.

43. Sachdev PS, Loo CK, Mitchell PB, et al. Repetitive transcranial magnetic stimulation for the treatment of obsessive compulsive disorder: a double-blind controlled investigation. Psychol Med 2007;37(11):1645-9.

44. Ruffini C, Locatelli M, Lucca A, et al. Augmentation effect of repetitive transcranial magnetic stimulation over the orbitofrontal cortex in drug-resistant obsessive-compulsive disorder patients: a controlled investigation. Prim Care Companion J Clin Psychiatry 2009;11(5):226-30.

45. Radhu N, de Jesus DR, Ravindran LN, et al. A meta-analysis of cortical inhibition and excitability using transcranial magnetic stimulation in psychiatric disorders. Clin Neurophysiol 2013;124(7):1309-20.

46. Mantovani A, Lisanby SH, Pieraccini F, et al. Repetitive transcranial magnetic stimulation (rTMS) in the treatment of obsessive-compulsive disorder (OCD) and Tourette's syndrome (TS). Int J Neuropsychopharmacol 2006;9(1):95-100.

47. Mantovani A, Simpson HB, Fallon BA, et al. Randomized sham-controlled trial of repetitive transcranial magnetic stimulation in treatment-resistant obsessive-compulsive disorder. Int J Neuropsychopharmacol 2010;13(2):217-27.

48. Kang JI, Kim CH, Namkoong K, et al. A randomized controlled study of sequentially applied repetitive transcranial magnetic stimulation in obsessive-compulsive disorder. J Clin Psychiatry 2009;70(12):1645-51.

49. Gomes P, Brasil-Neto J, Allam N, et al. A randomized, double-blind trial of repetitive transcranial magnetic stimulation in obsessive-compulsive disorder with three-month follow-up. J Neuropsychiatry Clin Neurosci 2012;24:437-43.

50. Mantovani A, Westin G, Hirsch J, et al. Functional magnetic resonance imaging guided transcranial magnetic stimulation in obsessive-compulsive disorder. Biol Psychiatry 2010;67(7):e39-40.

51. Slotema CW, Blom JD, Hoek HW, et al. Should we expand the toolbox of psychiatric treatment methods to include repetitive transcranial magnetic stimulation (rTMS)? A meta-analysis of the efficacy of rTMS in psychiatric disorders. J Clin Psychiatry 2010;71(7):873-84.

52. Mindus P, Rasmussen SA, Lindquist C. Neurosurgical treatment of refractory obsessive-compulsive disorder: implications for understanding frontal lobe function. J Neuropsychiatry Clin Neurosci 1994;6(4):467-77.

53. Nuttin B, Cosyns P, Demeulemeester H, et al. Electrical stimulation in anterior limbs of internal capsules in patients with obsessive-compulsive disorder. Separating in-utero and postnatal influences on later disease. Lancet 1999;354:1526.

54. Nuttin BJ, Gabriëls LA, Cosyns PR, et al. Long-term electrical capsular stimulation in patients with obsessive-compulsive disorder. Neurosurgery 2003;52(6): 1263-74.

55. Anderson D, Ahmed A. Treatment of patients with intractable obsessive-compulsive disorder with anterior capsular stimulation. Case report. J Neurosurg 2003;98(5):1104-8.

56. Abelson JL, Curtis GC, Sagher O, et al. Deep brain stimulation for refractory obsessive-compulsive disorder. Psychiatry Res 2005;200(2-3):1067-70.

57. Greenberg BD, Malone DA, Friehs GM, et al. Three-year outcomes in deep brain stimulation for highly resistant obsessive-compulsive disorder. Neuropsychopharmacology 2006;31(11):2384–93.
58. Greenberg B, Price L, Rauch S, et al. Neurosurgery for intractable obsessive-compulsive disorder and depression: critical issue. Neurosurg Clin N Am 2003;14(2):199–212.
59. Aouizerate B, Martin-Guehl C, Cuny E, et al. Deep brain stimulation for OCD and major depression. Am J Psychiatry 2005;162(11):2192.
60. Goodman WK, Foote KD, Greenberg BD, et al. Deep brain stimulation for intractable obsessive compulsive disorder: pilot study using a blinded, staggered-onset design. Biol Psychiatry 2010;67(6):535–42.
61. Greenberg BD, Gabriels LA, Malone DA, et al. Deep brain stimulation of the ventral internal capsule/ventral striatum for obsessive-compulsive disorder: worldwide experience. Mol Psychiatry 2010;15(1):64–79.
62. Roh D, Chang WS, Chang JW, et al. Long-term follow-up of deep brain stimulation for refractory obsessive-compulsive disorder. Psychiatry Res 2012; 200(2–3):1067–70.
63. Tsai H, Chang C, Pan J, et al. Pilot study of deep brain stimulation in refractory obsessive-compulsive disorder ethnic Chinese patients. Psychiatry Clin Neurosci 2012;66(4):303–12.
64. Sturm V, Lenartz D, Koulousakis A, et al. The nucleus accumbens: a target for deep brain stimulation in obsessive–compulsive and anxiety-disorders. J Chem Neuroanat 2003;26(4):293–9.
65. Huff W, Lenartz D, Schormann M, et al. Unilateral deep brain stimulation of the nucleus accumbens in patients with treatment-resistant obsessive-compulsive disorder: outcomes after one year. Clin Neurol Neurosurg 2010; 112(2):137–43.
66. Figee M, Luigjes J, Smolders R, et al. Deep brain stimulation restores frontostriatal network activity in obsessive-compulsive disorder. Nat Neurosci 2013;16(4): 386–7.
67. Fontaine D, Mattei V, Borg M, et al. Effect of subthalamic nucleus stimulation on obsessive-compulsive disorder in a patient with Parkinson disease. Case report. J Neurosurg 2004;100(6):1084–6.
68. Mallet L, Mesnage V, Houeto JL, et al. Compulsions, Parkinson's disease, and stimulation. Lancet 2002;360(9342):1302–4.
69. Mallet L, Polosan M, Jaafari N, et al. Subthalamic nucleus stimulation in severe obsessive-compulsive disorder. N Engl J Med 2008;359(20):2121–34.
70. Chabardès S, Polosan M, Krack P, et al. Deep brain stimulation for obsessive-compulsive disorder: subthalamic nucleus target. World Neurosurg 2013; 80(3–4):S31.e1–8.
71. Barcia JA, Reyes L, Arza R, et al. Deep brain stimulation for obsessive-compulsive disorder: is the side relevant? Stereotact Funct Neurosurg 2014; 92(1):31–6.
72. Jiménez F, Nicolini H, Lozano AM, et al. Electrical stimulation of the inferior thalamic peduncle in the treatment of major depression and obsessive compulsive disorders. World Neurosurg 2013;80(3–4):S30.e17–25.
73. Nair G, Evans A, Bear RE, et al. The anteromedial GPi as a new target for deep brain stimulation in obsessive compulsive disorder. J Clin Neurosci 2014;21: 815–21.
74. Fenoy AJ, Simpson RK. Risks of common complications in deep brain stimulation surgery: management and avoidance. J Neurosurg 2014;120(1):132–9.

75. Haq IU, Foote KD, Goodman WK, et al. A case of mania following deep brain stimulation for obsessive compulsive disorder. Stereotact Funct Neurosurg 2010;88(5):322–8.

76. Okun MS, Mann G, Foote KD, et al. Deep brain stimulation in the internal capsule and nucleus accumbens region: responses observed during active and sham programming. J Neurol Neurosurg Psychiatry 2007;78(3):310–4. http://dx.doi.org/10.1136/jnnp.2006.095315.

77. Luigjes J, Mantione M, van den Brink W, et al. Deep brain stimulation increases impulsivity in two patients with obsessive-compulsive disorder. Int Clin Psychopharmacol 2011;26(6):338–40.

78. Bergfeld IO, Mantione M, Hoogendoorn ML, et al. Cognitive functioning in psychiatric disorders following deep brain stimulation. Brain Stimul 2013;6(4):532–7.

79. Sakai Y, Narumoto J, Nishida S, et al. Corticostriatal functional connectivity in non-medicated patients with obsessive-compulsive disorder. Eur Psychiatry 2011;26(7):463–9.

80. Harrison BJ, Soriano-Mas C, Pujol J, et al. Altered corticostriatal functional connectivity in obsessive-compulsive disorder. Arch Gen Psychiatry 2009;66(11):1189–200.

81. Bishnoi RJ, Jhanwar VG. Extended trial of transcranial magnetic stimulation in a case of treatment-resistant obsessive-compulsive disorder. Asian J Psychiatr 2011;4(2):152.

82. Aouizerate B, Cuny E, Martin-Guehl C, et al. Deep brain stimulation of the ventral caudate nucleus in the treatment of obsessive-compulsive disorder and major depression: case report. J Neurosurg 2004;101:682–6.

83. Franzini A, Messina G, Gambini O, et al. Deep-brain stimulation of the nucleus accumbens in obsessive compulsive disorder: clinical, surgical and electrophysiological considerations in two consecutive patients. Neurol Sci 2010;31(3):353–9.

# Cognitive Behavior Therapy for Obsessive-Compulsive and Related Disorders

CrossMark

Adam B. Lewin, PhD, ABPP[a,b,c,]*, Monica S. Wu, BA[a,c],
Joseph F. McGuire, MA[a,c], Eric A. Storch, PhD[a,b,c]

## KEYWORDS

- OCD - Obsessive-compulsive disorder - CBT - Cognitive behavior therapy
- Exposure therapy

## KEY POINTS

- Behavioral therapies constitute a high-efficacy, minimal risk treatment of obsessive-compulsive disorder (OCD) and related disorders for individuals of all ages.
- Based primarily on the principles of extinction learning, cognitive behavior therapy (CBT) and related therapies (eg, habit reversal training) produce equivalent or superior outcomes to pharmacotherapy for OCD and obsessive-compulsive spectrum disorders with few associated adverse side effects.
- Although flexible in dosing (weekly vs intensively) and format (individual vs group; extent of family involvement), focus on exposure and response prevention therapy is central to improvement.
- Behavioral therapies are highly efficacious, durable, and acceptable interventions for obsessive-compulsive spectrum disorders.

Dr A.B. Lewin has received research support from the International OCD Foundation, Joseph Drown Foundation, and NARSAD, has an agreement for a publishing honorarium from Springer Publishing, speakers honorarium from the Tourette Syndrome Association, reviewer honorarium from Children's Tumor Foundation, travel support from Rogers Memorial Hospital, National Institute of Mental Health, and American Academy of Child and Adolescent Psychiatry, and consulting fees from Prophase LLC. Dr E.A. Storch has received research support from the National Institutes of Health (1R01MH093381-01A1) and Agency for Healthcare Research and Quality (1R18HS018665-01A1), author honorarium from Springer Publishing, American Psychological Association, Wiley Incorporated, travel and salary support from Rogers Memorial Hospital, and consulting fees from Prophase LLC. Mr J.F. McGuire and Ms M.S. Wu have no potential conflicts of interest to report.

[a] Department of Pediatrics, Rothman Center for Neuropsychiatry, University of South Florida, 880 6th Street South, Suite 460, Box 7523, St Petersburg, FL 33701, USA; [b] Department of Psychiatry and Behavioral Neurosciences, University of South Florida, 3515 East Fletcher Avenue, Tampa, FL 33616, USA; [c] Department of Psychology, University of South Florida, 4202 East Fowler Avenue, PCD 4118G, Tampa, FL 33620, USA
* Corresponding author. Rothman Center for Neuropsychiatry, USF Pediatrics, 880 6th Street South, Suite 460, Box 7523, St Petersburg, FL 33701.
E-mail address: alewin@health.usf.edu

Psychiatr Clin N Am 37 (2014) 415–445
http://dx.doi.org/10.1016/j.psc.2014.05.002
0193-953X/14/$ – see front matter © 2014 Elsevier Inc. All rights reserved.

psych.theclinics.com

| Abbreviations | |
|---|---|
| AACAP | American Academy of Child and Adolescent Psychiatry |
| BDD | Body dysmorphic disorder |
| CBIT | Comprehensive behavioral intervention for tics |
| CBT | Cognitive behavior therapy |
| DCS | D-Cycloserine |
| ERP | Exposure and response prevention |
| HRT | Habit reversal training |
| NMDA | $N$-Methyl-D-aspartate |
| OCD | Obsessive-compulsive disorder |
| POTS | Pediatric OCD Treatment Study |
| PST | Psychoeducation and supportive therapy |
| RCTs | Randomized controlled trials |
| SRIs | Serotonin reuptake inhibitors |
| TTM | Trichotillomania |
| YBOCS | Yale-Brown Obsessive-Compulsive Scale |

## OVERVIEW OF COGNITIVE BEHAVIOR TREATMENT OF OBSESSIVE-COMPULSIVE AND RELATED DISORDERS

Cognitive behavior therapy (CBT) with exposure and response prevention (ERP) for obsessive-compulsive disorder (OCD) is a well-established treatment, supported by randomized clinical trials among adults and youth. CBT is a durable, side effect–free intervention that consistently produces improvement in 60% to 83% of patients.[1,2] Studies consistently identify the efficacy of CBT with ERP, with response rates equivalent to or greater than multimodal treatment with pharmacotherapy.[3] With relapse rates considerably lower[4] and acceptability higher for CBT (compared with pharmacotherapy[5]), behavioral interventions for OCD are (at least in part) the first-line interventions for OCD across the lifespan.[6,7] The key element of CBT for OCD, exposure therapy with response prevention, is based on extinguishing the negative reinforcement paradigm between obsessions and compulsions. Extinction-based treatments for other obsessive-compulsive spectrum disorders, for example Tourette syndrome, are becoming increasingly well tested and part of core treatment recommendations.[8]

### OCD

OCD is a chronic neuropsychiatric illness affecting approximately 2% of the population, with a fluctuating severity course and the potential for marked distress and interference with functioning.[9,10] Beyond individual morbidity, untreated OCD contributes to significant societal cost, estimated at US$8.4 billion in 1990.[11] OCD is listed among the top 20 contributors toward disability by the World Health Organization.[12] Although untreated OCD is estimated to contribute a negative impact on quality of life that is comparable with schizophrenia,[13] the disparity between those who are estimated to have OCD in contrast with those who receive treatment (57%) is much higher than for other serious mental illnesses.[14] However, 2 evidence-based treatments are available for OCD: pharmacotherapy with serotonin reuptake inhibitors (SRIs) and CBT with ERP.[6,7] Despite the efficacy of the former, concerns about relapse following discontinuation, side effects, and safety limit enthusiasm (especially among parents of minors) and there is significant patient preference for CBT-oriented treatments.[5] Although most CBT outcome research is focused on OCD, an increasing number of well-controlled trials have been conducted for other obsessive-compulsive spectrum disorders (eg, Tourette syndrome, trichotillomania, body dysmorphic disorder [BDD], and hoarding disorder), which are generally based on a similar set of behavioral principals akin to ERP. This article (1) reviews the theoretic basis for CBT with ERP and related therapies (eg, habit reversal training) for obsessive-compulsive spectrum disorders, (2) describes core treatment procedures, and (3) provides an overview of empirical treatment outcome research.

## Cognitive Behavioral Model of OCD

Learning theory serves as the basis for the cognitive behavioral treatment model of OCD and related disorders. Behavioral treatments are based on the 2-factor model for the acquisition and maintenance of fear learning via classical and operant mechanisms.[15] Fears (obsessions) develop when a previously neutral stimuli (eg, a door handle) becomes paired with an aversive stimuli (eg, worries about being contaminated by a virus) via classical conditioning.[16] Thus, a previously neutral stimulus generates a conditioned fear response previously associated with the original aversive stimuli (eg, fear of touching a virus-contaminated door handle), becoming conditioned to elicit distress. As a result of the acquired fear, the individual engages in compulsive rituals to alleviate obsessional distress (eg, ritualized hand washing) and/or engages in avoidance of stimuli that trigger obsessional worries (eg, avoidance of contaminated door handles). The ritualistic behavior associated with distress reduction (eg, hand washing, avoidance) becomes negatively reinforced and leads to its strengthening or maintenance via negative reinforcement. Although rituals/compulsions temporarily alleviate distress, they persist and often prohibit new learning opportunities that would potentially extinguish the conditioning.

Cognitive models of OCD assert that obsessive symptoms develop from cognitive misappraisals (eg, dysfunctional schema, cognitive distortions) that lead to inaccurate evaluations of intrusive thoughts (eg, touching a door handle after a person coughed on it will lead to sickness and perhaps even death).[17] Individuals with OCD hold dysfunctional cognitive beliefs (eg, thought-action fusion, overestimation) that often result in their inaccurate evaluation of ostensibly innocuous intrusive thoughts, so they perceive these thoughts/worries as a cause for concern (eg, touching a public door handle will result in sickness).[18,19] These misappraisals cause an individual to experience increased anxiety and distress (eg, worries about death after exposure to a door handle). Avoidance prohibits the opportunity for new learning that may invalidate or weaken cognitive errors. In an attempt to neutralize feared outcomes, individuals initiate ritualistic behaviors (eg, ritualized hand washing) and/or engage in avoidance behaviors, which are negatively reinforced and lead to symptom persistence.

There is support for brain-based changes following CBT for OCD.[20] Using positron emission tomography, Baxter and colleagues[21] reported changes in caudate glucose metabolism rates following CBT (n = 9) with percent changes in OCD severity corresponding with glucose metabolism rates in the caudate. Similar findings have been reported subsequently.[22,23] Using structural magnetic resonance imaging, Hoexter and colleagues[24] found smaller gray matter volumes in the medial orbitofrontal cortex, putamen, and left anterior cingulate cortex in patients with OCD versus healthy controls. After treatment with CBT or fluoxetine (n = 26), there were volumetric differences between controls and subjects with OCD. More recently, proton magnetic resonance spectroscopic imaging was used to evaluate brain-based metabolic and putative neurotransmitter changes following 4 weeks of intensive CBT for OCD (all 8 subjects responded robustly to CBT).[25] Compared with controls, baseline levels of N-acetyl-aspartyl-glutamate in the right anterior cingulate cortex was significantly lower in patients with OCD but subsequently increased following only 4 weeks of CBT (with pretreatment levels of *N*-acetyl-aspartyl-glutamate correlating with change in OCD severity). Posttreatment reductions in glutamine anterior middle cingulate cortex were also reported.[25]

## Tourette Syndrome/Chronic Tic Disorders

The behavioral model postulates that internal factors (eg, premonitory urges, anxiety) and external factors (eg, specific activities, environmental cues) serve as antecedents that increase or decrease tics. The model suggests that corresponding consequences exist to internal and external factors that reinforce tic symptoms. For instance, many youth report experiencing an internal sensation/tension that precedes a tic, commonly referred to as a premonitory urge.[26,27] This premonitory urge is subsequently alleviated on the performance of the tic and/or multiple tics. The tic consequently becomes negatively reinforced because of the reduction in the premonitory urge. For external factors, some patients similarly report that they have difficulty controlling their tics when completing certain activities, which results in the disruption and/or early discontinuation of potentially aversive activities (eg, doing homework after school). Thus, tics during these activities become negatively reinforced because they result in early discontinuation of undesirable activities. Although the behavioral model acknowledges the biological/neurologic basis of tics,[28] it suggests that tic symptoms can be influenced through habituation to uncomfortable internal factors (eg, premonitory urges) and modifying consequences to external factors (eg, no early discontinuation and/or avoidance of homework).

## Hair Pulling Disorder

The general behavioral model for hair pulling disorder (also known as trichotillomania [TTM]) conceptualizes hair pulling symptoms as learned behaviors that are maintained through conditioning mechanisms. Through repetitive pairings, internal (eg, increasing tension, stress/anxiety, "not just right" experiences) and external (eg, environmental stimuli, specific situations) cues become associated with pulling behaviors. For example, an individual may experience increased internal tension akin to a premonitory urge.[29] In response to this internal trigger, an individual engages in hair pulling to reduce the unpleasant feeling, which negatively reinforces pulling behaviors (eg, pulling out hair until tension alleviates, removing hair that is perceived to be "not just right"). Classical conditioning plays an important role for external cues, because stimuli from pulling situations (eg, environment/setting, activity, mood/emotional state) become repeatedly paired with pulling behaviors. Over time and repeated pairings, these external factors can serve to trigger pulling behaviors, even in the absence of the initially reported internal cues. Thus, pulling behaviors can become habitual and occur outside the individual's awareness and under decreasing control.[30] Research suggests that focused hair pulling (characterized by pulling within an individual's awareness) is likely to be an attempt to decrease levels of negative affect and/or regulate internalized affective experiences (eg, anxiety, stress, specific worries, boredom) in contrast with automatic pulling (which generally occurs outside an individual's awareness).[30–32]

## Body Dysmorphic Disorder

The cognitive behavioral model for BDD suggests that people with BDD have dysfunctional cognitive schema (ie, core beliefs) about themselves (eg, that if they looked better their whole lives would improve) or others (eg, that people only like attractive people).[33] These dysfunctional cognitive schema result in misappraisal and/or interpretative biases of ambiguous social stimuli as negative and/or threatening.[34] These interpretative biases cause individuals with BDD to experience negative emotions (eg, fear, anxiety, depression, shame) when encountering ambiguous situations and/or experiencing negative appearance-related thoughts and beliefs. In an attempt to reduce these negative emotions and/or internalized distress, individuals with BDD engage in ritualistic behaviors and/or avoidance. Ritualistic behaviors can include mirror checking, skin picking, reassurance seeking, repeated plastic surgery, body comparisons, and excessive grooming.[33] Avoidance behaviors may include avoiding social contacts and/or other situations in which ambiguous social stimuli may be encountered. The temporary distress reduction that results from ritualistic behaviors and/or avoidance serves to negatively reinforce and maintain BDD-related behavior.

### Hoarding Disorder

The cognitive behavioral model of hoarding disorder suggests that the core features of hoarding behaviors result from information processing problems, emotional and/or dysfunctional beliefs regarding possessions, and distress and/or avoidance (usually precipitated by the two preceding factors).[35,36] Information processing problems (eg, inattention, difficulty categorizing, memory problems, impaired decision making) contribute to the development of clutter and disorganization, but are not linked to acquisition and/or difficulty discarding.[37] Along with impaired information processes, individuals who hoard have strong beliefs regarding possessions that centralize around themes of emotional attachment, memory-related concerns, desire for control, and responsibility.[36] These beliefs contribute to acquisition behaviors and saving behaviors, and limit discarding.[35] The information processing problems and strong beliefs/attachment to items elicit distress when valued possessions are discarded and/or not acquired. In an attempt to minimize distress and/or perceived negative outcomes, an individual engages in acquisition and saving behaviors, and avoids discarding possessions and/or making decisions regarding which possessions to discard. As acquisition and saving behaviors increase, and discarding decreases, clutter begins to accumulate. As acquisition and hoarding behaviors minimize distress, these behaviors become negatively reinforced, contributing to symptom persistence.

## PATIENT EVALUATION OVERVIEW FOR OCD

Before initiating CBT, a clinical assessment should be conducted to assess for diagnosis, symptom presentation and severity, illness course, functioning/impairment, comorbidity, treatment history, individual strengths, and social support.[6,38] It is important to differentiate obsessions and compulsions associated with OCD from similar symptoms associated with other neuropsychiatric illnesses that may present with ruminations, worries, ritualized behavior, or repetitive intrusive thoughts (eg, psychosis, depression, anxiety disorders, posttraumatic stress disorder, anorexia nervosa).[39–42] These disorders may necessitate prerequisite/concurrent treatment and may suggest attenuated CBT response. Further, it is recommended to assess for factors associated with reduced CBT response, including poor insight/beliefs that obsessive fears are real, severe depression, poor compliance with ERP, reduced treatment expectancies, severe family accommodation/conflict, or prior history of failed treatment.[1,43–47] Assessment can typically be accomplished via clinician interview but semistructured inventories and rating scales are recommended to complement the initial clinical assessment as well as for tracking treatment outcomes[38] (eg, response, remission, or clinically significant change[48–50]).

## MANAGEMENT GOALS IN OCD
### CBT for OCD

CBT has garnered much attention and empirical support for the treatment of OCD.[3,51-56] Although numerous treatment manuals are available,[57-64] CBT for OCD typically includes the following core therapeutic elements:

- Psychoeducation
- Symptom hierarchy development
- Cognitive training
- The core therapeutic component, ERP

Psychoeducation (central to CBT for any disorder) provides patients and/or families information about OCD, discusses the cognitive behavioral model of OCD (discussed earlier), and orients patients and families to the procedures and demands associated with treatment.

In symptom hierarchy development, therapists and patients collaboratively construct a stimulus hierarchy consisting of the patient's obsessive-compulsive symptoms (eg, obsessive thoughts, compulsive rituals, avoidance behaviors). Construction of a symptom hierarchy allows treatment initially to focus on symptoms that evoke less distress during ERP (ie, when the ritual is inhibited), and subsequently progressing upwards through the hierarchy as mastery over lower level obsessions/compulsions is achieved.

During cognitive training, patients learn cognitive strategies for resisting OCD (eg, identifying dysfunctional cognitions, thought evaluation, cognitive restructuring). Cognitive-based intervention focuses on modifying core OCD-related domains identified by the Obsessive Compulsive Cognitions Working Group[17]: threat estimation, responsibility, overimportance of thoughts, tolerance for ambiguity, control over thoughts, and perfectionism. Individuals with OCD tend to overestimate the risk of threat and the extent of the potential negative outcome, and underestimate mitigating factors. They similarly endorse excessive perceptions of responsibility and equate failing to prevent a negative event from happening with causing/intending deliberate harm. Individuals with OCD express a strong need to control their thoughts and may equate thinking with desiring (thought-action fusion). Tolerance for ambiguity tends to be poor, whereas drive for perfectionism is often excessive.[65] Cognitive strategies are included on a complementary basis together with ERP, with developmentally appropriate modifications of cognitive therapy when treating youth. It is intrinsically difficult to study the individual contributions of cognitive therapy versus ERP given that attempts at modifying cognitions may constitute an exposure. Although there is preliminary evidence for primarily using cognitive strategizes in adults as opposed to emphasizing in vivo ERP,[66] expert consensus[6,7] remains that the core psychotherapeutic component for both youth and adult OCD is ERP.[67] Although cognitive restructuring can be omitted from CBT with successful outcomes, removal of ERP is deleterious.[3]

The putative mechanism of ERP is extinction, whereby repeated presentations of a conditioned stimulus (eg, a butter knife), in the absence of a previously paired unconditioned stimulus (eg, harming someone with the knife), lead to reductions in the conditioned response (avoidance). During ERP, patients are repeatedly exposed to situational (eg, touching an object perceived as contaminated) and/or internal triggers (eg, thinking or imagining a forbidden thought) that elicit an anxious state and trigger compulsive rituals (eg, hand washing, ritualized avoidance, praying, seeking forgiveness). While completing these exposures, patients resist engaging in ritualized behaviors until habituation to the anxious state is achieved. As habituation to feared situations/stimuli is achieved via response prevention, the necessity/reliance on the compulsive rituals to produce reductions in distress is reduced (via extinction of the negative reinforcement paradigm). New learning occurs, weakening the relationship between the previously acquired fear (knives are dangerous) and worrisome consequence (holding a knife may result in severe injury). The patient learns that rituals are not required in order to reduce distress and, moreover, feared outcomes are inaccurate. The frequency and intensity of obsessions decrease over repeated ERP.

Over the course of ERP sessions, graduated exposures are implemented, typically beginning with less distressing exposures and progressing toward exposures to stimuli/situations associated with greater levels of distress/avoidance on the stimulus hierarchy. Via ERP, the individual experiences the feared situations and obsessional cues while refraining from engaging in rituals. Several mechanisms of action are engaged: the conditioned fear related to obsessions is extinguished and the need for rituals is depleted, dysfunctional beliefs are corrected, and self-efficacy is garnered by ceasing reliance on maladaptive behaviors such as avoidance.[52,68] Implementation of exposures can be in vivo or imaginal, depending on the content of the obsession; although some exposures can be completed in vivo within the treatment session (eg, touching a contaminated doorknob and refraining from excessive hand washing), some symptoms necessitate imaginal exposures (eg, vividly envisioning violent imagery stabbing a family member while refraining from compensatory ritualized praying). To generalize treatment gains, ERP is implemented in multiple contexts over time to prevent relapse, which can occur through spontaneous recovery or reacquisition of the original conditioned fear associations.[69]

*Pediatric OCD*

CBT is implemented similarly in the pediatric population, with ERP remaining as the key active ingredient, and minor modifications made to tailor the treatment to be developmentally appropriate.[70,71] For youth, cognitive strategies focus on externalizing OCD (ie, as a common adversary against whom the child, parent, and therapist will ally in order to combat), constructive self-talk (eg, patients declaring themselves to be stronger than OCD), and cognitive restructuring, with the goal of providing the child with cognitive strategies to use during later ERP tasks. Use of cognitive strategies is typically reduced in contrast with adult CBT and is contingent on the youth's developmental level, cognitive functioning, and insight into OCD symptoms. Another modification (as necessary to bolster compliance and participation) includes the frequent implementation of reward-based systems to encourage motivation to engage in therapy sessions and facilitate homework compliance,[72] which is an integral component of therapeutic outcome.[73] Furthermore, parental involvement is heavily encouraged in the treatment of pediatric OCD to ensure structured implementation of treatment outside therapy sessions (eg, completed exposures, reduced family accommodation[57–59]). Family members often benefit from observing therapy techniques implemented by the therapist, which are purposed to be used in a noncoercive and supportive manner (in contrast with blaming, reprimanding, or accommodating). ERP is well tolerated and efficacious even for very young children with OCD.[74,75] The American Academy of Child and Adolescent Psychiatry (AACAP) practice parameters explicitly state that the first-line treatment recommended for youth with mild to moderate symptoms of OCD should be CBT, with more moderate to severe cases of OCD to be treated with CBT in conjunction with pharmacotherapy.[7] International stepped-care investigations are also underway. CBT is used as the first-line treatment of all patients, followed by extended CBT for treatment nonresponders (rather than pharmacotherapy).[76] Pending results of this trial, combined with underwhelming support for pharmacotherapy augmentation of CBT, there is an initiative for studying additional/more intensive ERP following initial courses of CBT that produce suboptimal results. This initiative is of particular importance given patient and parental preference for behavioral treatments.

### Behavioral Treatments for Obsessive-Compulsive and Related Disorders

There is considerable evidence for using CBT and/or related behavior therapies to treat obsessive-compulsive spectrum disorders. Treatments generally emphasize extinction-based behavioral interventions that operate similarly to ERP (weakening the relationship between the target behavior and the maintaining contingencies). General descriptions of the treatment of each disorder are provided here.

#### Tourette syndrome/chronic tic disorders

Habit reversal training (HRT) is a behavioral intervention indicated for individuals who present with moderate or greater tic symptom severity and experience impairment caused by the tics.[8] Although HRT can include multiple therapeutic components (eg, relaxation training, contingency management, generalization training[77]), the core components are considered to be awareness training and competing response training.[78] A typical course of treatment begins with psychoeducation about Tourette syndrome/chronic tic disorders and orienting patients and/or their families to the behavioral model of treatment. Next, patients and therapists develop a list of current tics and rank them in order of most to least bothersome/frequent, with the most problematic tics typically serving as a starting point for treatment. Awareness training focuses on the detection of premonitory urges and/or early tic movements that precede a tic. Once awareness training is achieved for the targeted tic, competing response training is used to develop alternative behaviors (termed competing responses) that ideally are physically incompatible with the targeted tic. Competing responses are implemented on early tic detection (eg, premonitory urges, early tic movements) and are sustained until the urge to tic dissipates. Over repeated attempts, patients learn to break the premonitory urge-tic-relief cycle, which is posited to be maintained via a negative reinforcement paradigm. Differential reinforcement is used to build the competing response (via praise, reward, and so forth) for youth. In doing so, patients learn that the discomfort associated with the premonitory urge diminishes over time (even in the absence of performing the tic), thereby reducing tic symptoms. Inhibiting tics does not result in a worsening of tics (a tic rebound) or premonitory urges as feared by many patients.[79–81]

HRT serves as the core therapeutic component in the comprehensive behavioral intervention for tics (CBIT). This updated intervention integrates HRT with functional assessment and function-based intervention strategies designed to mitigate external influences that worsen tics. For instance, when specific situations are identified that maintain and/or exacerbate tics (eg, increased tics during homework assignments), antecedents and consequences of tics are identified and function-based interventions are implemented (eg, a child is not allowed to avoid homework because of tic symptoms). In addition, CBIT incorporates social support to help patients practice exercises outside of sessions.

#### Hair pulling disorder/trichotillomania

Behavioral interventions such as HRT have shown efficacy for reducing hair pulling behaviors among youth and adults with TTM. There are 3 core components across HRT trials: awareness training, stimulus control, and competing response training.[82] In general, treatment typically begins with psychoeducation about TTM, orientation to the cognitive behavioral treatment model, and a thorough assessment to identify symptom severity, comorbidity, and antecedents/consequences of pulling behaviors. Awareness training for TTM focuses on improving patients' awareness of internal factors (eg, internal tension/urges, anxiety, mood) and external factors (eg, early signs of pulling, specific environments/situations) that precipitate pulling behaviors. Once pulling triggers are identified, stimulus control involves the collaborative development of function-based strategies to reduce the likelihood that pulling behavior begins. For example, if a patient identified that pulling behaviors occurred while seated at the computer in the bedroom, stimulus control interventions may include moving the computer into a public place, leaving the door open to the room when on the computer, and/or keeping an object (eg, a stress ball) proximal to the computer to occupy the patient's free hands. Similar to HRT for tics, competing response training for TTM involves the implementation of alternative behaviors that are (preferably) physically incompatible with hair pulling, which are implemented on recognition of internal or external pulling cues/urges to pull. Although these elements serve as the core ingredients to HRT treatment packages for TTM, more recent studies have examined the incorporation of components from acceptance and commitment therapy[83] and dialectical behavior therapy.[84]

## BDD

CBT, including ERP, has been used with individuals with BDD. Similar to ERP in patients with OCD, patients with BDD begin treatment by constructing a hierarchy of specific body parts and feared situations that are avoided for fear of evaluation,[85] which serve as the basic structure of treatment progress. Exposures typically entail asking patients to direct their focus on the body part that is perceived as flawed, and to face situations that are typically avoided for fear of evaluation. Response prevention generally involves having the patient refrain from engaging in ritualistic behaviors, such as excessive checking of body parts in the mirror, reassurance seeking, or excessive grooming.[86] Cognitive restructuring is also commonly used in the treatment of BDD, which is focused on countering dysfunctional beliefs and replacing them with more adaptive and realistic cognitions.[87]

## Hoarding disorder

Several recent studies have examined CBT tailored specifically for those who hoard.[88,89] CBT for hoarding disorder most commonly includes development of decision-making skills, improved organizational skills, and tools for discarding items/decreasing clutter. Treatment begins by conducting a comprehensive assessment of hoarding behaviors and providing the patient with psychoeducation about the treatment model. Coaches are identified to be included in the therapeutic process to help patients implement the skills learned in therapy outside of sessions. In treatment, patients practice using decision-making and organizational skills to sort and discard clutter under a therapist's guidance. As patients develop competency with these skills in session, coaches are incorporated to help patients use these skills in home/other cluttered environments. Although not as central a treatment component as in CBT for OCD, ERP can be implemented, along with cognitive restructuring, to help correct dysfunctional beliefs about hoarding[88]; in ERP for hoarding, patients are gradually exposed to situations that elicit anxiety (eg, making decisions about certain possessions, throwing specific objects away, or being exposed to situations that trigger acquisition), and are then encouraged to refrain from further saving or avoidance behaviors.

### Evaluation of Outcome, Adjustment of Treatment, and Long-term Recommendations

#### Evaluation of outcome

Numerous randomized controlled trials (RCTs) show the efficacy and durability of CBT for OCD in adult (**Table 1**) and pediatric (**Table 2**) samples. Research studies meeting the following criteria were included for consideration: (1) RCTs, (2) greater than or equal to 20 subjects per treatment group, (3) conducted in 1970 or later, and (4) the use of CBT/ERP. Regarding obsessive-compulsive spectrum disorders, because of the relative paucity of research studies meeting the aforementioned criteria, studies beyond RCTs (eg, pilot studies) were included for consideration. **Table 3** summarizes key research studies for obsessive-compulsive spectrum disorders.

#### OCD

In the adult OCD literature, RCTs show strong support for CBT with ERP for treating OCD (see **Table 1**). McLean and colleagues[90] compared the effects of CBT, traditional ERP, and a delayed waitlist group in 76 treatment-seeking adults with OCD. Both active treatments received statistically significant reductions in OCD symptom severity and were both found to be superior to the waitlist group. Exposure and response prevention were marginally superior to CBT after treatment, and had significantly higher rates of adults achieving clinically significant improvement at the 3-month follow-up (44% for ERP, 13% for CBT), suggesting that the core behavioral (ie, exposure-based) components in treating OCD are critical for achieving durable improvement. In addition, Foa and colleagues[91] compared ERP alone, clomipramine alone, their combination (ERP plus clomipramine), and placebo in 122 adults with OCD. The addition of clomipramine to ERP did not reduce OCD symptom severity to a greater extent than ERP alone; both were superior to clomipramine alone. Eighty-six percent of ERP completers and 79% of combination (ERP plus clomipramine) treatment completers were considered treatment responders. Simpson and colleagues[92] investigated the relative efficacy of CBT versus stress management training in augmenting SRIs that had been associated with at least limited improvement. ERP was superior to stress management training in the magnitude of decreased OCD symptom severity, as well as in the achievement of minimal OCD symptoms (as defined by a Yale-Brown Obsessive Compulsive Scale [YBOCS][93] score less than 13). More recently, Simpson and colleagues[94] similarly investigated CBT versus risperidone and pill placebo in augmenting SRIs in 100 adults with OCD. Adults in the CBT group had significantly greater reductions in OCD symptom severity compared with participants taking risperidone or placebo (who did not differ), with more participants receiving responder status, achieving minimal symptoms, and having improved insight, functioning, and quality of life. Furthermore, a unique study investigating the relative efficacies of cognitive therapy alone, ERP alone, sequentially added cognitive therapy or ERP to fluvoxamine, and a waitlist control group was conducted with 117 adults with OCD.[95] Data showed no statistically significant difference between the active treatment groups, though all treatment groups were superior to the waiting list group and showed substantial decreases in OCD symptom severity. CBT/ERP has collectively received much empirical support for adults with OCD, with further investigations warranted for the comparative effects of adjunctive pharmacotherapy and management of complex and/or treatment-refractory cases.

Group administrations of CBT have also been investigated within the adult OCD literature. One trial[96] randomized 63 adults to receive 1 of 3 conditions: individual CBT, group CBT, or a waitlist control condition. After 10 weeks of treatment, both active treatment groups achieved significant reductions in OCD symptom severity, with no statistically significant difference observed between the two treatment groups.

**Table 1**
Key RCTs investigating CBT/ERP for adult OCD

| Investigators | Design | N | Duration | Outcomes/Key Findings |
|---|---|---|---|---|
| Anderson & Rees,[96] 2007 | RCT; ICBT vs GCBT vs WL | N = 63; ICBT (n = 25); GCBT (n = 21); WL (n = 17) | 10 wk | No differences between ICBT and GCBT on OCD severity after treatment. YBOCS ES (against WL): ICBT 1.03, GBT 0.77. Recovered (based on reliable and clinically significant change): ICBT 41%, GCBT 20%, WL 0% |
| Foa et al,[91] 2005 | RCT; ERP vs CME vs combination (ERP + CME) vs PBO | N = 122 ERP (n = 29); CME (n = 36); combination (n = 31); PBO (n = 26) | 15 sessions of ERP over 12 wk | YBOCS ES (against PBO): ERP 1.56, CME 0.56, combination 1.59. Response rates (completers): ERP 86% vs CME 48% vs combination 79% vs PBO 10% |
| McLean et al,[90] 2001 | RCT; CBT vs ERP vs WL (delayed) | N = 76; CBT (n = 34); ERP (n = 42); WL (n = 38) | 12 wk | YBOCS ES (against WL): ERP 1.62, CBT 0.98. Recovered (reliable and clinically significant change) for completers: ERP 38% vs CBT 16% |
| Simpson et al,[92] 2008 | RCT; CBT vs SMT (augment SRI) | N = 108; CBT (n = 56); SMT (n = 55) | 17 twice-weekly sessions | YBOCS ES: 1.31. Achieved minimal OCD symptoms: CBT 33% vs SMT 4% |
| Simpson et al,[94] 2013 | RCT; ERP vs RIS vs PBO (augment SRI) | N = 100 ERP (n = 40); RIS (n = 40) PBO (n = 20) | 17 twice-weekly sessions over 8 wk | YBOCS ES (against PBO): 1.55 ERP, 0.06 RIS |
| van Balkom et al,[95] 1998 | RCT; CT vs ERP vs FLV + CT vs FLV + ERP vs WL | N = 117 CT (n = 25); ERP (n = 22) FLV + CT (n = 24); FLV + ERP (n = 28); WL (n = 18) | 16 sessions over 16 wk (10 sessions over 8 wk for combined treatment groups) | Significant decreases in OCD severity across active treatment groups, no statistically significant difference between treatments (but all are superior to WL) |

All effect sizes reported are between-group comparisons after treatment; if ES was not explicitly reported in the manuscript, ES were calculated using the means and pooled standard deviations. Improvement was measured by the Clinical Global Impression Improvement Scale.

*Abbreviations:* CME, clomipramine; CT, cognitive therapy; ES, effect size; FLV, fluvoxamine; GCBT, group CBT; ICBT, individual CBT; PBO, placebo; RIS, risperidone; SMT, stress management training; WL, waitlist; YBOCS, Yale-Brown Obsessive Compulsive Scale.[93]

**Table 2**
**Key RCTs investigating CBT/ERP for pediatric OCD**

| Investigators | Design | N | Age Range (y) | Duration of Treatment | Outcomes/Key Findings |
|---|---|---|---|---|---|
| Barrett et al,[100] 2004 | RCT ICBT vs GCBT vs WL | N = 77 ICBT (n = 24) GCBT (n = 29) WL (n = 24) | 7–17 | 14 sessions over 14 wk | CYBOCS ES: ICBT 2.75, GCBT 2.65. OCD diagnosis free: ICBT 88%, GCBT 76%, WL 0% |
| Piacentini et al,[99] 2011 | RCT CBT vs PRT | N = 71 CBT (n = 49) PRT (n = 22) | 8–17 | 12 sessions over 14 wk | CYBOCS ES: 0.4. Completer response rates: CBT 68.3% vs PRT 35.3%. Clinical remission rates: CBT 42.5% vs 17.6% PRT |
| POTS,[98] 2004 | RCT CBT vs SRT vs CBT + SRT vs PBO | N = 112 CBT (n = 28) SRT (n = 28) CBT + SRT (n = 28) PBO (n = 28) | 7–17 | CBT 14 sessions over 12 wk | CYBOCS ES: CBT 0.97, SRT 0.67, CBT + SRT 1.4 Clinical remission: CBT 39.3% vs SRT 21.4% vs CBT + SRT 53.6% vs PBO 3.6% |
| Storch et al,[101] 2007 | RCT Weekly CBT vs intensive CBT | N = 40 Weekly CBT (n = 28) Intensive CBT (n = 28) | 7–17 | Weekly: 14 1 × weekly Intensive: 14 daily sessions over 3 wk | CYBOCS ES: 0.42 (intensive favored) Remission: weekly CBT 50% vs intensive CBT 75% Improvement: weekly CBT 65% vs intensive CBT 90% |

All effect sizes reported are between-group comparisons after treatment; if ES was not explicitly reported in the manuscript, ES were calculated using the means and pooled standard deviations. Improvement was measured by the Clinical Global Impression Improvement Scale.[158]
*Abbreviations:* BT, behavior therapy; CYBOCS, Children's Yale-Brown Obsessive Compulsive Scale[159]; MAC, minimal attention control; POTS, Pediatric OCD Treatment Study; PRT, psychoeducation plus relaxation training; SRT, sertraline.

**Table 3**
**Summary of research studies investigating psychotherapy for obsessive-compulsive–related disorders**

| Disorder | Investigators | Design | N | Age Range (If Reported) | Duration of Treatment | Outcomes/Key Findings |
|---|---|---|---|---|---|---|
| TS/CTD | Azrin & Peterson,[160] 1990 | RCT HRT vs WL | N = 10 HRT (n = 5) WL (n = 5) | 6–36 | M = 20 sessions (range 13–30) over 8–11 mo | ES of percent change scores on tics: Z corrected, 2.19 |
| TS/CTD | O'Connor et al,[161] 2001 | RCT Cognitive behavior HRT vs WL | N = 47 HRT (n = 25) WL (n = 22) | Adults | 14–16 wk | Significant changes in tic frequency, intensity, and control over tic for HRT group and not WL |
| TS/CTD | CBIT child[103] | RCT CBIT vs PST | N = 126 CBIT (n = 61) PST (n = 65) | 9–17 | 8 sessions over 10 wk | YGTSS ES: 0.68, improvement: CBIT 52.5% vs PST 18.5% |
| TS/CTD | Verdellen et al,[162] 2004 | RCT HRT vs ERP | N = 43 HRT (n = 22) ERP (n = 21) | 7–55 | HRT 10 weekly sessions, ERP 12 weekly sessions | YGTSS ES: −0.25. Clinically significant improvements: HRT 83% vs ERP 95% |
| TS/CTD | CBIT adult[102] | RCT CBIT vs PST | N = 122 CBIT (n = 63) PST (n = 59) | 16–69 | 8 sessions over 10 wk | YGTSS ES: 0.6. Improvement: CBIT 38.1% vs PST 13.9% |
| TS/CTD | Wilhelm et al,[163] 2003 | RCT HRT vs ST | N = 29 HRT (n = 16) ST (n = 13) | Adults | 14 sessions (first 8, weekly; last 6, twice monthly) | YGTSS ES: 0.84. Improvement M (SD): HRT 2.13 (0.93) vs ST 3.55 (1.19) |
| TTM | Azrin et al,[164] 1980 | RCT HRT vs NPT | N = 34 HRT (n = 19) NPT (n = 15) | 13–48 | 1 session (2 h) | Number of hair pulling episodes per day ES: 0.66 |
| TTM | Diefenbach et al,[107] 2006 | RCT Group BT vs ST | N = 24 BT (n = 12) ST (n = 12) | Adults | 8 sessions over 8 wk | MGH-HPS ES: 0.25. Clinically significant change: BT 16.7% vs ST 25% |

*(continued on next page)*

**Table 3**
*(continued)*

| Disorder | Investigators | Design | N | Age Range (If Reported) | Duration of Treatment | Outcomes/Key Findings |
|---|---|---|---|---|---|---|
| TTM | Keuthen et al,[84] 2010 | RCT DBT-enhanced HRT vs MAC | N = 38 HRT (n = 20) MAC (n = 18) | Adults | 11 sessions over 11 wk | MGH-HPS ES: 1.78. NIMH-TIS: 0.93. Treatment responders: HRT 55% vs MAC 5.56% |
| TTM | Franklin et al,[108] 2011 | RCT BT vs MAC | N = 24 BT (n = 12) MAC (n = 12) | 7–17 | 8 sessions over 8 wk | NIMH-TSS ES: 1.25. Improvement: 75% BT vs 0% MAC |
| TTM | Ninan et al,[109] 2000 | RCT CBT/HRT vs CME vs PBO | N = 16 CBT/HRT (n = 5) CME (n = 6) PBO (n = 5) | 22–53 | 9 sessions over 9 wk | Treatment responders for completers: CBT/HRT 100% vs CME 67% vs placebo 0% |
| TTM | van Minnen et al,[106] 2003 | RCT BT vs FLU vs WL | N = 40 BT (n = 14) FLU (n = 11) WL (n = 15) | 17–57 | 6 sessions over 12 wk | MGH-HPS ES: FLU 1.63, WL 1.10. Clinically significant change: BT 64% vs FLU 9% vs WL 20% |
| TTM | Woods et al,[83] 2006 | RCT ACT/HRT vs WL | N = 25 ACT/HRT (n = 12) WL (n = 13) | Adults | 10 sessions over 12 wk | MGH-HPS ES: 1.72. NIMH-TIS ES: 1.36. Clinically significant change: ACT/HRT 66%, WL 8% |
| BDD | McKay et al,[112] 1997 | RCT ERP + MP vs ERP – MP | N = 10 ERP + MP (n = 5) ERP – MP (n = 5) | 21–45 | 5 sessions over 5 wk | BDD-YBOCS before to after: t(9) = 5.48, P<.001 (no difference between groups) |
| BDD | Rosen et al,[110] 1995 | RCT CBT vs no Tx | N = 54 CBT (n = 27) No Tx CBT (n = 27) | 20–61 | 8 sessions over 8–12 wk | BDDE[165] ES: 2.29. Clinically significant change: CBT 81.5% vs no Tx 7.4% |

| BDD | Veale et al,[111] 1996 | RCT CBT vs WL | N = 19 CBT (n = 9) WL (n = 10) | Adults | 12 sessions over 12 wk | BDDE ES: 2.72. Subclinical symptoms: CBT 77.78% vs WL 0% |
|---|---|---|---|---|---|---|
| BDD | Wilhelm et al,[114] 1999 | Case series for group CBT | N = 13 | 18–48 | 12 sessions over 12 wk | BDD-YBOCS[166] before to after: t(10) = 3.94, P<.01 |
| BDD | Wilhelm et al,[115] 2011 | Pilot (open trial) for modular CBT | N = 12 18 sessions (n = 5) 22 sessions (n = 7) | Adults | Weekly sessions over 18 or 22 wk | BDD-YBOCS ES (completer before to after): 3.82. Treatment responders (completers): 80% |
| Hoarding | Muroff et al,[117] 2009 | Pilot (open trial) GCBT | N = 32 | 38–65 | M number of sessions: 16.6 (16 wk, n = 27; 20 wk, n = 5; 2 individual sessions, n = 32) | SI-R ES (before to after): partial $\eta^2$ = .38, t(23) = 3.76, P<.001 |
| Hoarding | Steketee et al,[118] 2000 | Pilot (open trial) Group + individual CBT vs individual CBT alone | N = 7 Group + individual CBT (n = 6) Individual CBT alone (n = 1) | 36–61 | 20 wk (n = 3 continued on for 14 individual sessions over 28 more wk) | YBOCS ES (before to after): 0.73, t(5) = 3.29, P<.03 |
| Hoarding | Steketee et al,[89] 2010 | RCT CBT vs WL | N = 46 CBT (n = 23) WL (n = 23) | Adults | 26 sessions over M = 44.8 wk | SI-R ES: 1.07. Clinically significant change: 41% CBT |
| Hoarding | Tolin et al,[119] 2007 | Pilot (open trial) of CBT | N = 14 (n = 10 completers) | Adults | 26 sessions over 7–12 mo | SI-R ES (before to after): partial $\eta^2$ = .49. Clinically significant change: 60%. Improvement: 50% |
| Hoarding | Turner et al,[120] 2010 | Pilot (open trial) of CBT | N = 11 (n = 6 completers) | 56–87 | M sessions completed: 35.3 (approximately weekly) | Clutter image rating[167] before to after: t(5) = 6.14, P<.002 |

All effect sizes reported are between-group comparisons after treatment; if ES was not explicitly reported, numbers reported in the table were calculated using the means and pooled standard deviations. Improvement was measured by the Clinical Global Impression Improvement Scale.

*Abbreviations:* ACT, acceptance and commitment therapy; BDDE, Body Dysmorphic Disorder Examination[165]; CTD, chronic tic disorder; DBT, Dialectical Behavior Therapy; FLU, fluoxetine; MGH-HPS, Massachusetts General Hospital Hair Pulling Scale[171]; M, mean; MP, maintenance program; NIMH-TSS, NIMH Trichotillomania Severity Scale[169]; NPT, negative practice training; PST, psychoeducation and supportive therapy; SD, standard deviation; SI-R, Saving Inventory - Revised[170]; ST, supportive therapy; TS, Tourette syndrome; Tx, treatment; YGTSS, Yale Global Tic Severity Scale.[168]

However, when considering recovery rates (based on reliable and clinically significant change), 41% of adults in the individual CBT group achieved recovered status, compared with 20% of the adults in the CBT group. By follow-up, differences had largely attenuated and no differences were observed thereafter. Further investigation into the modality of group treatments is warranted.

### Pediatric OCD

Several RCTs offer supporting evidence in favor of the efficacy and durability of CBT for youth with OCD (see **Table 2**).[97] The Pediatric OCD Treatment Study (POTS) team[98] conducted a multisite trial investigating the efficacy of CBT alone, sertraline alone, the combination of CBT and sertraline, and placebo in 112 youth (aged 7–17 years) with OCD. Results indicated that remission rates for CBT alone (39.3%) were statistically significantly superior to placebo. A large effect size of 0.97 was found for individuals receiving CBT alone compared with patients receiving placebo treatment, supporting the relative efficacy of CBT in pediatric OCD treatment. Piacentini and colleagues[99] compared a family-based CBT protocol with psychoeducation and relaxation training in 71 youth aged 8 to 17 years. Patients receiving CBT yielded a significantly higher response rate (68.3%) than those receiving psychoeducation and relaxation training (35.3%). In addition, 6-month follow-up data suggested that treatment gains were largely maintained, showing the durability of CBT for pediatric OCD. Barrett and colleagues[100] similarly implemented a family-based CBT protocol, comparing the relative efficacy of individual CBT, group CBT, and a brief waitlist group in 77 youth (aged 7–17 years). Statistically significant decreases in OCD severity were observed for both CBT conditions, although no differences were found between the CBT treatments. Both CBT groups showed superiority compared with the waitlist group, with 88% and 76% of the individual and group CBT participants classified as treatment responders, respectively, compared with 0% of waitlist group participants. Three-month and 6-month follow-up assessments confirmed the durability of CBT for pediatric OCD, showing the maintenance of treatment gains. In addition, Storch and colleagues[101] investigated the relative efficacy of weekly versus intensive family-based CBT in 40 youth (aged 7–17 years) with OCD. Both treatment groups had most participants rated as treatment responders after treatment (90% intensive CBT, 65% weekly CBT), and large percentages of participants achieving remission (75% intensive CBT, 50% weekly CBT). Although treatment group differences were seen immediately after the acute treatment phase, differences largely attenuated at the 3-month follow-up assessment. Comparable with previous studies, treatment gains were maintained at follow-up, providing further support for the efficacy and durability of CBT for pediatric OCD.

### Tourette syndrome/chronic tic disorders

HRT and CBIT, collectively referred to as behavioral interventions for tics, have received empirical support in RCTs[102,103] and show similar efficacy across tic symptom profiles.[104] The 2 large, multicenter RCTs of CBIT compared with psychoeducation and supportive therapy (PST) were conducted in a pediatric[103] and adult sample.[102] These trials showed statistically significant tic symptom improvement in favor of CBIT, with 52.5% of the pediatric sample and 38.1% of the adult sample showing clinical improvement. Moreover, a recent meta-analysis of behavioral interventions for tics (eg, HRT, CBIT) identified a large treatment effect for these interventions that was comparable with treatment effects observed in RCTs of antipsychotic medications,[105] but without the potential for deleterious side effects. The durability of CBIT was shown by the maintenance of treatment gains determined through 3-month and 6-month follow-up assessments with treatment responders. Other key RCTs investigating the efficacy of behavioral interventions for tics are summarized in **Table 3**.

### Hair pulling disorder/trichotillomania

A small number of research studies have shown the preliminary efficacy of HRT in treating TTM. In an RCT comparing behavior therapy, fluoxetine, and a waitlist control group, van Minnen and colleagues[106] found behavior therapy to be superior to fluoxetine and the control group in decreasing pulling. In addition, Diefenbach and colleagues[107] compared behavior therapy with supportive therapy, in which statistically significant reductions in hair pulling symptoms were found for the behavior therapy group but not the supportive therapy group. In the only pediatric RCT for TTM published to date,[108] investigators examined behavior therapy versus a minimal attention control group. Behavior therapy was superior to the minimal attention control group with regard to decreases in TTM symptom severity, and treatment gains were still maintained 8 weeks following the acute treatment phase. Furthermore, various studies have investigated the relative efficacy of enhanced HRT protocols, with core components of dialectical behavior therapy,[84] acceptance and commitment therapy,[83] and CBT[109] incorporated into the treatment of trichotillomania. Compared with minimal attention controls, waitlist, or placebo, enhanced HRT protocols showed comparable superiority to the control groups, with higher treatment responses and decreases in hair pulling severity. The added benefit of these additional therapies remains unclear. Key RCTs investigating the efficacy of behavioral interventions for TTM (inclusive of the aforementioned studies) are summarized in **Table 3**; larger replication studies remain warranted, especially in children and adolescents with TTM given the lack of evidence-based pharmacotherapy for TTM.

### BDD

Few RCTs have been conducted to date for treatment of BDD. Extant literature showed preliminary support for CBT/ERP in treating BDD symptoms. Two RCTs[110,111] compared CBT versus no treatment or a waitlist control group, respectively. Both trials showed large posttreatment effect sizes between the treatment groups, favoring CBT more than either control condition with regard to decreases in BDD symptoms. Follow-up assessments suggest treatment durability for CBT, with 77% of the CBT group no longer meeting diagnostic criteria for BDD.[110] McKay and colleagues[112] examined the relative efficacy of ERP with and without a 6-month maintenance program for the treatment of BDD. Results showed statistically significant decreases in BDD symptoms after the acute phase of treatment, and gains were maintained at the 6-month follow-up assessment for both groups (with no significant differences in BDD symptoms between groups). Although patients receiving ERP without the maintenance program reported significantly more lapses at the 2-year follow-up than patients in the ERP treatment group with the maintenance program, both groups remained significantly improved regarding acute BDD symptoms, emphasizing the overall efficacy of ERP for BDD.[113] A case series[114] showed large effect sizes for decreases in BDD symptom severity before and after receiving group CBT, and a pilot trial of a modularized CBT treatment[115] has shown similar promise in finding substantial decreases in BDD symptoms. The key studies investigating the efficacy of cognitive behavioral interventions for BDD are summarized in **Table 3**.

### Hoarding disorder

Empirical support for the treatment of hoarding disorder is sparse, because hoarding has only recently been conceptualized as a separate disorder from OCD. Much of the extant literature on treatment of hoarding is often conducted within the general context of patients with OCD, resulting in poor generalization and low representation of individuals primarily with hoarding disorder without OCD. Several studies examining the efficacy of CBT specifically designed to target compulsive hoarding have recently emerged. However, to the best of our knowledge, only 1 RCT has been conducted[89] that compared CBT against a waiting list control, with statistically significantly greater reductions in the severity of hoarding symptoms during and after treatment, in favor of the CBT group. Forty-one percent of treatment completers eventually satisfied criteria for clinically significant improvement, and treatment gains were maintained up to the 12-month follow-up assessment.[116] Other open trials of CBT for hoarding have been piloted, with investigations of group CBT[117,118] and individual CBT[89,119,120] showing similar decreases in various hoarding symptoms. However, the pilot studies have yielded conflicting results regarding improvements in various hoarding symptoms; improvements have been reported in excessive acquiring, difficulty discarding, and clutter,[119] but mixed findings are found for organizing.[118,120] Key studies investigating the efficacy of cognitive behavioral interventions for hoarding disorder are summarized in **Table 3**.

## Adjustment of Treatment

### Timing and modality of treatment

Although CBT for OCD is typically administered in a weekly and individual format, several variations of the treatment have been evaluated empirically. For instance, CBT with ERP can be implemented in a more time-intensive format, which typically entails daily treatment sessions. In 2 studies, intensive ERP was compared with weekly[101] or twice-weekly ERP[51]; comparisons immediately after treatment revealed trends toward greater treatment gains for the sample receiving intensive ERP, but differences between the groups largely attenuated by the follow-up phases. Intensive CBT formats may be most appropriate for individuals without access to a local provider or to patients who have failed to maximally benefit from weekly CBT.[59,121] In addition, ERP can be administered via a group format, with therapists implementing CBT with several patients simultaneously. There are limited data on the relative efficacy of treatment gains between patients receiving individual CBT and group CBT, although preliminary results suggest support.[96,122]

### Involvement of others in treatment

When implementing CBT for OCD, it is common for family members and/or spouses/partners to be involved in treatment. Formal incorporation of significant others in CBT for OCD has growing empirical support,[123] with preliminary data showing sizable decreases in OCD severity, along with improvements in relationship factors that may indirectly affect OCD symptoms.[124,125] Incorporation of family members is paramount for the pediatric population (including adolescents), and extant research has provided strong support for the efficacy and acceptability of family-based CBT in the treatment of pediatric OCD.[74,99,101,122,126]

### D-Cycloserine augmentation of CBT

D-Cycloserine (DCS) is an antibiotic that serves as a partial agonist of the N-methyl-D-aspartate (NMDA) receptor in the amygdala. Based on previous research studies showing the effects of DCS on fear extinction and learning in animals and humans, there has been a recent increase in interest regarding its potential for enhancing the efficacy of CBT for OCD. When DCS is used in conjunction with CBT, it is postulated to instigate treatment effects earlier in the course of ERP,[127] and/or show a faster and greater reduction in OCD symptoms after treatment. Although extant literature on the effects of DCS combined with ERP for OCD has yielded mixed findings, preliminary results suggest that individuals using DCS in conjunction with CBT showed faster decreases in OCD symptoms earlier in treatment[128–131] compared with placebo plus CBT, but significant differences between groups tended to dissipate after treatment.[132] A meta-analysis[133] suggests that treatment effects may be modulated by the timing and number of DCS administrations.

### Long-term Recommendations

Few studies have examined relapse and recovery of OCD symptoms longitudinally, and the extant investigations are largely heterogeneous because of variable assessment instruments, timing of follow-up assessments, statistical analysis variability, and methodology (eg, naturalistic vs follow-up of clinical sample receiving a specific treatment modality). As such, this article focuses on the empirical research examining relapse and recovery within samples that specifically received CBT for OCD.

O'Sullivan and colleagues[134] followed up with patients 6 years after receiving exposure therapy with clomipramine or placebo. Results suggest that neither clomipramine nor the placebo had significant effects on treatment outcome, but more ERP, better homework compliance, and improvement at the end of treatment were associated with better treatment outcomes. A 1-year follow-up after group CBT revealed that 35.5% (n = 11) had relapsed, with full remission and intensity of improvement serving as predictors for nonrelapsing during the follow-up period.[25] In another follow-up study[135] patients were largely maintaining treatment gains 2 years after treatment, with 21.4% (n = 9) fully remitted, 52.4% (n = 22) partially remitted, and 26.2% (n = 11) unchanged in OCD symptom severity. Full remission similarly served as a protective factor for relapse after 2 years.[135] In contrast, Rufer and colleagues[20] did not find short-term treatment outcome to be linked to long-term treatment outcome when the investigators followed up with patients 7 years after receiving CBT with fluvoxamine or placebo. Reductions in OCD symptoms were largely maintained at the follow-up assessment, with 60% achieving treatment responder status and 27% (n = 8) achieving full remission. Individuals not achieving full remission typically had longer histories of OCD, which was confirmed in a subsequent study.[136] Jakubovski and colleagues[136] followed up with patients 2 years after being randomized to receive group CBT or fluoxetine, although treatment nonresponders were able to receive combinations of these treatments or other medications; poorer prognosis was linked to the duration of the OCD, at least one comorbid disorder, and the presence of a depressive disorder. Given the extant research suggesting the deleterious effects of comorbid depression on treatment response, Anholt and colleagues[137] investigated the impact of depression on treatment outcome 5 years after treatment; depression did not predict treatment response in patients receiving behavior or cognitive therapy for OCD, necessitating further investigation into this factor. Overall, initial outcome seems to be the strongest predictor of longer-term outcome.

A meta-analysis investigating the long-term outcomes of pediatric OCD largely corroborated much of what has been found in the adult literature[138]; specifically, earlier age of onset, longer duration of OCD, and inpatient versus outpatient status predicted persistence of sustained OCD symptoms, whereas comorbidity and poor response to initial treatment were linked to poor prognosis. Furthermore, a 7-year follow-up of 38 individuals receiving a family-based CBT protocol found that between 79% and 95% of participants no longer met diagnostic criteria for OCD.[139] More long-term follow-up studies are needed, especially tracking youth outcomes prospectively, with additional focus on the factors influencing relapse and recovery in patients specifically receiving CBT for OCD.

## COMBINATION THERAPIES: CBT AND PHARMACOTHERAPY

There are several studies of CBT in combination with pharmacotherapy (or as an augmenting agent). As described earlier, in a double-blind RCT, Foa and colleagues[91] examined the relative efficacy of ERP, clomipramine, their combination, and a pill placebo in 122 adults. ERP alone and ERP with clomipramine were both superior to clomipramine alone, with no differences between ERP alone and ERP with clomipramine. In other trials directly comparing CBT and pharmacotherapy, results have been mixed, with some studies indicating no differences in treatment outcomes,[24,125] whereas others indicate superiority of CBT alone.[140] Taken together, when considering the adverse effect profile of medications as well as strong patient preference for psychotherapy,[5] ERP may be efficacious as a monotherapy for some individuals and should be considered before recommending concurrent medications.

Despite its efficacy, CBT is often not received as the initial intervention. Thus, recent studies have investigated the potential augmenting effect of CBT for patients concurrently taking medication. Simpson and colleagues[94] recently investigated the relative efficacy of ERP, risperidone, or pill placebo in augmenting SRIs in 100 adults with OCD. After participants received 8 weeks of each treatment, results indicated that ERP was superior to both risperidone and pill placebo in augmenting SRIs with regard to decreases in OCD symptom severity, achieving minimal OCD symptoms, and improved insight, functioning, and quality of life. Given the lesser negative adverse effect profile and greater efficacy of ERP, ERP is recommended to be implemented before antipsychotic medications to augment concurrent SRI use.[94]

Similar trials and results have been observed in the pediatric OCD literature. The largest randomized trial to date conducted by the POTS[98] team showed that CBT combined with sertraline was superior to CBT alone when considering OCD symptom severity, although remission rates did not differ between the two treatment groups. A significant treatment condition by site interaction effect complicates the interpretation of this study. As a result, the study investigators recommended that youth should receive combination treatment (CBT plus sertraline) or CBT alone before using sertraline alone, although more recent AACAP practice parameters indicate use of CBT alone first for mild to moderate cases, with combination therapies reserved for more severe cases of pediatric OCD.[7] Recent data for sequential sertraline and CBT found no significant effects relative to CBT and pill placebo in children with OCD.[141] In addition, in the only pediatric trial investigating the augmenting effect of CBT or brief CBT instructions on medication management for concurrent SRIs,[142] significantly more youth in the CBT treatment group achieved treatment responder status versus youth receiving brief CBT instructions or medication management alone. ERP seems to be similarly efficacious and is recommended for use in pediatric OCD as well, whether as an adjunct to concurrent medications or alone.

## TREATMENT RESISTANCE/COMPLICATIONS/DISEASE RECURRENCE
### OCD

Despite the efficacy of CBT for OCD, at least 30% of individuals do not achieve significant symptom improvement or complete remission.[143,144] Several clinical factors have been implicated in explaining treatment-refractory cases.[43,46] First, comorbid disorders have been associated with poorer treatment response in both pediatric and adult populations; specifically, depressive, schizotypal personality, and disruptive behavior, and attention-deficit/hyperactivity disorders (ADHDs) have shown deleterious effects on treatment response.[1,145] Poor insight into OCD symptoms has also been linked to poorer treatment response.[146,147] In addition, individuals with higher baseline severity of OCD symptoms[148,149] as well as different subtypes of OCD symptoms, such as hoarding and sexual and religious obsessions,[20,143,150,151] have shown poorer treatment response. Poorer treatment adherence and homework compliance have been linked to poorer outcomes in treatment as well.[152,153] Furthermore, several family factors have also been implicated in treatment resistance, such as increased family dysfunction and poorer family functioning,[44] as well as increased levels of family accommodation.[154] In youth with OCD, treatment expectancies were linked to treatment response.[47]

### Obsessive-Compulsive Spectrum Disorders

Although multiple RCTs have been conducted across obsessive-compulsive spectrum disorders, there has been limited examination of factors associated with an attenuated response to treatment. For individuals with Tourette syndrome/chronic tic disorders, a meta-analysis identified that RCTs with a greater percentage of ADHD showed attenuated treatment effects.[105] In comparison, large treatment effects were still observed in RCTs with a high and low percentage of co-occurring ADHD, suggesting that individuals with comorbid ADHD can still greatly benefit from behavioral interventions. For individuals with TTM, clinicians are recommended to glean the function and type (ie, focused or automatic) of pulling behaviors in order to fine-tune psychotherapeutic procedures. It has been suggested that automatic pulling behaviors may be more responsive to the traditional components of HRT[82] (eg, awareness training, competing response), whereas focused pulling may benefit more from treatment protocols enhanced with dialectical behavior therapy[84] or acceptance and commitment therapy,[83] which are designed to address the cognitive/affective antecedents to pulling behaviors more directly. However, there is insufficient evidence to offer strong support for either of these adjunctive treatments. Developmental level is postulated to also play a role in treatment response, which may be caused by the higher prevalence of automatic pulling behaviors in youth,[155] leading to improved treatment response in pediatric trials.[142] For patients with BDD, there has been no empirical evaluation of factors associated with poor treatment response to CBT. Despite the lack of empirical investigation, preliminary findings and clinical experience suggest that poor insight can complicate treatment.[147,156,157] For patients with hoarding disorder, preliminary evidence suggests that pretreatment hoarding symptom severity, gender, perfectionism, and social anxiety are associated with worse outcomes for CBT.[116,117] A relationship between homework compliance and hoarding symptom improvement has also been observed in a pilot CBT trial.[119] In considering the geriatric population, a pilot study[120] remarked that treatment of hoarding was complicated by safety risks (eg, fire hazards) and physical limitations (eg, inability to organize belongings alone), eliciting the need for problem solving and modifications to individual treatment protocols. Overall, these preliminary findings should be interpreted with caution, because limited empirical research on factors associated with treatment refractoriness has been conducted on obsessive-compulsive spectrum disorders to date.

### SUMMARY

CBT with ERP is an effective and well-tolerated first-line treatment of OCD and spectrum disorders. Compared with medication, CBT with ERP has consistently produced equivalent or superior outcomes. CBT is a highly acceptable treatment and therapeutic gains are more durable following discontinuation of treatment. Nevertheless, accessibility and dissemination remain barriers. Too few practitioners specialize in exposure-based therapies, with an even greater disparity for patients seeking behavioral therapy (eg, HRT, CBIT, CBT for hoarding) for obsessive-compulsive spectrum disorders. Efforts to improve availability, reduce costs, maximize efficiency, and better personalize treatments are therefore needed. Enhanced understanding of the quantity/intensity of therapy required, optimal sequencing of treatments, determining sufficient response/need for continuation, and larger scale long-term follow-ups are needed. In particular, larger replication studies (with long-term follow-up) are needed for the less-researched obsessive-compulsive spectrum disorders, in particular hoarding disorder, BDD, and TTM. Nevertheless, extinction-based behavioral therapy has been extended across obsessive-compulsive spectrum disorders to individuals of all ages with growing support of neurobiological change accompanying treatment response.

## REFERENCES

1. Baer L, Minichiello WE. Behavior therapy for obsessive-compulsive disorder. In: Jenike MA, Baer L, Minichiello WE, editors. Obsessive-compulsive disorders. St Louis (MO): Mosby; 1998. p. 337–67.
2. DeVeaugh-Geiss J, Landau P, Katz R. Preliminary results from a multicenter trial of clomipramine in obsessive-compulsive disorder. Psychopharmacol Bull 1989; 25(1):36–40.
3. Franklin ME, Foa EB. Cognitive behavioral treatments for obsessive compulsive disorder. In: Nathan PE, Gorman JM, editors. A guide to treatments that work, vol. 2. Oxford (United Kingdom): Oxford University Press; 2002. p. 367–86.
4. Pato MT, Zohar-Kadouch R, Zohar J, et al. Return of symptoms after discontinuation of clomipramine in patients with obsessive-compulsive disorder. Am J Psychiatry 1988;145(12):1521–5.
5. Patel SR, Simpson HB. Patient preferences for obsessive-compulsive disorder treatment. J Clin Psychiatry 2010;71(11):1434–9.
6. Koran LM, Hanna GL, Hollander E, et al, the Work Group on Obsessive-Compulsive Disorder. Practice guideline for the treatment of patients with obsessive-compulsive disorder. Am J Psychiatry 2007;164:5–53.
7. Geller DA, the American Academy of Child and Adolescent Psychiatry Committee on Quality Issues. Practice parameter for the assessment and treatment of children and adolescents with obsessive-compulsive disorder. J Am Acad Child Adolesc Psychiatry 2012;51(1):98–113.
8. Murphy TK, Lewin AB, Storch EA, et al, the American Academy of Child and Adolescent Psychiatry Committee on Quality Issues. Practice parameter for the assessment and treatment of children and adolescents with tic disorders. J Am Acad Child Adolesc Psychiatry 2013;52(12):1341–59.
9. Hollander E. Obsessive-compulsive disorder: the hidden epidemic. J Clin Psychiatry 1997;58(Suppl 12):3–6.
10. Jenike MA. Obsessive-compulsive and related disorders: a hidden epidemic. N Engl J Med 1989;321(8):539–41.
11. DuPont RL, Rice DP, Shiraki S, et al. Economic costs of obsessive-compulsive disorder. Med Interface 1995;8(4):102–9.
12. Organization WH. The newly defined burden of mental problems, Fact Sheet No. 217. Geneva (Switzerland); 1999.
13. Bobes J, Gonzalez MP, Bascaran MT, et al. Quality of life and disability in patients with obsessive-compulsive disorder. Eur Psychiatry 2001;16(4):239–45.
14. Kohn R, Saxena S, Levav I, et al. The treatment gap in mental health care. Bull World Health Organ 2004;82(11):858–66.

15. Mowrer OH. A stimulus-response analysis of anxiety and its role as a reinforcing agent. Psychol Rev 1939;46:553–66.
16. Dollard J, Miller NE. Personality and psychotherapy: an analysis in terms of learning, thinking and culture. New York: McGraw-Hill; 1950.
17. Obsessive Compulsive Cognitions Working Group. Cognitive assessment of obsessive-compulsive disorder. Behav Res Ther 1997;35(7):667–81.
18. Salkovskis PM. Obsessional-compulsive problems: a cognitive-behavioural analysis. Behav Res Ther 1985;23(5):571–83.
19. Rachman S. A cognitive theory of obsessions. Behav Res Ther 1997;35(9): 793–802.
20. Rufer M, Hand I, Alsleben H, et al. Long-term course and outcome of obsessive-compulsive patients after cognitive-behavioral therapy in combination with either fluvoxamine or placebo: a 7-year follow-up of a randomized double-blind trial. Eur Arch Psychiatry Clin Neurosci 2005;255(2):121–8.
21. Baxter LR Jr, Schwartz JM, Bergman KS, et al. Caudate glucose metabolic rate changes with both drug and behavior therapy for obsessive-compulsive disorder. Arch Gen Psychiatry 1992;49(9):681–9.
22. Schwartz JM, Stoessel PW, Baxter LR Jr, et al. Systematic changes in cerebral glucose metabolic rate after successful behavior modification treatment of obsessive-compulsive disorder. Arch Gen Psychiatry 1996;53(2):109–13.
23. Nakatani E, Nakgawa A, Ohara Y, et al. Effects of behavior therapy on regional cerebral blood flow in obsessive-compulsive disorder. Psychiatry Res 2003; 124(2):113–20.
24. Hoexter MQ, de Souza Duran FL, D'Alcante CC, et al. Gray matter volumes in obsessive-compulsive disorder before and after fluoxetine or cognitive-behavior therapy: a randomized clinical trial. Neuropsychopharmacology 2012;37(3):734–45.
25. O'Neill J, Gorbis E, Feusner JD, et al. Effects of intensive cognitive-behavioral therapy on cingulate neurochemistry in obsessive-compulsive disorder. J Psychiatr Res 2013;47(4):494–504.
26. Leckman JF, Walker DE, Cohen DJ. Premonitory urges in Tourette's syndrome. Am J Psychiatry 1993;150(1):98–102.
27. Woods DW, Piacentini J, Himle MB, et al. Premonitory Urge for Tics Scale (PUTS): initial psychometric results and examination of the premonitory urge phenomenon in youths with tic disorders. J Dev Behav Pediatr 2005;26(6):397–403.
28. Felling RJ, Singer HS. Neurobiology of Tourette syndrome: current status and need for further investigation. J Neurosci 2011;31(35):12387–95.
29. Woods DW, Flessner C, Franklin ME, et al. Understanding and treating trichotillomania: what we know and what we don't know. Psychiatr Clin North Am 2006; 29(2):487–501, ix.
30. Christenson GA, Ristvedt SL, Mackenzie TB. Identification of trichotillomania cue profiles. Behav Res Ther 1993;31(3):315–20.
31. Diefenbach GJ, Mouton-Odum S, Stanley MA. Affective correlates of trichotillomania. Behav Res Ther 2002;40(11):1305–15.
32. Begotka AM, Woods DW, Wetterneck CT. The relationship between experiential avoidance and the severity of trichotillomania in a nonreferred sample. J Behav Ther Exp Psychiatry 2004;35(1):17–24.
33. Wilhelm S, Phillips KA, Steketee G. Cognitive-behavioral therapy for body dysmorphic disorder: a treatment manual. New York: Guildford Press; 2012.
34. Buhlmann U, McNally RJ, Wilhelm S, et al. Selective processing of emotional information in body dysmorphic disorder. J Anxiety Disord 2002;16(3):289–98.

35. Frost RO, Hartl TL. A cognitive-behavioral model of compulsive hoarding. Behav Res Ther 1996;34(4):341–50.
36. Steketee G, Frost R. Compulsive hoarding: current status of the research. Clin Psychol Rev 2003;23(7):905–27.
37. Fitch KE, Cougle JR. Perceived and actual information processing deficits in nonclinical hoarding. J Obsessive Compuls Relat Disord 2013;2(2):192–9.
38. Lewin AB, Piacentini J. Evidence-based assessment of child obsessive compulsive disorder: recommendations for clinical practice and treatment research. Child Youth Care Forum 2010;39(2):73–89.
39. Lewin AB, Menzel J, Strober M. Assessment and treatment of comorbid anorexia nervosa and obsessive compulsive disorder. In: Storch EA, McKay D, editors. Handbook of treating variants and complications in anxiety disorders. New York: Springer; 2013. p. 337–48.
40. Rodowski MF, Cagande CC, Riddle MA. Childhood obsessive-compulsive disorder presenting as schizophrenia spectrum disorders. J Child Adolesc Psychopharmacol 2008;18(4):395–401.
41. Thomsen PH. Obsessive-compulsive disorder in adolescence. Differential diagnostic considerations in relation to schizophrenia and manic-depressive disorder: a comparison of phenomenology and sociodemographic characteristics. Psychopathology 1992;25(6):301–10.
42. Poyurovsky M, Koran LM. Obsessive-compulsive disorder (OCD) with schizotypy vs. schizophrenia with OCD: diagnostic dilemmas and therapeutic implications. J Psychiatr Res 2005;39(4):399–408.
43. Storch EA, Bjorgvinsson T, Riemann B, et al. Factors associated with poor response in cognitive-behavioral therapy for pediatric obsessive-compulsive disorder. Bull Menninger Clin 2010;74(2):167–85.
44. Peris TS, Sugar CA, Bergman RL, et al. Family factors predict treatment outcome for pediatric obsessive-compulsive disorder. J Consult Clin Psychol 2012;80(2):255–63.
45. Santana L, Fontenelle JM, Yucel M, et al. Rates and correlates of nonadherence to treatment in obsessive-compulsive disorder. J Psychiatr Pract 2013;19(1): 42–53.
46. Lewin AB. Tractable impediments to cognitive behavioral therapy for pediatric obsessive compulsive disorder. In: McKay D, Storch EA, editors. Obsessive-compulsive disorder and its spectrum: a lifespan approach. Washington, DC: American Psychological Association Press; 2014. p. 81–96.
47. Lewin AB, Peris TS, Bergman RL, et al. The role of treatment expectancy in youth receiving exposure-based CBT for obsessive compulsive disorder. Behav Res Ther 2011;49(9):536–43.
48. Lewin AB, De Nadai AS, Park J, et al. Refining clinical judgment of treatment outcome in obsessive-compulsive disorder. Psychiatry Res 2011;185(3):394–401.
49. Tolin DF, Abramowitz JS, Diefenbach GJ. Defining response in clinical trials for obsessive-compulsive disorder: a signal detection analysis of the Yale-Brown obsessive compulsive scale. J Clin Psychiatry 2005;66(12):1549–57.
50. Storch EA, Lewin AB, De Nadai AS, et al. Defining treatment response and remission in obsessive-compulsive disorder: a signal detection analysis of the Children's Yale-Brown Obsessive Compulsive Scale. J Am Acad Child Adolesc Psychiatry 2010;49(7):708–17.
51. Abramowitz JS, Foa EB, Franklin ME. Exposure and ritual prevention for obsessive-compulsive disorder: effects of intensive versus twice-weekly sessions. J Consult Clin Psychol 2003;71(2):394–8.

52. Abramowitz JS, Taylor S, McKay D. Obsessive-compulsive disorder. Lancet 2009;374(9688):491–9.
53. Lewin AB, Storch EA, Adkins J, et al. Current directions in pediatric obsessive-compulsive disorder. Pediatr Ann 2005;34(2):128–34.
54. Olatunji BO, Davis ML, Powers MB, et al. Cognitive-behavioral therapy for obsessive-compulsive disorder: a meta-analysis of treatment outcome and moderators. J Psychiatr Res 2013;47(1):33–41.
55. Rosa-Alcazar AI, Sanchez-Meca J, Gomez-Conesa A, et al. Psychological treatment of obsessive-compulsive disorder: a meta-analysis. Clin Psychol Rev 2008;28(8):1310–25.
56. Thomsen PH. Obsessive-compulsive disorders. Eur Child Adolesc Psychiatry 2013;22(Suppl 1):S23–8.
57. March JS, Mulle K. OCD in children and adolescents: a cognitive-behavioral treatment manual. New York: Guilford Press; 1998.
58. Piacentini J, Langley A, Roblek T. Overcoming childhood OCD: a therapist's guide. New York: Oxford University Press; 2007.
59. Lewin AB, Storch EA, Merlo LJ, et al. Intensive cognitive behavioral therapy for pediatric obsessive compulsive disorder: a treatment protocol for mental health providers. Psychol Serv 2005;2(2):91–104.
60. Freeman JB, Garcia AM. Family-based treatment for young children with OCD workbook. New York: Oxford University Press; 2009.
61. Steketee G. Treatment of obsessive compulsive disorder. New York: Guilford Press; 1993.
62. Kozak MJ, Foa EB. Mastery of obsessive-compulsive disorder: a cognitive-behavioral approach. Therapist guide. San Antonio (Texas): The Psychological Corporation; 1997.
63. Foa EB, Yadin E, Lichner TK. Exposure and response (ritual) prevention for obsessive-compulsive disorder: therapist guide. New York: Oxford University Press; 2012.
64. Abramowitz A. Therapist manual for twice-weekly exposure and ritual prevention treatment of obsessive-compulsive disorder. Philadelphia: University of Pennsylvania; 1998.
65. Steketee GS, Frost RO, Rheaume J, et al. Cognitive theory and treatment of obsessive-compulsive disorder. In: Jenike MA, Baer L, Minichiello WE, editors. Obsessive-compulsive disorders. St Louis (MO): Mosby; 1998. p. 368–99.
66. Wilhelm S, Steketee G, Fama JM, et al. Modular cognitive therapy for obsessive-compulsive disorder: a wait-list controlled trial. J Cognit Psychother 2009;23(4): 294–305.
67. Olatunji BO, Rosenfield D, Tart CD, et al. Behavioral versus cognitive treatment of obsessive-compulsive disorder: an examination of outcome and mediators of change. J Consult Clin Psychol 2013;81(3):415–28.
68. Lewin AB, Storch EA, Geffken GR, et al. A neuropsychiatric review of pediatric obsessive-compulsive disorder: etiology and efficacious treatments. Neuropsychiatr Dis Treat 2006;2(1):21–31.
69. Craske MG, Kircanski K, Zelikowsky M, et al. Optimizing inhibitory learning during exposure therapy. Behav Res Ther 2008;46(1):5–27.
70. Lewin AB, Piacentini J. Obsessive-compulsive disorder in children. In: Sadock BJ, Sadock VA, Ruiz P, editors. Kaplan & Sadock's comprehensive textbook of psychiatry, vol. 2, 9th edition. Philadelphia: Lippincott Williams & Wilkins; 2009. p. 3671–8.
71. Lewin AB, Storch EA, Adkins JW, et al. Update and review on pediatric obsessive-compulsive disorder. Psychiatr Ann 2005;35:745–51.

72. Lewin AB. Parent training for childhood anxiety. In: McKay D, Storch EA, editors. Handbook of child and adolescent anxiety disorders. New York: Springer; 2011. p. 405–18.

73. Park JM, Small BJ, Geller DA, et al. Does D-cycloserine augmentation of CBT improve therapeutic homework compliance for pediatric obsessive-compulsive disorder? J Child Fam Stud 2013;23:863–71.

74. Freeman JB, Garcia AM, Coyne L, et al. Early childhood OCD: preliminary findings from a family-based cognitive-behavioral approach. J Am Acad Child Adolesc Psychiatry 2008;47(5):593–602.

75. Lewin AB, Park JM, Jones AM, et al. Family-based exposure and response prevention therapy for preschool-aged children with obsessive-compulsive disorder: a pilot randomized controlled trial. Behav Res Ther 2014;56:30–8.

76. Thomsen PH, Torp NC, Dahl K, et al. The Nordic long-term OCD treatment study (NordLOTS): rationale, design, and methods. Child Adolesc Psychiatry Ment Health 2013;7(1):41.

77. Piacentini J, Chang S. Habit reversal training for tic disorders in children and adolescents. Behav Modif 2005;29(6):803–22.

78. Miltenberger RG, Fuqua RW, Woods DW. Applying behavior analysis to clinical problems: review and analysis of habit reversal. J Appl Behav Anal 1998;31(3): 447–69.

79. Specht MW, Woods DW, Nicotra CM, et al. Effects of tic suppression: ability to suppress, rebound, negative reinforcement, and habituation to the premonitory urge. Behav Res Ther 2013;51(1):24–30.

80. Himle MB, Woods DW. An experimental evaluation of tic suppression and the tic rebound effect. Behav Res Ther 2005;43(11):1443–51.

81. Woods DW, Himle MB, Miltenberger RG, et al. Durability, negative impact, and neuropsychological predictors of tic suppression in children with chronic tic disorder. J Abnorm Child Psychol 2008;36(2):237–45.

82. Franklin ME, Zagrabbe K, Benavides KL. Trichotillomania and its treatment: a review and recommendations. Expert Rev Neurother 2011;11(8):1165–74.

83. Woods DW, Wetterneck CT, Flessner CA. A controlled evaluation of acceptance and commitment therapy plus habit reversal for trichotillomania. Behav Res Ther 2006;44(5):639–56.

84. Keuthen NJ, Rothbaum BO, Welch SS, et al. Pilot trial of dialectical behavior therapy-enhanced habit reversal for trichotillomania. Depress Anxiety 2010; 27(10):953–9.

85. Rosen JC. Body dysmorphic disorder: assessment and treatment. In: Thompson JK, editor. Body image, eating disorders and obesity. Washington, DC: American Psychological Association; 1996. p. 149–70.

86. Cororve MB, Gleaves DH. Body dysmorphic disorder: a review of conceptualizations, assessment, and treatment strategies. Clin Psychol Rev 2001;21(6): 949–70.

87. Schmidt NB, Harrington P. Cognitive-behavioral treatment of body dysmorphic disorder: a case report. J Behav Ther Exp Psychiatry 1995;26(2):161–7.

88. Saxena S, Maidment KM. Treatment of compulsive hoarding. J Clin Psychol 2004;60(11):1143–54.

89. Steketee G, Frost RO, Tolin DF, et al. Waitlist-controlled trial of cognitive behavior therapy for hoarding disorder. Depress Anxiety 2010;27(5):476–84.

90. McLean PD, Whittal ML, Thordarson DS, et al. Cognitive versus behavior therapy in the group treatment of obsessive-compulsive disorder. J Consult Clin Psychol 2001;69(2):205–14.

91. Foa EB, Liebowitz MR, Kozak MJ, et al. Randomized, placebo-controlled trial of exposure and ritual prevention, clomipramine, and their combination in the treatment of obsessive-compulsive disorder. Am J Psychiatry 2005;162(1): 151–61.
92. Simpson HB, Foa EB, Liebowitz MR, et al. A randomized, controlled trial of cognitive-behavioral therapy for augmenting pharmacotherapy in obsessive-compulsive disorder. Am J Psychiatry 2008;165(5):621–30.
93. Goodman WK, Price LH, Rasmussen SA, et al. The Yale-Brown Obsessive Compulsive Scale. I. Development, use, and reliability. Arch Gen Psychiatry 1989;46(11):1006–11.
94. Simpson HB, Foa EB, Liebowitz MR, et al. Cognitive-behavioral therapy vs risperidone for augmenting serotonin reuptake inhibitors in obsessive-compulsive disorder: a randomized clinical trial. JAMA Psychiatry 2013; 70(11):1190–9.
95. van Balkom AJ, de Haan E, van Oppen P, et al. Cognitive and behavioral therapies alone versus in combination with fluvoxamine in the treatment of obsessive compulsive disorder. J Nerv Ment Dis 1998;186(8):492–9.
96. Anderson RA, Rees CS. Group versus individual cognitive-behavioural treatment for obsessive-compulsive disorder: a controlled trial. Behav Res Ther 2007;45(1):123–37.
97. Lewin AB, Park JM, Storch EA. Obsessive compulsive disorder in children and adolescents. In: Vasa RA, Roy AK, editors. Pediatric anxiety disorders - a clinical guide. New York: Humana Press; 2013. p. 151–75.
98. Pediatric OCD Treatment Study (POTS) Team. Cognitive-behavior therapy, sertraline, and their combination for children and adolescents with obsessive-compulsive disorder: the Pediatric OCD Treatment Study (POTS) randomized controlled trial. JAMA 2004;292(16):1969–76.
99. Piacentini J, Bergman RL, Chang S, et al. Controlled comparison of family cognitive behavioral therapy and psychoeducation/relaxation training for child obsessive-compulsive disorder. J Am Acad Child Adolesc Psychiatry 2011; 50(11):1149–61.
100. Barrett P, Healy-Farrell L, March JS. Cognitive-behavioral family treatment of childhood obsessive-compulsive disorder: a controlled trial. J Am Acad Child Adolesc Psychiatry 2004;43(1):46–62.
101. Storch EA, Geffken GR, Merlo LJ, et al. Family-based cognitive-behavioral therapy for pediatric obsessive-compulsive disorder: comparison of intensive and weekly approaches. J Am Acad Child Adolesc Psychiatry 2007;46(4):469–78.
102. Wilhelm S, Peterson AL, Piacentini J, et al. Randomized trial of behavior therapy for adults with Tourette syndrome. Arch Gen Psychiatry 2012;69(8):795–803.
103. Piacentini J, Woods DW, Scahill L, et al. Behavior therapy for children with Tourette disorder: a randomized controlled trial. JAMA 2010;303(19):1929–37.
104. McGuire JF, Nyirabahizi E, Kircanski K, et al. A cluster analysis of tic symptoms in children and adults with Tourette syndrome: clinical correlates and treatment outcome. Psychiatry Res 2013;210(3):1198–204.
105. McGuire JF, Piacentini J, Brennan E, et al. A meta-analysis of habit reversal training for chronic tic disorders. J Psychiatr Res 2014;50:106–12.
106. van Minnen A, Hoogduin KA, Keijsers GP, et al. Treatment of trichotillomania with behavioral therapy or fluoxetine: a randomized, waiting-list controlled study. Arch Gen Psychiatry 2003;60(5):517–22.
107. Diefenbach GJ, Tolin DF, Hannan S, et al. Group treatment for trichotillomania: behavior therapy versus supportive therapy. Behav Ther 2006;37(4):353–63.

108. Franklin ME, Edson AL, Ledley DA, et al. Behavior therapy for pediatric tricho-tillomania: a randomized controlled trial. J Am Acad Child Adolesc Psychiatry 2011;50(8):763–71.
109. Ninan PT, Rothbaum BO, Marsteller FA, et al. A placebo-controlled trial of cognitive-behavioral therapy and clomipramine in trichotillomania. J Clin Psychiatry 2000;61(1):47–50.
110. Rosen JC, Reiter J, Orosan P. Cognitive-behavioral body image therapy for body dysmorphic disorder. J Consult Clin Psychol 1995;63(2):263–9.
111. Veale D, Gournay K, Dryden W, et al. Body dysmorphic disorder: a cognitive behavioural model and pilot randomised controlled trial. Behav Res Ther 1996; 34(9):717–29.
112. McKay D, Todaro J, Neziroglu F, et al. Body dysmorphic disorder: a preliminary evaluation of treatment and maintenance using exposure with response prevention. Behav Res Ther 1997;35(1):67–70.
113. McKay D. Two-year follow-up of behavioral treatment and maintenance for body dysmorphic disorder. Behav Modif 1999;23(4):620–9.
114. Wilhelm S, Otto MW, Lohr B, et al. Cognitive behavior group therapy for body dysmorphic disorder: a case series. Behav Res Ther 1999;37(1):71–5.
115. Wilhelm S, Phillips KA, Fama JM, et al. Modular cognitive-behavioral therapy for body dysmorphic disorder. Behav Ther 2011;42(4):624–33.
116. Muroff J, Steketee G, Frost RO, et al. Cognitive behavior therapy for hoarding disorder: follow-up findings and predictors of outcome. Depress Anxiety 2013. [Epub ahead of print].
117. Muroff J, Steketee G, Rasmussen J, et al. Group cognitive and behavioral treatment for compulsive hoarding: a preliminary trial. Depress Anxiety 2009;26(7): 634–40.
118. Steketee G, Frost RO, Wincze J, et al. Group and individual treatment of compulsive hoarding: a pilot study. Behav Cogn Psychother 2000;28:259–68.
119. Tolin DF, Frost RO, Steketee G. An open trial of cognitive-behavioral therapy for compulsive hoarding. Behav Res Ther 2007;45(7):1461–70.
120. Turner K, Steketee G, Nauth L. Treating elders with compulsive hoarding: a pilot program. Cognitive and Behavioral Practice 2010;17:449–59.
121. Bjorgvinsson T, Hart AJ, Wetterneck C, et al. Outcomes of specialized residential treatment for adults with obsessive-compulsive disorder. J Psychiatr Pract 2013;19(5):429–37.
122. Barrett P, Farrell L, Dadds M, et al. Cognitive-behavioral family treatment of childhood obsessive-compulsive disorder: long-term follow-up and predictors of outcome. J Am Acad Child Adolesc Psychiatry 2005;44(10):1005–14.
123. Baxter LR Jr, Saxena S, Brody AL, et al. Brain mediation of obsessive-compulsive disorder symptoms: evidence from functional brain imaging studies in the human and nonhuman primate. Semin Clin Neuropsychiatry 1996;1(1): 32–47.
124. Abramowitz JS, Baucom DH, Wheaton MG, et al. Enhancing exposure and response prevention for OCD: a couple-based approach. Behav Modif 2013; 37(2):189–210.
125. Hoexter MQ, Dougherty DD, Shavitt RG, et al. Differential prefrontal gray matter correlates of treatment response to fluoxetine or cognitive-behavioral therapy in obsessive-compulsive disorder. Eur Neuropsychopharmacol 2013;23(7):569–80.
126. Peris TS, Piacentini J. Optimizing treatment for complex cases of childhood obsessive compulsive disorder: a preliminary trial. J Clin Child Adolesc Psychol 2013;42(1):1–8.

127. Chasson GS, Buhlmann U, Tolin DF, et al. Need for speed: evaluating slopes of OCD recovery in behavior therapy enhanced with D-cycloserine. Behav Res Ther 2010;48(7):675–9.
128. Kushner MG, Kim SW, Donahue C, et al. D-cycloserine augmented exposure therapy for obsessive-compulsive disorder. Biol Psychiatry 2007;62(8):835–8.
129. Wilhelm S, Buhlmann U, Tolin DF, et al. Augmentation of behavior therapy with D-cycloserine for obsessive-compulsive disorder. Am J Psychiatry 2008;165(3): 335–41 [quiz: 409].
130. Storch EA, Murphy TK, Goodman WK, et al. A preliminary study of D-cycloserine augmentation of cognitive-behavioral therapy in pediatric obsessive-compulsive disorder. Biol Psychiatry 2010;68(11):1073–6.
131. Farrell LJ, Waters AM, Boschen MJ, et al. Difficult-to-treat pediatric obsessive-compulsive disorder: feasibility and preliminary results of a randomized pilot trial of D-cycloserine-augmented behavior therapy. Depress Anxiety 2013;30(8): 723–31.
132. Storch EA, Merlo LJ, Bengtson M, et al. D-cycloserine does not enhance exposure-response prevention therapy in obsessive-compulsive disorder. Int Clin Psychopharmacol 2007;22(4):230–7.
133. Norberg MM, Krystal JH, Tolin DF. A meta-analysis of D-cycloserine and the facilitation of fear extinction and exposure therapy. Biol Psychiatry 2008; 63(12):1118–26.
134. O'Sullivan G, Noshirvani H, Marks I, et al. Six-year follow-up after exposure and clomipramine therapy for obsessive compulsive disorder. Journal of Clinical Psychiatry 1991;52(4):150–5.
135. Braga DT, Manfro GG, Niederauer K, et al. Full remission and relapse of obsessive-compulsive symptoms after cognitive-behavioral group therapy: a two-year follow-up. Rev Bras Psiquiatr 2010;32(2):164–8.
136. Jakubovski E, Diniz JB, Valerio C, et al. Clinical predictors of long-term outcome in obsessive-compulsive disorder. Depress Anxiety 2013;30(8):763–72.
137. Anholt GE, Aderka IM, van Balkom AJ, et al. The impact of depression on the treatment of obsessive-compulsive disorder: results from a 5-year follow-up. J Affect Disord 2011;135(1–3):201–7.
138. Stewart SE, Geller DA, Jenike M, et al. Long-term outcome of pediatric obsessive-compulsive disorder: a meta-analysis and qualitative review of the literature. Acta Psychiatr Scand 2004;110(1):4–13.
139. O'Leary EM, Barrett P, Fjermestad KW. Cognitive-behavioral family treatment for childhood obsessive-compulsive disorder: a 7-year follow-up study. J Anxiety Disord 2009;23(7):973–8.
140. Sousa MB, Isolan LR, Oliveira RR, et al. A randomized clinical trial of cognitive-behavioral group therapy and sertraline in the treatment of obsessive-compulsive disorder. J Clin Psychiatry 2006;67(7):1133–9.
141. Storch EA, Bussing R, Small BJ, et al. Randomized, placebo-controlled trial of cognitive-behavioral therapy alone or combined with sertraline in the treatment of pediatric obsessive-compulsive disorder. Behav Res Ther 2013;51(12): 823–9.
142. Franklin ME, Sapyta J, Freeman JB, et al. Cognitive behavior therapy augmentation of pharmacotherapy in pediatric obsessive-compulsive disorder: the Pediatric OCD Treatment Study II (POTS II) randomized controlled trial. JAMA 2011;306(11):1224–32.
143. Ferrao YA, Shavitt RG, Bedin NR, et al. Clinical features associated to refractory obsessive-compulsive disorder. J Affect Disord 2006;94(1–3):199–209.

144. McGuire JF, Lewin AB, Geller DA, et al. Advances in the treatment of pediatric obsessive-compulsive D-cycloserine with exposure and response prevention. Neuropsychiatry (London) 2012;2(4):291–300.

145. Storch EA, Larson MJ, Keely ML, et al. Comorbidity of pediatric obsessive-compulsive disorder and anxiety disorders: impact on symptom severity and impairment. J Psychopathol Behav Assess 2008;30(2):111–20.

146. Foa EB, Abramowitz JS, Franklin ME, et al. Feared consequences, fixity of belief, and treatment outcome in patients with obsessive-compulsive disorder. Behav Ther 1999;30:717–24.

147. Lewin AB, Bergman RL, Peris TS, et al. Correlates of insight among youth with obsessive-compulsive disorder. Journal of Child Psychology and Psychiatry 2010;51(5):603–11.

148. Ginsburg GS, Kingery JN, Drake KL, et al. Predictors of treatment response in pediatric obsessive-compulsive disorder. J Am Acad Child Adolesc Psychiatry 2008;47(8):868–78.

149. McGuire JF, Storch EA, Lewin AB, et al. The role of avoidance in the phenomenology of obsessive-compulsive disorder. Compr Psychiatry 2012;53(2):187–94.

150. Abramowitz JS, Franklin ME, Schwartz SA, et al. Symptom presentation and outcome of cognitive-behavioral therapy for obsessive-compulsive disorder. J Consult Clin Psychol 2003;71(6):1049–57.

151. Mataix-Cols D, Marks IM, Greist JH, et al. Obsessive-compulsive symptom dimensions as predictors of compliance with and response to behaviour therapy: results from a controlled trial. Psychother Psychosom 2002;71(5):255–62.

152. Simpson HB, Maher MJ, Wang Y, et al. Patient adherence predicts outcome from cognitive behavioral therapy in obsessive-compulsive disorder. Journal of Consulting and Clinical Psychology 2011;79(2):247–52.

153. Abramowitz JS, Franklin ME, Zoellner LA, et al. Treatment compliance and outcome in obsessive-compulsive disorder. Behav Modif 2002;26(4):447–63.

154. Merlo LJ, Lehmkuhl HD, Geffken GR, et al. Decreased family accommodation associated with improved therapy outcome in pediatric obsessive-compulsive disorder. J Consult Clin Psychol 2009;77(2):355–60.

155. Franklin ME, Flessner CA, Woods DW, et al. The Child and Adolescent Trichotillomania Impact Project: descriptive psychopathology, comorbidity, functional impairment, and treatment utilization. J Dev Behav Pediatr 2008;29(6):493–500.

156. Gelhorn HL, Sexton CC, Classi PM. Patient preferences for treatment of major depressive disorder and the impact on health outcomes: a systematic review. Prim Care Companion CNS Disord 2011;13(5).

157. McHugh RK, Whitton SW, Peckham AD, et al. Patient preference for psychological vs pharmacologic treatment of psychiatric disorders: a meta-analytic review. J Clin Psychiatry 2013;74(6):595–602.

158. Guy W. Clinical global impressions. ECDEU assessment manual for psychopharmacology. Vol Revised DHEW Pub. (ADM). Rockville (MD): National Institute for Mental Health; 1976. p. 218–22.

159. Scahill L, Riddle MA, McSwiggin-Hardin M, et al. Children's Yale-Brown Obsessive Compulsive Scale: reliability and validity. J Am Acad Child Adolesc Psychiatry 1997;36(6):844–52.

160. Azrin NH, Peterson AL. Treatment of Tourette syndrome by Habit reversal - a waiting-list control-group comparison. Behav Ther 1990;21(3):305–18.

161. O'Connor KP, Brault M, Robillard S, et al. Evaluation of a cognitive-behavioural program for the management of chronic tic and habit disorders. Behav Res Ther 2001;39(6):667–81.

162. Verdellen CW, Keijsers GP, Cath DC, et al. Exposure with response prevention versus habit reversal in Tourettes's syndrome: a controlled study. Behav Res Ther 2004;42(5):501–11.

163. Wilhelm S, Deckersbach T, Coffey BJ, et al. Habit reversal versus supportive psychotherapy for Tourette's disorder: a randomized controlled trial. Am J Psychiatry 2003;160(6):1175–7.

164. Azrin NH, Nunn RG, Frantz SE. Habit reversal training versus negative practice treatment of nervous tics. Behav Ther 1980;11:169–78.

165. Rosen JC, Reiter J. Development of the body dysmorphic disorder examination. Behav Res Ther 1996;34(9):755–66.

166. Phillips KA, Hollander E, Rasmussen SA, et al. A severity rating scale for body dysmorphic disorder: development, reliability, and validity of a modified version of the Yale-Brown Obsessive Compulsive Scale. Psychopharmacol Bull 1997; 33(1):17–22.

167. Frost RO, Steketee G, Tolin DF, et al. Development and validation of the Clutter Image Rating. J Psychopathol Behav Assess 2008;32:401–17.

168. Leckman JF, Riddle MA, Hardin MT, et al. The Yale Global Tic Severity Scale: initial testing of a clinician-rated scale of tic severity. J Am Acad Child Adolesc Psychiatry 1989;28(4):566–73.

169. Swedo SE, Leonard HL, Rapoport JL, et al. A double-blind comparison of clomipramine and desipramine in the treatment of trichotillomania (hair pulling). N Engl J Med 1989;321(8):497–501.

170. Frost RO, Steketee G, Grisham J. Measurement of compulsive hoarding: saving inventory-revised. Behav Res Ther 2004;42(10):1163–82.

171. Keuthen NJ, O'Sullivan RL, Ricciardi JN, et al. The Massachusetts General Hospital (MGH) Hairpulling Scale: 1. Development and factor analyses. Psychother Psychosom 1995;64(3–4):141–5.

# Index

Note: Page numbers of article titles are in **boldface** type.

## A

Acceptance-enhanced behavior therapy, for trichotillomania, 311
ADHD, characterization of, 275
  comorbid with Tourette syndrome, 275
  tic disorders and, 281
Anxiety disorders, comorbid with Tourette syndrome, 275–276

## B

Behavioral model, in hair-pulling disorder, 418
Body dysmorphic disorder (BDD), **287–300**
  CBT for, 418–419
  CBT with exposure and response prevention for, 423, 431
  clinical features of, delusionality, 288–289
    suicidality, 289
  cognitive behavioral therapy for, 293–294
    modular form, 294
  combination therapies for, 294
  cosmetic treatments of, 295
  epidemiology of, course and outcome in, 291
    gender differences in, 291
    prevalence in, 290–291
  etiology of, biological factors in, 289
    cognitive and socioenvironmental factors in, 290
    heritability in, 289
  exposure and response prevention therapy for, 294
  in *DSM III* and revisions, 287–288
  long-term recommendations for, 295–296
  neurosurgery for, 295
  nosologic issues in, delusionality, 292–293
    eating disorders, 291–292
    OCD, 291
    social anxiety disorder, 291–292
  pharmacologic treatment of, SRIs in, 292–293, 295–296
    SSRIs, 293
  surgical treatments of, 294–295
  treatment resistance in, 295
  twin studies and heritability of, 323

## C

CANS (childhood acute neuropsychiatric symptoms), criteria for, 356
Clomipramine, for OCD, 377–378

Psychiatr Clin N Am 37 (2014) 447–454
http://dx.doi.org/10.1016/S0193-953X(14)00067-7
0193-953X/14/$ – see front matter © 2014 Elsevier Inc. All rights reserved.

# Moving?

## Make sure your subscription moves with you!

To notify us of your new address, find your **Clinics Account Number** (located on your mailing label above your name), and contact customer service at:

**Email: journalscustomerservice-usa@elsevier.com**

**800-654-2452** (subscribers in the U.S. & Canada)
**314-447-8871** (subscribers outside of the U.S. & Canada)

**Fax number: 314-447-8029**

**Elsevier Health Sciences Division**
**Subscription Customer Service**
**3251 Riverport Lane**
**Maryland Heights, MO 63043**

*To ensure uninterrupted delivery of your subscription, please notify us at least 4 weeks in advance of move.